PANCREATITIS AND ITS COMPLICATIONS

CLINICAL GASTROENTEROLOGY

GEORGE Y. WU, SERIES EDITOR

PANCREATITIS AND ITS COMPLICATIONS

Edited by

CHRIS E. FORSMARK, MD

University of Florida College of Medicine, Gainesville, FL

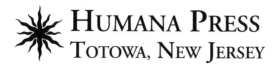

HUMANA PRESS
TOTOWA, NEW JERSEY

PREFACE

Diseases of the pancreas have been extremely difficult to study. Until relatively recently, the pancreas was viewed by surgeons as an organ to be avoided, given its deep retroperitoneal location and the sometimes severe consequences of manipulation. Similar difficulties have plagued careful study of the pancreas. In humans, only infrequently have we had the opportunity to evaluate the evolution of diseases of the pancreas; instead, we are confronted with end-stage chronic pancreatitis or acute pancreatitis with extensive necrosis of the gland.

Within the past decade, revolutionary techniques in molecular biology, genetics, and animal models have begun to give us dramatic new insights into pancreatic disease. Coupled with these advances has been a slow but steady progress in the development of our clinical tools for diagnosing and treating pancreatic diseases. These advances place us on the threshold of a much more complete understanding of pancreatic diseases, opening up new opportunities for novel therapies and preventive measures.

Pancreatitis and Its Complications brings together many of the world's experts in pancreatic diseases. These "pancreatologists" include basic scientists, endoscopists, gastroenterologists, and surgeons. The chapters have been organized to provide a comprehensive discussion of acute and chronic pancreatitis, with up-to-date discussions of pathophysiology, epidemiology, diagnostic strategies, treatment, and complications of disease. It is hoped that this text will serve as a useful reference for clinicians as well as provide a clinical background for scientists with an interest in pancreatic or related diseases.

I would like to thank all the contributors for their outstanding contributions and the staff at Humana Press for its superbly competent support.

Chris E. Forsmark, MD

CONTENTS

CONTRIBUTORS

JOHN BAILLIE, MB, ChB, FRCP • *Division of Gastroenterology, Department of Medicine, Duke University Medical Center, Durham, NC*

FRANK R. BURTON, MD • *Division of Gastroenterology and Hepatology, St Louis University, Saint Louis, MO*

MICHAEL F. BYRNE, MA, MB, ChB, MRCP • *Division of Gastroenterology, Department of Medicine, Duke University Medical Center, Durham, NC*

JONATHAN E. CLAIN, MD • *Division of Gastroenterology and Hepatology, Mayo Clinic, Rochester, MN*

ELIAS DEGIANNIS, MD • *Department of Surgery, University of the Witwatersrand, Johannesburg, South Africa*

EUGENE P. DIMAGNO, MD • *Division of Gastroenterology and Hepatology, Department of Internal Medicine, Mayo Clinic, Rochester, MN*

PETER DRAGANOV, MD • *Division of Gastroenterology, Hepatology, and Nutrition, University of Florida College of Medicine, Gainesville, Fl*

CHRIS E. FORSMARK, MD • *Division of Gastroenterology, Hepatology, and Nutrition, University of Florida College of Medicine, Gainesville, Fl*

FRED S. GORELICK, MD • *Department of Medicine and Cell Biology, Yale University School of Medicine, New Haven, CT*

MICHAEL L. KENDRICK, MD • *Department of Surgery, Mayo Clinic, Rochester, MN*

MATTHIAS KRAFT, MD • *Department of Gastroenterology, Endocrinology and Nutrition, Ernst-Moritz-Arndt-Universität, Greifswald, Germany*

GLEN LEHMAN, MD • *Division of Gastroenterology and Hepatology, Indiana University Medical Center, Indianapolis, IN*

MARKUS M. LERCH, MD, FRCP, FACG • *Department of Gastroenterology, Endocrinology and Nutrition, Ernst-Moritz-Arndt Universität, Greifswald, Germany*

ALBERT B. LOWENFELS, MD • *Department of Surgery, New York Medical College, Valhalla, NY*

PATRICK MAISONNEUVE, ING • *Unit of Clinical Epidemiology, European Institute of Oncology, Milan, Italy*

LEE MCHENRY, MD • *Division of Gastroenterology and Hepatology, Indiana University Medical Center, Indianapolis, IN*

MICHAEL MORELLI, MD • *Division of Digestive Diseases, Department of Medicine, University of Cincinnati, Cincinnati, OH*

ANIL B. NAGAR, MD • *Department of Internal Medicine, Yale University School of Medicine, New Haven, CT*

JOHN PETERSEN, DO, FACP, FACG • *Division of Gastroenterology, Hepatology, and Nutrition, University of Florida College of Medicine, Gainesville, FL*

SUPOT PONGPRASOBCHAI, MD • *Division of Gastroenterology and Hepatology, Mayo Clinic, Rochester, MN*

MICHAEL G. SARR, MD • *Department of Surgery, Mayo Medical School and Department of Surgery, Mayo Clinic, Rochester, MN*

STUART SHERMAN, MD • *Department of Medicine and Radiology, Indiana University Medical Center, Indianapolis, IN*

MARTIN D. SMITH, MD • *Department of Surgery, University of the Witwatersrand, Johannesburg, South Africa*

LEHEL SOMOGYI, MD • *Division of Digestive Diseases, Department of Medicine, University of Cincinnati, Cincinnati, OH,*

PHILLIP P. TOSKES, MD • *Division of Gastroenterology, Hepatology and Nutrition, University of Florida College of Medicine, Gainesville, FL*

CHARLES D. ULRICH, II, MD, FACP, FACG • *Texas Digestive Disease Consultants, Lewisville, TX*

SELWYN M. VICKERS, MD • *Division of Gastrointestinal Surgery, Department of Surgery, University of Alabama, Birmingham, AL*

DAVID C. WHITCOMB, MD, PhD • *Division of Gastroenterology, Hepatology, and Nutrition, Department of Medicine, University of Pittsburgh, Pittsburgh, PA*

I ACUTE PANCREATITIS

1 Epidemiology and Pathophysiology of Acute Pancreatitis

Anil B. Nagar, MD
and Fred S. Gorelick, MD

CONTENTS

INTRODUCTION
ETIOLOGY AND CLASSIFICATION
EPIDEMIOLOGY
NATURAL HISTORY
PATHOPHYSIOLOGY
CONCLUSION
REFERENCES

INTRODUCTION

Acute pancreatitis (AP) is an acute inflammatory process of the pancreas with variable involvement of the pancreas, regional tissues around the pancreas, or remote organ systems. The clinical course may range from mild discomfort with minimal pancreatic inflammation to severe necrotizing pancreatitis, complicated by multiorgan system failure and death. The most common etiologies are gallstones and alcohol abuse. The natural history is dependent on the degree of inflammation and necrosis. Following an acute attack, there is usually complete recovery of function if the offending agent is identified and removed. The pathogenesis of AP involves discrete intracellular events that prematurely activate intra-acinar zymogen granules and generate the release of proinflammatory and proapoptotic mediators. Understanding

From: *Pancreatitis and Its Complications*
Edited by: C. E. Forsmark © Humana Press Inc., Totowa, NJ

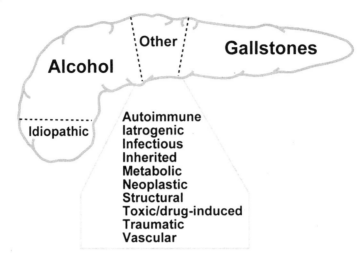

Fig. 1. Etiology of acute pancreatitis.

the natural history and specific roles of these cytokines may help develop therapies that can alter the course of severe pancreatitis and decrease its complications.

ETIOLOGY AND CLASSIFICATION

AP may be classified based on pathology, etiology, severity of disease, or the presence of necrosis. Risk factors are summarized in Fig. 1. In approximately 10–20% of patients, no etiology is identified. Some of these patients may have microlithiasis and/or sphincter of Oddi dysfunction (SOD) as the etiology of AP. With the increasing knowledge and understanding of the role of genetic abnormalities in hereditary and idiopathic chronic pancreatitis (CP), it is possible that these abnormalities will be implicated in idiopathic AP. Furthermore, polymorphisms in inflammatory mediators may influence disease severity.

Clinically, AP may be classified as mild or severe disease *(1)*. Severe acute pancreatitis (SAP) is associated with organ failure and/or local complications, such as necrosis, abscess, or pseudocyst. Approximately 10–20% of patients develop severe disease. Various clinical criteria (e.g., Ranson's or Acute Physiology And Chronic Health Evaluation [APACHE]), serum markers (e.g., interleukin [IL]-6, C-reactive protein, and trypsinogen activation peptide) and imaging modalities (contrast-enhanced computed tomography [CT] scan) have been used to predict severity. Complicated courses are more common in SAP with mortality rates from 5 to 20% *(2)*. In contrast, mild AP is the more frequent presentation and is associated with minimal or transient organ dysfunction and uneventful recovery.

The presence of pancreatic necrosis is the single best predictor of outcome during AP. Pancreatic necrosis is a diffuse or focal area of nonviable pancreatic parenchyma, typically associated with peripancreatic fat necrosis, which is observed as nonenhanced pancreatic parenchyma on a contrast CT scan. The degree of necrosis can predict morbidity and mortality. Approximately 30% of patients with pancreatic necrosis develop infected necrosis with a mortality of 6 to 40% and a morbidity of more than 80%.

Specific Etiologies

GALLSTONES

Gallstones are implicated in the majority of AP cases. Although gallstones are common, they rarely cause pancreatitis. It is estimated that over a 20- to 30-year period, the risk of developing biliary pancreatitis in patients with asymptomatic gallstones is approximately 2%. Small gallstones, particularly those smaller than 5 mm in size, increase the risk of AP. Additionally, a long common channel at the junction of the bile and pancreatic ducts may increase this risk. The specific mechanism by which gallstones produce pancreatitis is still debated, but most biliary pancreatitis is precipitated by the transient or persistent obstruction of the ampulla by gallstones. In the vast majority of patients, these stones pass into the intestine. Bile crystals, like stones, can cause AP. Patients with microlithiasis may present with recurrent "idiopathic" AP. The diagnosis is suggested by transient abnormalities in aminotransferases and the evidence of microscopic crystals in bile. Treatment by cholecystectomy eliminates the risk of recurrence.

ALCOHOL

Alcoholic pancreatitis presents as AP, although in most patients, it occurs in the presence of already established chronic pancreatitis (CP). It is the most common cause of recurrent pancreatitis. The incidence of alcoholic pancreatitis is low (about 5%) in alcohol abusers. This estimate suggests that in addition to alcohol ingestion, other factors, such as genetic background or environmental influences, may affect patient susceptibility. Several major physiological mechanisms may contribute to the development of alcoholic pancreatitis, including abnormal SOD spasm, obstruction of the small ducts by proteinaceous material, and direct toxic effect of alcohol and its metabolites.

HYPERLIPIDEMIA

Hyperlipidemia is a cause of AP and CP. Triglyceride levels greater than 1000 mg/dL are usually required for the development of pancreatitis.

The probable disease mechanism is generation of toxic-free fatty acids by the action of lipase on high triglyceride levels in the pancreatic capillary beds, which leads to endothelial damage with the recruitment of inflammatory cells, thrombosis, and ischemia. Following a bout of AP, patients require lipid-lowering medication, as well as treatment of concomitant diabetes and alcohol cessation.

DRUGS

Drugs are a rare cause of AP. Various medications have been implicated in AP. Azathioprine, 6-mercaptopurine, and 2′, 3′-dideoxyinosine appear to have an unquestionable association. Other drugs like angiotensin-converting enzyme inhibitors, and tetracycline have a weaker association. The relationship to AP is uncertain in such medications as corticosteroids, aminosalicylic acid, and methyldopa.

ENDOSCOPIC RETROGRADE CHOLANGIOPANCREATOGRAPHY

AP is the most common complication of endoscopic retrograde cholangiopancreatography (ERCP). Prospective studies have documented an incidence of approximately 5% with most cases being mild pancreatitis. Risk factors include young age, normal pancreatic ducts, operator inexperience, multiple injections of the pancreatic duct with acinarization, pancreatic sphincterotomy, SOD, and biliary or pancreatic sphincter manometry. Several strategies might reduce the incidence of this complication, including the use of protease inhibitors (gabexate mesilate), somatostatin, IL-6 antibodies, and temporary pancreatic duct stenting.

STRUCTURAL

A variety of conditions that obstruct the pancreatic duct chronically or intermittently may cause AP and include SOD, pancreas divisum, and benign and malignant pancreatic duct strictures. SOD is determined by measuring pressures through the sphincter segment at the time of ERCP. This condition is considered when all other possible etiologies have been eliminated, because performing ERCP with sphincter manometry is also likely to precipitate an attack of AP. Pancreas divisum is a condition in which there is failure of fusion of the dorsal and ventral pancreas during development. Therefore, the secretion of the larger dorsal pancreas drains through the small minor papilla. This common variant occurs in 7% of the population, and very few of these patients develop pancreatitis. In a very small subset, AP may develop. Finally, patients with pancreatic adenocarcinoma may rarely present with unexplained AP, which has led to the recommendation that patients older than 45 years of age with unexplained pancreatitis should undergo an ERCP or endoscopic ultrasonography to evaluate for the possibility of an underlying malignancy.

EPIDEMIOLOGY

Studies on the epidemiology of AP differ considerably in the incidence of AP, secondary to inadequate reporting, difficulty in making the diagnosis, difference in patient populations and prevalence of alcohol intake, and tertiary care referral bias. In fact, because patients with mild pancreatitis may never be diagnosed, the true incidence of AP may be higher than that suggested in the literature. Several studies have observed an increase in the incidence of AP in North America and Western Europe. Some of this increase may be explained by the improvement of diagnostic methods, but studies after 1985 have confirmed an increasing incidence, indicating that improved diagnosis is not the only explanation. The incidence of AP ranges from 10 to 50 per 100,000 per year. Studies from the United Kingdom from the 1970s suggested an incidence of 5.4 to 9.4 per 100,000 per year. A report from Scotland describes an increasing incidence of discharges with AP from hospitals between 1961 and 1985: 11-fold in male and 4-fold in female with an annual incidence of 23.3 per 100,000 per year (3). The low incidence reported from older studies in the United Kingdom is true first-attack incidences, as the inclusion of recurrent attacks in other studies lead to much higher rate. Swedish and Finnish studies have documented a high annual rate of 40 per 100,000 and 50 per 100,000, respectively. These studies have a high proportion of alcohol-induced pancreatitis. A recent 10-year retrospective study from Sweden that reviewed first attacks in a defined population observed an annual incidence of 23.4 per 100,000; when relapses were included, this estimate was 38.2 per 100,000 (4). A report from the Netherlands confirmed an increasing incidence of AP from 12.4/100,000 person years in 1985 to 15.9/100,000 in 1995. Although the incidence of AP may be rising, multiple studies have documented a stable or reduced mortality from AP. In a recent analysis from 1999, the number of AP cases that required hospitalization in the United States was between 166,000 and 252,000 (5). Incidence rates in the United States have been reported as being as high as 50 per 100,000 per year (6,7). Gallstone disease is identified as the most common etiology of the first attack, accounting for 30–50%. Alcohol association is between 20 and 40% of patients with AP (8). Worldwide, the main etiology is biliary tract disease (41%) and alcohol abuse (31.7%). There is a strong association between gender and age with the incidence of AP, being higher in men than women and increasing with age. The peak incidence of alcoholic pancreatitis is in the third and fourth decade; for gallstone pancreatitis, it is the seventh decade.

Acute Biliary Pancreatitis

Gallstones account for between 30 and 50% of AP *(9)*. It is the most frequent cause of the first AP episode. Most studies exclude patients with microlithiasis; thus, the incidence is likely higher. The wide variation in incidence is noted within and between countries, dependent on the population studied and extent of alcohol use in the community. Gallstone pancreatitis is most common in women between the ages of 50 and 70. However, AP occurs more frequently in males than in females with gallstone disease. The risk for severe disease is similar to that observed for other etiologies, but some studies suggest biliary patients have a higher mortality than alcoholic pancreatitis. This higher mortality may be secondary to the increased risk of cholangitis and the older age of presentation. Biliary pancreatitis may be recurrent if the gallstones are left untreated, although it is not a cause of CP. Recurrence rates are uncertain but may be as high as 30% in the absence of cholecystectomy or biliary sphincterotomy.

Acute Alcoholic Pancreatitis

Excess alcohol intake is the most common etiology of AP in males. Overall, it is the second most common etiology for AP (30%), yet several studies from North America suggest that it may be the most common etiology of AP in the continent. Because alcohol causes recurrent AP, it becomes the predominant etiology when relapses are included in the analysis. Although the incidence of AP is increasing, recent studies do not show any increase in the incidence of alcoholic pancreatitis. Most attacks of acute alcoholic pancreatitis represent an acute attack on CP; however, in most cases, the structural and functional aspects of the pancreas are unknown and the attacks are therefore assumed to be AP. Despite the fact that alcoholic pancreatitis is complicated by severe disease, it is a less common cause of fatal pancreatitis.

Other Etiologies

Other etiologies identified include pancreatic cancer in 1% of cases, post-ERCP in 2–3%, medications in 1%, miscellaneous causes in 2%, and unknown causes in 15–23% of first attacks of AP.

Recurrent Acute Pancreatitis

Bouts of recurrent AP are most commonly alcohol-related (60%); other etiologies include unknown causes (17%) and untreated gallstones (19%). Recurrent AP appears to be relatively benign and is associated with a low mortality rate.

NATURAL HISTORY

Natural History and Long-Term Outcome

The majority of patients with mild pancreatitis recover uneventfully and once the etiological factor is identified and removed, there are no long-term complications or recurrences. An estimate of 10–20% of patients with AP develop severe disease and have a complicated hospital course. The incidence of necrosis is between 6 and 20%. Approximately 33% of patients with pancreatic necrosis develop infected necrosis and have the highest mortality and morbidity with nearly 90% of these patients developing failure of at least one organ system *(10)*. In patients with necrotizing pancreatitis, long-term follow-up has demonstrated pancreatic ductal changes on ERCP, although the clinical significance of this evidence is uncertain *(11)*. Following necrosectomy for necrotizing pancreatitis, approximately 50% of patients will develop long-term pancreatic exocrine and endocrine dysfunction, yet most preserve a good overall functional status *(12)*. The development of pancreatic insufficiency varies with the extent of pancreatic necrosis and resection.

Mortality

The mortality of AP is reported in the literature as being between 1.3 and 10%. A range of 2–5% likely represents a true mortality because the higher rates are indicated in studies from referral centers and probably do not include patients with mild disease. Overall, studies suggest a reduction in mortality in the last decade. Gender is not an independent risk factor for severity in AP. When necrotizing pancreatitis is considered, the mortality rate is between 14 and 30%. Approximately half of this mortality is seen in the first 2 weeks. Mortality appears to be influenced by age, etiology (higher in patients with idiopathic, post-ERCP pancreatitis, and gallstone), presence of organ failure on admission and, most importantly, the presence of pancreatic necrosis. Additionally, patients with severe pancreatitis transferred to tertiary care facilities for management have higher mortalities *(13)*. Most studies suggest that approximately 10–20% of fatal pancreatitis is missed with the diagnosis only being made at autopsy. The missed diagnosis appears in patients who present without abdominal pain, with acute respiratory failure or neurological changes, and/or normal serum enzymes or pancreatic imaging.

PATHOPHYSIOLOGY

The syndrome of AP represents a series of pathological events. The initial pathology is likely to involve either the acinar cell or reduced

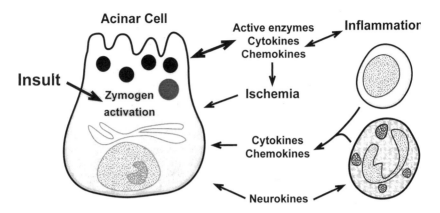

Fig. 2. Early and late cellular events in the pathogenesis of acute pancreatitis.

blood flow. Thus initiated, the process can involve the whole pancreas, surrounding tissues, and cause a systemic reaction that harms many organs. Because human pathological material is rarely available from early AP, much of our information is derived from experimental animal studies.

Acinar Cell Events

Pancreatic acinar cells form approximately 95% of the exocrine mass. In response to an initiating insult, the acinar cell mounts three key pathological responses: intracellular zymogen activation, inhibited secretion, and the generation and release of proinflammatory and proapoptotic mediators (Fig. 2).

ZYMOGEN ACTIVATION AND INHIBITION OF SECRETION

The majority of pancreatic digestive enzymes, including all proteases, are synthesized and stored as inactive proeznymes or zymogens. Within the first minutes to hours of AP, zymogens become activated within the pancreatic acinar cell *(14)*. At later disease stages, zymogens that have leaked into the interstitium may also be activated. The cellular mechanisms responsible for the acinar cell activation have not been fully defined; however, experimental models have consistently identified several factors. Elevations in cytosolic calcium mediate many of the physiological responses of the acinar cell to neurohumoral stimuli. A pathologically high level of cytosolic calcium may be a key component of the acinar cell response to an insult. Pathological elevations in cytosolic calcium have been linked to the activation of zymogens, but the basis for this association is unknown. One possible explanation is that excessive calcium causes fusion between different classes of organelles and thus generates novel organelles that support the conditions for zymogen activation. In the normal state, zymogens are sequentially activated in the small intestine. The brush border enzyme, enterokinase, first converts trypsinogen to trypsin, and then the other zymogens are activated by trypsin. As the pancreas does not contain enterokinase, another mechanism must be responsible for activation. The leading candidates are activation of trypsinogen by the lysosomal enzyme, cathepsin B, or trypsinogen autoactivation *(15)*. Several mechanisms may permit cathepsin B to mix with trypsinogen. First, although lysosomal enzymes are usually separated from digestive zymogens in the Golgi complex, the pancreas directs some lysosomal enzymes to the secretory compartment. Second, organelles containing the two enzyme families may fuse *(16)*. Enzyme activation alone may not be sufficient to cause acinar cell damage, and the decreased secretion of proteins from the acinar cell observed at the onset of pancreatitis may have a critical role in disease. The reduced secretion may result from the disruption of the apical actin cytoskeleton. Conditions that cause zymogen activation but leave secretion intact do not cause acinar cell injury or pancreatitis. Thus, both enzyme activation and retention of enzymes in the acinar cell may be required to initiate disease.

The acinar cell has several safety mechanisms to avoid the damaging effects of active intracellular enzymes. Packaged within the zymogen granule is the pancreatic secretory trypsin inhibitor. It is estimated that the amount of inhibitor is sufficient to block approximately 15% of trypsin activity within the acinar cell. Thus, extensive levels of activation could overwhelm the trypsin inhibitor. The low pH value of the zymogen granule and condensation of content proteins may also limit enzyme activity. When these protective mechanisms are overwhelmed, active enzymes escape their membrane-bound organelles, degrade cell proteins, and cause cell death. This process has been called "autodigestion," but involves the release of many detrimental substances. Although the blood has numerous effective protease inhibitors, some active enzymes may reach and damage other tissues. The release of trypsin into the interstitium may have a unique role in causing the severe pain associated with AP. Trypsin may specifically stimulate protease-activated receptors on nerves that carry pain sensation. Because zymogen activation appears to be a very early feature of disease, the therapeutic use of protease inhibitors may be limited to prophylaxis (e.g., for ERCP-induced pancreatitis). The importance of zymogen activation in the pathogenesis of pancreatitis is underscored by the observation that some forms of hereditary pancreatitis are caused by mutations in cationic trypsinogen that might enhance its activation or prolong its activity *(17)*.

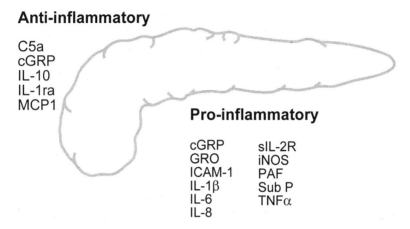

Anti-inflammatory

C5a
cGRP
IL-10
IL-1ra
MCP1

Pro-inflammatory

cGRP	sIL-2R
GRO	iNOS
ICAM-1	PAF
IL-1β	Sub P
IL-6	TNFα
IL-8	

Fig. 3. Cytokines, chemokines, and neurokines implicated in organ dysfunction in acute pancreatitis (AP). C5a, complement component C5a; ICAM, intracellular adhesion molecule 1; IL, interleukin; IL-1ra, interleukin-1 receptor antagonist; iNOS, inducible nitric oxide; PAF, platelet-activating factor; sIL-2R, soluble interleukin-2 receptor; Sub P, substance P; TNF-α, tumor necrosis factor-α; MCP1, monocyte chemotactic protein-1; GRO, growth-related oncogene.

CYTOKINE AND CHEMOKINE GENERATION

Two key features of AP are inflammation and cell death. Neutrophil recruitment and activation are early features of disease and correlate with the severity of disease. Soluble factors, such as tumor necrosis factor (TNF)-α and platelet-activating factor, are generated by the acinar cells and stimulate inflammation. Endothelial expression of intracellular adhesion molecule-1 and selectins promotes inflammatory cell adhesion. Neurokines, like substance P may also have a key role in disease. Even in acute disease, mononuclear cells may contribute to injury. Cytokines generated by the acinar cell (e.g., TNF-α) can also induce programmed cell death (apoptosis). Release of these soluble factors from the pancreas may also be responsible for the lung injury associated with severe pancreatitis *(18,19)*. Multiple cytokines that cause distinct patterns of organ injury are released (Fig. 3), which makes it unlikely that inhibition of a single pathway will be an effective disease treatment.

Pancreatic and Peripancreatic Events

EDEMA

Increased capillary permeability and potentially increased tissue oncotic pressure lead to early pancreatic edema. Such changes may contribute to decreased pancreatic blood by the compression of vascular structures and diminishing intravascular volume.

VASCULAR CHANGES AND FREE RADICAL GENERATION

Endothelial injury, vasospasm, and vascular thrombosis can all occur in AP. Changes in pancreatic perfusion can have two deleterious outcomes. Vasospasm with later increases in circulation can lead to perfusion–reperfusion injury and free radical generation. Ischemia and loss of perfusion can lead directly to cell death. Although there is a strong theoretical and experimental basis for implicating free radicals in AP, there has been little clinical support for the use of antioxidant therapy.

CHANGES IN PARACELLULAR CELL PERMEABILITY

Loss of the cell structures that form tight seals, known as "tight junctions," may occur in the acinar and duct cells. This early event (first 30 minutes) is associated with the breakdown of the actin cytoskeleton, an anchor for the tight junctions. Such disruptions allow the pancreatic duct contents to leak into the interstitial space. These changes may contribute to the very rapid increases in serum levels of pancreatic enzymes and rapid decrease in pancreatic secretion observed at the onset of disease. Furthermore, zymogens that enter the interstitial space may undergo activation.

Cell Death

Two general mechanisms of cell death are observed in AP: necrosis and programmed cell death or apoptosis. The factors that mediate the two mechanisms of death are not clearly understood. However, more severe forms of pancreatitis may be more strongly associated with necrotic death than apoptotic cell death. In humans, necrosis is the earliest and most prominent in adipose tissue. Injured adipocytes may be a rich source of harmful cytokines (TNF-α) and provide substrates (triglcyerides) for the generation of harmful free fatty acids. The acinar cell undergoes a unique form of necrosis after injury; instead of dying, the cell may respond to injury by pinching off their apical zymogen granule-rich region. This leaves acini filled with flattened cells—these glandular structures are known as "tubular complexes." Such a response may provide a scaffold for rapid regeneration. Similarly, the high levels of the pancreatitis-associated protein (PAP) and the pancreatic stone protein (PSP/reg) generated during the initial days of AP may have a role in reconstitution. Generally, endocrine and exocrine structure and function fully recovers from an AP episode. However, with severe disease, some deficiency in function may be detected for 1 year.

Systemic Events

Two major processes lead to death in AP: early deaths are caused by multiorgan failure and later deaths by organ failure and/or infected necrosis. The systemic inflammatory response syndrome (SIRS) is also associated with severe pancreatitis. The lungs are particularly sensitive to this injury, and the development of adult respiratory distress syndrome often indicates severe disease. SIRS and organ failure can be present upon admission but are often reversible. Although the presence of some organ failure or SIRS upon admission has a worse prognosis, the highest mortality is observed among those patients with deteriorating organ function or persistent SIRS. These systemic effects are felt to be caused by the release of these inflammatory cytokines, chemokines, and neurokines.

CONCLUSION

In conclusion, there appears to be an increasing incidence of AP with a stable or reduced mortality. Biliary pancreatitis is the most common etiology worldwide followed by alcohol. Most cases of AP are mild with full functional recovery following an acute attack. Following an initiating event, there is intracellular zymogen activation, followed by the release of proinflammatory mediators, which results in local and systemic injury. Research continues to provide new insights into the earliest changes within the cell during AP. Treatment and prevention of AP will be influenced by the effectiveness in targeting specific cytokines that have been demonstrated to produce local and systemic inflammatory responses.

REFERENCES

1. Bradley EL. A clinical based classification system for acute pancreatitis. Arch Surg 1993; 128: 586–590.
2. Beger HG. Surgical management of necrotizing pancreatitis. Surg Clin North Am 1989; 69: 529–549.
3. Wilson C, Imrie CW. Changing patterns of incidence and mortality from acute pancreatitis in Scotland, 1961–1985. Br J Surg 1990; 77: 731–734.
4. Appelros S, Brogstrom B. Incidence, etiology and mortality rate of acute pancreatitis over 10 years in a defined population in Sweden. Br J Surg 1999; 86: 465–470.
5. Grendell JH. Clinical and economic impact of acute pancreatitis in the United States. Pancreas 1999; 19(Abstract): 422.
6. Go VLW. Etiology and epidemiology of pancreatitis in the United States. In: Bradley III EL, ed. Acute Pancreatitis: Diagnosis and Therapy. Raven Press, NY, 1994: 235–239.
7. Chwistek M, Ingram R, Amoateng-Adjepong Y. Gallstone pancreatitis: A community teaching hospital experience. J Clin Gastroenterol 2001; 33: 41–44.
8. Thomson SR, Hendry WS, McFarlane GA, Davison AL. Epidemiology and outcome of acute pancreatitis. Br J Surg 1987; 74: 398–401.
9. Forsmark CE. The clinical problem of biliary acute necrotizing pancreatitis: epidemiology, pathophysiology, and diagnosis of biliary necrotizing pancreatitis. J Gastrointest Surg 2001; 5: 235–239.

10. Isenmann R, Beger HG. Natural history of acute pancreatitis and the role of infection. Best Practice & Research in Clin Gastroenterol 1999; 13: 291–301.
11. Angelini G, Cavallini G, Pederzoli P, et al. Long-term outcome of acute pancreatitis: Prospective study with118 patients. Digestion 1993; 54: 143–147.
12. Tsiotos GG, Luque-De Leon E, Sarr MG. Long-term outcome of necrotizing pancreatitis treated by necrosectomy. Br J Surg 1998; 85: 1650–1653.
13. De Beaux AC, Palmer KR, Carter DC. Factors influencing morbidity and mortality in acute pancreatitis; an analysis of 279 cases. Gut 1995; 37: 12–126.
14. Leach S, Modlin I, Scheele G, Gorelick F. Intracellular activation of digestive zymogens in rat pancreatic acini: stimulation by high doses of cholecystokinin. J Clin Invest 1991; 87: 362–366.
15. Halangk W, Lerch MM, Brandt-Nedelev B, et al. Role of cathepsin B in intracellular trypsinogen activation and the onset of acute pancreatitis. J Clin Invest 2000; 106: 773–781.
16. Otani T, Chelpinko S, Grendell J, Gorelick F. In vivo trypsinogen activation in distinct subcellular compartments of the pancreatic acinar cell. Am J Physiol 1998; 275: G999–G1009.
17. Whitcomb DC, Gorry MC, Preston RA, et al. Hereditary pancreatitis is caused by a mutation in the cationic trypsinogen gene. Nat Genet 1996; 14: 141–145.
18. Steinle AU, Weidenbach H, Wagner M, et al. NF-kappaB/Rel activation in cerulein pancreatitis. Gastroenterology 1999; 116: 420–430.
19. Frossard JL, Saluja A, Bhagat L, et al. The role of intercellular adhesion molecule 1 and neutrophils in acute pancreatitis and pancreatitis-associated lung injury. Gastroenterology 1999; 116: 694–701.

2 Diagnosis and Risk Stratification of Acute Pancreatitis

Frank R. Burton, MD

DIAGNOSIS OF ACUTE PANCREATITIS

Patients with acute pancreatitis (AP) usually present with sudden onset of abdominal pain, nausea, and vomiting. Approximately 80% of patients have interstitial pancreatitis with mild-to-moderate symptoms, and 20% have life-threatening necrotizing disease. Careful clinical assessment and the judicial use of biochemical tests and radiological imaging enables the practitioner to differentiate AP from other causes of acute abdomen and to assess the severity of disease (1–7).

History and Physical Exam

AP is typically characterized by abdominal pain located in the epigatsric or supraumbilical regions, often radiating to the mid-thoracic portion of the back. Pain usually reaches maximum intensity within 20 minutes but may have a more gradual onset. The pain from AP is usually sharp, constant, lasts hours to days, and is severe enough to force the patient to visit the emergency room. In mild AP, the pain may decrease when sitting or leaning forward in comparison to lying flat.

From: *Pancreatitis and Its Complications*
Edited by: C. E. Forsmark © Humana Press Inc., Totowa, NJ

Nausea and vomiting with or without low-grade fever are the most commonly associated symptoms (1,4,5).

A recent history of binge drinking may be frequently elicited in patients with alcohol-induced pancreatitis. The concomitant presence of jaundice and high-grade fever strongly suggests choledocholithiasis as the etiology of AP, complicated by coexistent cholangitis (1–6). Less commonly, respiratory failure, confusion, and even coma are the main presenting features, which are frequently manifestations of severe necrotizing pancreatitis. In rare cases, abdominal pain may be absent, leading to a delayed or missed diagnosis (1).

The usual findings on a physical examination are abdominal distension, tenderness, guarding, and absent bowel sounds. Fever associated with AP is generally low grade. High-grade temperature may indicate the development of infected pancreatic necrosis and associated fluid collection or cholangitis, particularly if jaundice is present (1,2,5,6).

Severe acute pancreatitis (SAP) is often complicated by massive loss of fluid into the retroperitoneal spaces. Tachycardia and hypotension are some of the earliest clues for a moderate-to-severe attack of pancreatitis and are markers for significant early depletion of intravascular volume. These may soon progress to hypovolemic shock caused by increased vascular permeability, vasodilatation, and hemorrhage (1). Tachnypnea and dyspnea are also common in severe pancreatitis, owing to splinting from the subdiaphragmatic inflammatory process, associated pleural effusions, or pulmonary capillary leak syndrome (adult respiratory distress syndrome). Pleural effusions are mainly found on the left side but can be bilateral.

Rare clinical findings include ecchymoses of the umbilicus or flanks, peripheral subcutaneous fat necrosis, and polyarthritis. Classically, dark skin discoloration of the flanks and periumbilical areas because of hemorrhage is described with severe and hemorrhagic pancreatitis; however these physical findings may result from any type of retroperitoneal bleeding (6).

Laboratory Tests

The diagnosis of AP is usually suspected based on the appropriate clinical features and is confirmed by laboratory and imaging tests. Leakage of pancreatic enzymes into the circulation is a hallmark of AP. Although amylase and lipase constitute a small fraction of all pancreatic enzymes, they are the easiest and the quickest enzymes to measure. Typically, the elevation of serum amylase in AP is above threefold of the normal values. Amylase levels are usually increased within a few hours of disease onset, but they may be cleared from the serum rather quickly. Serum amylase usually remains elevated for 3–5 days in uncomplicated

Table 1
Causes of Increased Serum Amylase Activity

Pancreatic diseases
   Acute pancreatitis
   Pancreatic cancer
Abdominal emergencies
   Acute cholecystitis
   Common bile duct obstruction
   Perforated viscous
   Intestinal ischemia
   Acute appendicitis
   Ruptured ectopic pregnancy and acute salpingitis
Salivary gland diseases
Renal insufficiency
Macroamylasemia
Diabetic ketoacidosis
HIV infection/AIDS
Sphincter Oddi stenosis or spasm
Drugs: Morphine

AP. Because many conditions can cause hyperamylasemia (Table 1), the specificity of elevated serum amylase level is less than 70%. Very high elevations of serum amylase (more than fivefold normal), however, are rarely associated with diseases other than AP. Elevations of three- to fivefold normal are commonly seen in the absence of acute pancreatitis in patients with renal failure, as a result of decreased clearance of the enzyme. Measurements of urinary amylase and the amylase-to-creatinine ratio may be helpful to distinguish AP from other causes of hyperamylasemia, but such measurements are infrequently employed *(2–6)*.

Serum amylase isoenzyme measurements may improve the diagnostic accuracy of serum amylase alone. In healthy people, less than half of all circulating amylase originates in the pancreas, whereas the remainder is of salivary origin. Serum pancreatic isoamylase (P-isoamylase) accounts for the elevated total serum amylase level in AP and tends to persist for several days. However, pancreatic isoamylase can be elevated in some other gastrointestinal disorders and in renal insufficiency, making it difficult to diagnose AP based on P-isoamylase levels alone without additional diagnostic parameters *(2,5,8)*.

The elevation of serum lipase generally parallels the serum amylase level in AP. However, the serum lipase level often remains elevated longer, making it more useful to diagnose pancreatitis after symptoms have subsided. Lipase is considered more specific than amylase for pancreatic tissue injury, despite that lipase is also produced by numerous other gastrointestinal tissues. Another potential advantage of lipase is that it is generally not elevated in diabetic ketoacidosis or macroamylasemia *(1)*.

Both amylase and lipase are widely available and are, in general, rapidly available from hospital laboratories. In practice, combining the measurement of serum amylase and lipase somewhat enhances the diagnostic accuracy for AP. A normal amylase or lipase level makes the diagnosis of AP unlikely, except in the presence of hyperlipidemia. Very high levels of serum triglyceride (one of the causes of AP) can interfere with the laboratory assay for both amylase and lipase; dilution of the serum may be necessary in this situation to reliably measure the elevations of amylase or lipase. In some patients with chronic pancreatitis, acute abdominal pain can be the result of focal acute inflammation of the gland, and serum amylase and lipase levels may remain normal *(5,6)*. It is important to note that a correlation has not been found between the degree or trend of serum amylase and lipase elevation with the amount of structural damage of the pancreas or severity of AP *(9)*.

Pancreatic enzymes, such as serum trypsin, chymotrypsin, elastase, ribonuclease, and phospholipase A_2 have been all reported to be elevated in AP, but assays to measure these enzymes are not readily available for clinical use, and their specificity has not been defined *(2,5,6,9)*.

The use of other clinically available laboratory tests may have a role in determining the etiology of AP. For example, elevated bilirubin and hepatic transaminases, particularly alanine aminotransferase more than 80 IU/L should raise the suspicion of gallstone pancreatitis *(1–5;* *see* Chapter 3).

Imaging

ULTRASONOGRAPHY

Transabdominal ultrasonography is widely available, relatively inexpensive, and quite safe. Unfortunately, pancreatic imaging by ultrasound has limitations from overlying bowel gas and surrounding fat planes, which tend to be exaggerated in the acutely inflamed pancreas owing to ileus and peripancreatic edema. Thus the sensitivity and specificity of this modality for diagnosing AP is low *(1)*. Nonetheless, transabdominal ultrasonography is useful in the early stages of AP to search for gallbladder stones or sludge, evaluate for dilation of the common bile duct caused by choledocholithiasis, and analyze for other possible causes of severe abdominal pain.

COMPUTED TOMOGRAPHY SCAN

The computed tomography (CT) scan, particularly when done with helical or multidetector technology, is a valuable tool in the diagnosis and management of AP. However, not every patient with AP requires a CT scan. CT is mainly indicated if the initial diagnosis is in doubt or for prognostic purposes in severely ill patients as in the section on Risk Stratification *(4)*. The role of CT is both to document the appropriate findings that confirm the diagnosis of AP and to exclude other intra-abdominal catastrophes that can mimic AP (e.g., a perforated viscus). CT scan findings, which support the diagnosis of AP, include diffuse or segmental enlargement of the pancreas, irregularity of the pancreatic contour with obliteration of the peripancreatic fat planes, areas of decreased density within the pancreas, and ill-defined fluid collections in the pancreas or outside the gland in the lesser sac or pararenal spaces. The frequency of these findings varies according to the severity of pancreatitis, and these findings do not require intravenous administration of contrast material to be identified.

Intravenous contrast-enhanced computed tomography (CECT) is mainly used to differentiate pancreatic necrosis from interstitial pancreatitis or to monitor for pancreatitis complications in selected cases (i.e., to assist in estimating prognosis or managing patients with AP, rather than simply confirming a diagnosis). Normal CT findings have been reported in 24–67% of patients with mild AP *(2)*.

Controversy exists as to whether intravenous contrast early in the clinical course exacerbates the severity of AP. Although deleterious effects of intravenous contrast have been observed in animal models of experimental pancreatitis, studies in humans have yielded conflicting results *(10)*. Many authors agree that CECT scans are unneccessary in patients with mild AP (*see* Risk Stratification in Acute Pancreatitis section) and should be reserved for those pateints with a more complicated clinical course. Additionally, early CECT may underestimate the degree of pancreatic necrosis that may develop over time from the disruption of pancreatic microvascular circulation that usually occurs in the first 12–24 hours of SAP *(11,12)*. At present, it is recommended that CECT be obtained 3–4 days after the onset of SAP for optimal assessment of pancreatic necrosis *(8)*.

MAGNETIC RESONANCE IMAGING

Currently, magnetic resonance imaging (MRI) has no advantage over CT scan in the management of AP. MRI has a comparable specificity and sensitivity for diagnostic and severity assessment of AP *(1,2)*. Its cost, availability, and contraindication in patients with metallic implants has limited the application of MRI in AP to date.

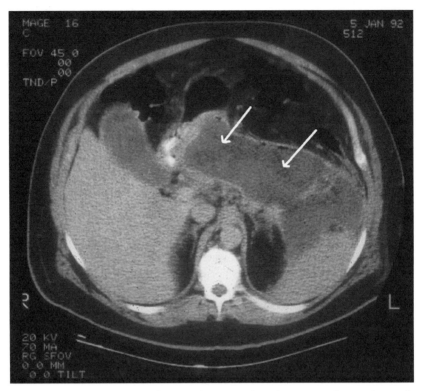

Fig. 1. A computed tomography scan demonstrating a large area of necrosis as evidenced by the lack of contrast enhancement (arrows) after intravenous contrast administration.

ENDOSCOPIC RETROGRADE CHOLANGIOPANCREATOGRAPHY

Endoscopic retrograde cholangiopancreatography (ERCP) has no role in diagnosing AP. Therapeutic application of ERCP in moderate-to-severe acute gallstone pancreatitis has been shown by several controlled clinical trials to lower morbidity and mortality when compared to traditional medical treatment alone (*see* Chapter 3). ERCP is also utilized in the differential diagnosis and elective treatment of recurrent unexplained pancreatitis secondary to sphincter Oddi dysfunction, pancreatic divisum, and microlithiasis *(13–15)*.

ENDOSCOPIC ULTRASOUND

The diagnostic role of endoscopic ultrasound (EUS) in AP is still evolving; it is not readily available in all institutions. In recent studies, the immediate application of EUS for suspected biliary AP may aid in the diagnosis of gallstone pancreatitis, thereby helping to triage patients for therapeutic ERCP with endoscopic sphincterotomy and stone removal *(16)*.

RISK STRATIFICATION IN ACUTE PANCREATITIS

Early evaluation of AP severity is essential to allow the clinician to predict the patient's clinical course, estimate prognosis, and determine the need for intensive care unit admission. Severe pancreatitis can be defined by various systems that predict complications and mortality or by the development of the complication itself. Thus, there is a difference between a predictive system that suggests complications may develop and the actual development of a complication. (This issue is discussed in more detail in Chapter 6.) This section focuses on methods to predict morbidity and mortality. Severe pancreatitis can be predicted by clinical criteria, multiple factor scoring systems, serum markers, and radiographic features. The ability of a seasoned clinician's ability to detect severe pancreatitis is similar to the accuracy of the multiple factor scoring systems. Several of these scoring systems have been developed to assist the clinician in the assessment of the severity of AP. The most commonly used systems are the Ranson criteria, the modified Glasgow scoring system, and the Acute Physiology And Chronic Health Evaluation II (APACHE II; *2,8,16–19*).

The Ranson Criteria and the Modified Glasgow System rely on a collection of clinical and biochemical variables measured within the first 48 hours of admission, as shown in Table 2. Clearly, from looking at these systems, many of the variables are factors that any clinician would be attuned to in managing a critically ill patient, and the scoring systems merely place these variables within a numerical framework. Using these systems, it is only possible to predict severity after 48 hours have passed. Higher Ranson or Glasgow scores predict severe disease with reasonable sensitivity. Mortality is less than 5% in patients with Ranson score of 0, in comparison to 10% for those with a criteria of 3–5, and 60% for those with a Ranson score greater than 6. Thus, many patients with higher Ranson scores do not die and, in fact, do not develop organ failure or other complications. The same is true for the modified Glasgow scoring system. Therefore, the Ranson and modified Glasgow scoring systems lack specificity. It should also be noted that there are separate Ranson scoring systems for alcohol-induced and biliary pancreatitis, and the total score cannot be calculated unless all factors are measured after 48 hours of observation. The most important roles of the Ranson and Glasgow scoring may be to exclude severe disease. A Glasgow or Ranson score of 0 or 1 virtually guarantees that complications will not develop and that mortality will be negligible. A second

Table 2
Variables of the Ranson Criteria and Modified Glasgow System

Ranson Criteria		Modified Glasgow System	
For Acute Non-Gallstone Pancreatitis			
Upon admission:		Arterial PO$_2$	<60 mmHg
1. Age	>55 years	Serum albumin	<3.2 g/dL
2. WBC	>16,000/mm^3	Serum Ca	<8 mg/dL
3. Glucose	>200 mg/dL	WBC	>15,000/mm^3
4. LDH	>350 IU/L	AST	>200 IU/L
5. AST	>250 IU/L	LDH	>600 IU/L
Within 48 hours:		Glucose	>180 mg/dL
1. Drop in HCT	>10%	BUN	>45 mg/dL
2. Serum Ca	<8 mg/dL		
3. Base deficit	>4 mEq/L		
4. Increase BUN	>5 mg/dL		
5. Fluid deficit	>6 L		
6. Arterial PO$_2$	<60 mmHg		
For Acute Gallstone Pancreatitis			
Upon admission:			
1. Age	>70 years		
2. WBC	>18,000/mm^3		
3. Glucose	>220 mg/dL		
4. LDH	>400 IU/L		
5. AST	>440 IU/L		
Within 48 hours:			
1. Drop in HCT	>10%		
2. Serum Ca	<8 mg/dL		
3. Base deficit	>5 mEq/L		
4. Increase BUN	>2 mg/dL		
5. Fluid deficit	>6 L		
6. Arterial PO$_2$	<60 mmHg		

HCT, hemoconcentration; WBC, white blood count; LDH, lactate dehydrogenase; AST, aspartate aminotransferase; BUN, blood urea nitrogen.

important use of these scoring systems is for clinical research, in characterizing disease severity for comparison between studies.

The APACHE II scoring system is considered more specific and accurate when compared to clinical assessment and Ranson/modified Glasgow system (Table 3). The APACHE II may be applied at any time point in the course of disease, which is an advantage over the Ranson and Glasgow criteria. The APACHE II system is quite complex (9), making it unwieldy for everyday clinical use. Many free downloadable programs for PDA use are available on the Web, which has markedly

Table 3
The APACHE II Severity of Disease Classification System

Physiologic variable	High abnormal range				0	Low abnormal range				Points
	+4	+3	+2	+1	0	+1	+2	+3	+4	
Temperature–rectal (°C)	≥41°	39–40.9°		38.5–38.9°	36–38.4°	34–35.9°	32–33.9°	30–31.9°	≤29.9°	
Mean arterial pressure–mmHg	≥160	130–159	110–129		70–109		50–69		≤49	
Heart rate (ventricular response)	≥180	140–179	110–139		70–109		55–69	40–54	≤39	
Respiratory rate (nonventilated or ventilated)	≥50	35–49		25–34	12–24	10–11	6–9		≤5	
Oxygenation: A-aDO$_2$ or PaO$_2$ (mmHg) a. FIO$_2$ ≥ 0.5 record A-aDO$_2$	≥500	350–499	200–349		<200					
b. FIO$_2$ < 0.5 record PaO$_2$					PO$_2$ >70	PO$_2$ 61–70		PO$_2$ 55–60	PO$_2$ <55	
Arterial pH (preferred)	≥7.7	7.6–7.69		7.5–7.59	7.33–7.49		7.25–7.32	7.15–7.24	<7.15	
Serum HCO$_3$ (venous mEq/L) (not preferred, but may use if no ABGs)	≥52	41–51.9		32–40.9	22–31.9		18–21.9	15–17.9	<15	
Serum sodium (mEq/L)	≥180	160–179	155–159	150–154	130–149		120–129	111–119	≤110	
Serum potassium (mEq/L)	≥7	6–6.9		5.5–5.9	3.5–5.4	3–3.4	2.5–2.9		<2.5	
Serum creatinine (mg/dL) Double point score for acute renal failure	≥3.5	2–3.4	1.5–1.9		0.6–1.4		<0.6			
Hematocrit (%)	≥60		50–59.9	46–49.9	30–45.9		20–29.9		<20	

Continued

Table 3 (Continued)

Physiologic variable	High abnormal range				0	Low abnormal range				Points
	+4	+3	+2	+1		+1	+2	+3	+4	
White blood count (total/mm^3) (in 1000s)	≥40		20–39.9	15–19.9	3–14.9		1–2.9		<1	
Glasgow coma score (GCS) Score = 15 minus actual GCS										
A. Total acute physiology score (sum of 12 above points)										
B. Age points (years)	≤44 = 0;		45–54 = 2;	55–64 = 3;	65–74 = 5;	≥75 = 6				
C. Chronic health points (see below)										
Total APACHE II score (add together the points from A + B + C)										

Chronic Health Points: If the patient has a history of severe organ system insufficiency or is immunocompromised as defined below, assign points as follows:

    5 points for nonoperative or emergency postoperative patients

    2 points for elective postoperative patients

Definitions: organ insufficiency or immunocompromised state must have been evident prior to this hospital admission and conform to the following criteria: *Liver*—biopsy proven cirrhosis and documented portal hypertension; episodes of past upper gastrointestinal bleeding attributed to portal hypertension; or prior episodes of hepatic failure/encephalopathy/coma. *Cardiovascular*—New York Heart Association Class IV. *Respiratory*—Chronic restrictive, obstructive, or vascular disease resulting in severe exercise restriction (i.e., unable to climb stairs or perform household duties; or documented chronic hypoxia, hypercapnia, secondary polycythemia, severe pulmonary hypertension (>40 mmHg), or respirator dependency. *Renal*—receiving chronic dialysis. *Immunocompromised*—the patient has received therapy that suppresses resistance to infection (e.g., immunosuppression, chemotherapy, radiation, long term or recent high-dose steroids, or has a disease that is sufficiently advanced to suppress resistance to infection, e.g., leukemia, lymphoma, AIDS).

Interpretation of score

0–4 = ~4% death rate	10–14 = ~15% death rate	20–24 = ~40% death rate	30–34 = ~75% death rate
5–9 = ~8% death rate	15–19 = ~25% death rate	25–29 = ~55% death rate	Over 34 = ~85% death rate

ABGs, arterial blood gases.

Table 4
Computed Tomography Grading System

Grade A:	Normal findings
Grade B:	Focal or diffuse pancreatic enlargement
Grade C:	Inflammation of the pancreas and pancreatic fat
Grade D:	Peripancreatic fluid collection in single location usually within the anterior para-renal space
Grade E:	Two or more fluid collections or the presence of peripancreatic gas

improved the ease in using the APACHE II scoring system. Predicted SAP is defined by a Ranson score of 3 or greater or an APACHE II score of 8 or greater (8,9). Actual SAP is defined by the presence of organ failure or local pancreatic complications (e.g., necrosis, infected necrosis, pseudocyst, and abscess).

CT has also become routinely used in the prediction and determination of disease severity. The initial CT grading system, which did not require intravenous contrast administration, was developed by Balthazar and Ranson (Table 4; 20). However, using CT alone also has a relatively high false-positive rate (i.e., many patients with grade C and even D pancreatitis recover without developing organ failure or dying). Combining the CT grading system with Ranson prognostic signs further improves the prognostic capacity when compared to either system alone. Patients with grade D or E are almost certain to develop complications, and they have a significantly increased risk of mortality, and this risk is augmented by the coexistence of a high Ranson score. Those patients with grade C pancreatitis and a Ranson score less than 3 routinely do well, whereas those with grade C pancreatitis and a Ranson score more than 3 are much more likely to develop complications and/or die. A grade of A or B strongly predicts an uncomplicated outcome (1,20). These grading systems are based on non-CECT scans. CECT can also be used to determine the presence of pancreatic necrosis. Interstitial pancreatitis (the absence of necrosis) is defined by homogeneous and uniform intravenous contrast enhancement of the pancreas, which requires rapid scanning over the pancreas timed to the infusion of intravenous contrast. Necrosis is defined by inhomogeneous enhancement with intravenous contrast, especially when large areas of the pancreas are entirely devoid of enhancement. Pancreatic necrosis per se is not always associated with other clinical features of severe disease (e.g., organ failure or infected necrosis), but the presence of necrosis markedly increases the chance of developing these severe clinical markers. Particularly, pancreatic necrosis puts patients at risk for infection of the devitalized tissue, one of the most severe complications of AP (*see* Chapter 7). CT scans with intravenous contrast enhancement is our only method currently available to identify necrosis.

Given that the multiple factor scoring systems are complex and that CT scans are expensive, there has been continued interest in identifying simpler or less expensive methods to predict severity. Several clinical and serum markers of disease severity have been proposed, which include routine laboratory tests and novel markers of disease severity. Despite the diagnostic importance of elevated serum amylase and lipase in AP, numerous studies have demonstrated that elevated levels of these enzymes have no prognostic value in AP *(2,8,9)*. This is the reason why they are excluded in any AP severity scoring system. Hemoconcentration more than 44% at presentation has been demonstrated by several investigators to be a reasonably accurate early marker that predicts pancreatic necrosis and organ failure *(21–23)*. In contrast, Whitcomb et al. showed that an admission hematocrit of 40% or below predicts a low risk of pancreatic necrosis and may reduce the need for diagnostic CT scans *(24)*.

More novel serum tests have also been evaluated. C-reactive protein (an acute-phase reactant) is cheap, widely available, and commonly used in Europe as a measure of severity. A level of 150 mg/L of C-reactive protein has been proposed as a criterion for distinguishing mild AP from SAP *(9)*. Other markers, such as trypsinogen activation peptide, interleukin-6, and polymorphonuclear elastase, have been shown in research studies to be of value to predict severe necrotizing pancreatitis, but commercial assays are not yet available for clinical use *(2–7)*.

Clinical or demographic features may also predict disease severity. Obesity has been shown in several studies to be a risk factor for the severe outcome of AP, and it is associated with an increased risk of mortality *(9)*. Advanced age and comorbid diseases are also risk factors for morbidity and mortality from AP. Other clinical parameters like hypovolemic shock, massive pleural effusion, prolonged hypoxia, and body echymosis are indicative of a complicated course and a higher risk of mortality *(1)*.

Many steps have already been taken to guide the clinician's goal of predicting the severity of AP. The ability to accurately predict outcome would allow the improved use of intensive and intermediate care unit beds and would allow specific therapy (once available) to be directed at those patients most likely to benefit. However, the ideal grading system or the predictive marker of choice does not yet exist. Careful and repeated clinical evaluation by skillful clinicians remains an important part of detecting complications early. Multiple factor scoring systems are useful adjuncts but remain complex, difficult to use, and all have a high false-positive rate. CT scans are widely used and seem to provide the best addition to clinical assessment, both to confirm the diagnosis and/or rule out alternative diagnoses and estimate the disease severity.

REFERENCES

1. Topazian M, Gorelick F. Acute pancreatitis. In: Yamada T, ed. Textbook of Gastroenterology 3rd ed. Lippincott, Philadelphia, PA, 1999: 2121–2150.
2. Ranson JHC. Diagnostic standards for acute pancreatitis. World J Surg 1997; 21: 136–142.
3. Beger HG, Rau B, Mayer J, Pralle U. Natural course of acute pancreatitis. World J Surg 1997; 21: 130–135.
4. Mergener K, Baillie J. Acute pancreatitis. BMJ 1998; 316: 44–48.
5. Banks P. Acute and chronic pancreatitis. In: Feldman M, Scharschmidt B, Sleisenger M, eds. Sleisenger & Fordtran's Gastrointestinal and Liver Disease 6th ed. Saunders, Philadelphia, PA, 1998: 809–862.
6. Levitt MD, Eckfeldt JH. Diagnosis of acute pancreatitis. In: Go V, Dimango E, Gardner J, et al., eds. The Pancreas: Biology, Pathophysiology and Disease 2nd ed. Raven Press, NY, 1993: 613–635.
7. Steinberg W, Tenner S. Acute pancreatitis. N Engl J Med 1994; 330: 1198–1210.
8. Banks PA. Practice guidelines in acute pancreatitis. Am J Gastroenterol 1997; 92: 377–386.
9. Triester SL, Kowdley KV. Prognostic factors in acute pancreatitis. J Clin Gastroenterol 2002; 34: 167–176.
10. Foitzik T, Bassi DG, Schmidt J, et al. Intravenous contrast medium accentuates the severity of acute necrotizing pancreatitis in the rat. Gastroenterology 1994; 106: 207–214.
11. Baron T, Morgan D. Acute necrotizing pancreatitis. N Engl J Med 1999; 340: 1412–1417.
12. Nuutinen P, Kivisaari L, Schroder T. Contrast-enhanced computed tomography and microangiography of the pancreas in acute human hemorrhagic/necrotizing pancreatitis. Pancreas 1988; 3: 53–60.
13. Baillie J. Treatment of acute biliary pancreatitis. N Engl J Med 1997; 336: 286–287.
14. Frakes J. Biliary pancreatitis: A review. J Clin Gastroenterol 1999; 28: 97–109.
15. Neoptolemos JP, Carr-Locke DL, Baily IA, et al. Controlled trial of urgent endoscopic retrograde cholangiopancreatography and endoscopic sphincterotomy versus conservative treatment for acute pancreatitis due to gallstones. Lancet 1988; 2: 979–983.
16. Prat F, Edery J, Meduri B, et al. Early EUS of the bile duct before endoscopic sphincterotomy for acute biliary pancreatitis. Gastrrointest Endosc 2001; 54: 724–729.
17. Ranson JHC. Etiological and Prognostic factors in human acute pancreatitis: A review. Am J Gastroenterol 1982; 77: 633–638.
18. Balthazar E, Ranson JHC, Naidich DP, et al. Acute pancreatitis: Prognostic value of CT. Radiology 1985; 156: 767–772.
19. Balthazar E, Robinson DL, Meigibow AJ, Ranson JHC. Acute pancreatitis: value of CT in establishing prognosis. Radiology 1990; 174: 331–336.
20. Balthazar E. Acute pancreatitis: Assessment of severity with clinical and CT evaluation. Radiology 2002; 223: 603–613.

21. Brown A, Orav J, Banks PA. Hemoconcentration is an early marker for organ fail-
    ure and necrotizing pancreatitis. Pancreas 2000; 20: 367–372.
22. Lankisch PG, Mahlke R, Blum T, et al. Hemoconcentration: An early marker of
    severe and/or necrotizing pancreatitis? A critical appraisal. Am J Gastroenterol
    2001; 96: 2081–2086.
23. Baron T. Predicting the severity of acute pancreatitis: Is it time to concentrate on
    hematocrit?. Am J Gastroenterol 2001; 96: 1960–1961.
24. Whitcomb DC, Pederso MRA, Oliva J, et al. An admission hematocrit of 40 or less
    predicts a low risk of pancreatic necrosis and may reduce the need for diagnostic
    CT scans. Gastroenterology 1999; 116: A1176.

3 Gallstone Pancreatitis

Matthias Kraft, MD
and Markus M. Lerch, MD, FRCP, FACG

Contents

INTRODUCTION

Acute pancreatitis (AP) is a disease of great social impact with an incidence of approximately 20/100,000 population per year. The mild form, which accounts for 75–80% of cases, has virtually no mortality and benefits from simple symptomatic treatment. In contrast, the severe form is characterized by local and systemic complications, may lead to multi-organ failure, and is burdened by a mortality rate between 5 and 20%.

The most frequent form of AP is acute biliary pancreatitis, which in published reports accounts for a range between 16 and 70% of all cases in most Western countries. Also, there is evidence that up to one-third of AP cases that had previously been thought to be idiopathic are, in fact, caused by microlithiasis or bile crystals.

From: *Pancreatitis and Its Complications*
Edited by: C. E. Forsmark © Humana Press Inc., Totowa, NJ

In recent years, there have been many changes in the management of patients suffering from AP. Improvements include the general availability of contrast-enhanced (dynamic) computed tomography (CECT) scanning, magnetic resonance imaging, interventional procedures like endoscopic retrograde cholangiopancreatography (ERCP) and endoscopic sphinctero-tomy (EST), a better understanding of the underlying pathophysiology, and improved standards of intensive care, as well as a more aggressive surgical approach in patients with infected pancreatic necrosis. All of these advances have only minimally reduced the overall mortality (~10–15%) during the last two decades. The improved medical and sur-gical care of these patients has been counterweighed by the increase in age and comorbid medical conditions of patients.

The purpose of this chapter is to review the principal pathophysio-logical mechanisms of gallstone pancreatitis and to provide clinical guidelines for the care of patients with gallstone-induced pancreatitis.

ETIOLOGY AND PATHOGENESIS

Since the 1856 discovery by Claude Bernard *(1)* that bile is an agent that can cause pancreatitis when injected into the pancreatic duct of lab-oratory animals, many studies have been performed to elucidate the pathophysiology of gallstone pancreatitis. Several conflicting hypothe-ses have later been proposed to explain how the passage of gallstones through the biliary tract triggers disease onset. In 1901, Eugene Lindsey Opie initially postulated that the impairment of pancreatic outflow owing to obstruction of the pancreatic duct causes pancreatitis *(2;* Fig. 1). This initial "duct obstruction" hypothesis was somewhat forgotten when Opie published his second "common channel" hypothesis in the same year *(3).* This second hypothesis predicted that an impacted gallstone at the papilla of Vater creates a communication between the pancreatic and bile duct (i.e., the common channel), through which bile flows into the pancreatic duct and causes pancreatitis.

Although Opie's common channel hypothesis seems rational from a mechanistic point of view and had become one of the most accepted theories in this field, some experimental and clinical evidence is incompatible with its assumptions *(4,5).* Anatomical studies have shown that the communication between the pancreatic duct and com-mon bile duct is much too short (<6 mm) to permit biliary reflux into the pancreatic duct *(6),* and an impacted gallstone would more likely obstruct both the common bile duct and the pancreatic duct *(7).* Even in the event of an existing anatomical communication, pancreatic secre-tory pressure would still exceed biliary pressure, and pancreatic juice would flow into the bile duct rather than bile flowing into the pancreatic

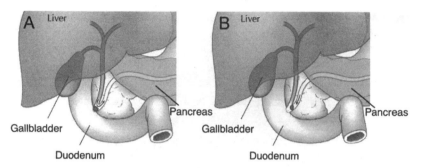

Fig. 1. The two "Opie hypotheses" for the pathogenesis of gallstone-induced pancreatitis, both reported in 1901, according to Lerch et al. *(97)* with permission. **(A)** The "common channel" reflux hypothesis. A gallstone, impacted at the duodenal papilla, creates a communication between the pancreatic duct and common bile duct. Behind it, bile can flow through this common channel into the pancreatic duct and would trigger the onset of acute pancreatitis (AP). **(B)** The pancreatic "duct obstruction" hypotheses. A gallstone on its passage through the biliary tract obstructs the pancreatic duct. The intraductal pressure rises and trigger acinar cell damage that leads to necrosis. Whether or not the common bile duct is also obstructed is immaterial to the triggering mechanism of pancreatitis, but it may determine later disease severity.

duct *(8,9)*. As a result of this gradient, bile flow into the pancreatic duct would not occur until 24–48 hours after complete obstruction, a time point at which necrotic cell damage in the pancreas has already been established *(5)*. Bilio-pancreatic reflux from a loss of barrier function of the damaged pancreatic ductal epithelium in the later stages of the disease may explain the observation of a bile-stained necrotic pancreas at the time of surgery. However, this is not evidence for the assumption that reflux of bile into the pancreas is an initial triggering event for the disease. Experiments performed on the opossum, an animal model that is anatomically well-suited to test the common channel hypothesis, have revealed that neither a common channel nor biliopancreatic reflux is required for the development of acute necrotizing pancreatitis *(5)*. This does not eliminate the possibility that bile acids can reach the pancreas by a systemic route and impair cellular Ca^{2+} signaling in pancreatic acinar cells through specific membrane transporters, as recently reported *(10)*. Another mechanism through which bile might aggravate pancreatitis is when its passage into the gut is obstructed by a gallstone. Obstruction of bile flow may lead to an impairment of the reticuloendothelial system in the liver, a factor that is known to affect the severity of pancreatitis *(11)*.

The potential communication between the pancreatic and bile duct through the common channel is controlled by the sphincter of Oddi. The data regarding function of the sphincter of Oddi in gallstone pancreatitis are conflicting, and both hypotonic *(12)* and hypertonic *(13)* sphincter of Oddi pressures have been reported in up to 72% of cases with recurrent AP of unknown origin *(14)*. Another hypothesis that might explain the pathogenesis of gallstone pancreatitis—reflux of duodenal contents into the pancreatic duct through an incompetent sphincter after the passage of a gallstone—has been conclusively ruled out as the cause of human biliary pancreatitis *(15)*. Perfusion of sterile bile through the pancreatic duct has been shown to be completely harmless *(16)*. However, it is still possible that an influx of infected bile into the pancreas after prolonged obstruction at the papilla, when the pressure gradient between the pancreatic duct (higher) and the bile duct (lower) is reversed *(17,18)*, may represent an aggravating factor of the course of pancreatitis or a risk factor for infected pancreatic necrosis.

It is now clear that the initial pathophysiological events during the course of gallstone-induced pancreatitis affect acinar cells *(19)* and are triggered by the obstruction or impairment of flow from the pancreatic duct *(20)*. Bacterial contamination of bile or reflux of bile into the pancreatic duct are not involved or required for pancreatitis to occur but may represent aggravating factors in the later course of disease and could possibly be important in determining the severity and prognosis of acute gallstone pancreatitis.

DIAGNOSIS

Since 1929, the diagnosis of AP has been based on the cardinal symptoms of abdominal pain and vomiting in combination with a significantly elevated serum amylase (or lipase) activity. A distinction between biliary pancreatitis and other etiological varieties is more difficult but should be made within 48–72 hours following hospital admission to permit effective and timely endoscopic intervention. Therefore, one goal of an initial diagnostic work-up is to distinguish AP from other life-threatening intraabdominal conditions that begin with acute abdominal pain (e.g., aortic aneurysm, visceral ischemia, and perforated ulcer). The approach to diagnosis is reviewed in Chapter 2. The second goal is defining the distinction between gallstone-induced pancreatitis and other etiological varieties of the disease and is the focus of this discussion.

Clinical Assessment

The common clinical findings of AP are often a diffuse abdominal tenderness, upper abdominal pain, and vomiting. Body ecchymosis is rarely evident (Cullens sign, and Grey-Turner's sign; *21*). Clinical findings alone are often unreliable in determining the diagnosis or etiology of AP because these features may be found in association with several

other acute abdominal conditions, especially after abdominal operations
(22). In the particular case of acute gallstone pancreatitis, a history of
previous gallstone-induced illness may be elicited, such as recurrent
right upper pain or a history of obstructive jaundice. A previous case of
drug or alcohol abuse does not always eliminate gallstone-induced pancreatitis but is suggestive of other etiologies. In patients who have had
recurrent pancreatitis, particularly if they are less than 25 years of age
or have a positive family history of pancreatitis, the hereditary variety of
pancreatitis associated with trypsinogen mutations must be considered
(23–25). Although helpful, history alone is never sufficient to distinguish
acute gallstone from nongallstone pancreatitis.

Laboratory Studies

Biochemical findings, such as serum amylase or lipase activity of
three times the upper limit, predict the diagnosis of AP with an accuracy
of approximately 95% *(26)*. If available, the advantages of measuring
serum lipase are that its activity will remain increased for a longer period
than amylase and that it is somewhat more specific than serum amylase
(27,28). Rarely, serum lipase concentrations may be within the normal
range in patients with pancreatitis when the pancreas is instantaneously
cut off from its entire blood supply (e.g., appoplexy and infarction).

Elevations in liver chemistries (bilirubin, alkaline phosphatase, and
transaminases) can occur when a gallstone transiently obstructs at the
ampulla and are useful markers for gallstone-induced AP. Serum bilirubin
measurements are one of the most reliable laboratory assays to differentiate a biliary cause of pancreatitis from other etiologies. Levels
greater than twofold the normal value are highly suggestive of a biliary
cause of AP. Similarly, levels of transaminases, particularly alanine
aminotransferase more than 60–80 IU/L (depending on the study) are predictive of a biliary etiology. Elevations in alkaline phosphatase are less
helpful in identifying gallstone pancreatitis. A very suggestive pattern
is a sharp increase in liver chemistries at the onset of attack, followed by
a rather prompt decrease over 1–2 days. Persistent elevations of liver
chemistries suggest a persistently obstructing common bile duct stone,
a condition that usually merits ERCP with removal of stones (*see*
below). Further laboratory findings (e.g., white cell count, blood glucose,
blood urea nitrogen, arterial pO_2, albumin, calcium, and C-reactive protein [CRP]) are important for severity stratification, although they do
not directly contribute to the diagnosis of pancreatitis nor the identification of gallstones as the etiology.

Several more novel tests show promise for diagnosis and risk stratification but are not widely available or used. A novel urinary test strip that
identifies the presence of trypsinogen-2 may have a role in establishing

the diagnosis of AP in the future *(29–32)*. Quantification of trypsinogen activation peptide in serum and urine has been found to determine the disease severity of AP with great accuracy *(33)* and may be widely used once the assay becomes available as a urinary test strip. Many other laboratory tests that have been purported to assist in establishing the severity of AP, such as antiprotease levels, polymorphonuclear elastase, complement factors, and interleukin and chemokine levels, have never been used in routine clinical practice. However, these novel tests do not appear to have any ability to distinguish gallstone from non-gallstone pancreatitis.

Ultrasound

Ultrasound (US) examination of the abdomen is a cheap and very reliable method to detect gallstones within the gallbladder. The finding of gallstones within the gallbladder is highly suggestive of a biliary cause of pancreatitis. Dilatation of the common bile duct or stones within the common bile duct, as well as edema and necrosis within the pancreas, can also be detected, albeit with less accuracy than gallbladder stones. Additionally, the US can be useful in assessing for other intra-abdominal disorders like aortic aneurysm, appendicitis, and abscess formation *(34–36)*. The accuracy of abdominal US is limited in AP because of the common presence of overlying intestinal gas. Along with providing information on the presence of gallstones, US can also help in selecting patients for urgent therapy. If a patient presents with a history of gall-stones and has either persistently elevated levels of serum bilirubin or a dilated bile duct on ultrasound, they will generally require urgent ERCP. In many European countries where abdominal ultrasound is performed as a real-time and bedside imaging technique by physicians, the technique is regarded as an initial diagnostic tool for patients with pancreatitis *(37)*. It is less popular in North America where radiologists prefer to assess computed tomography (CT) films over ultrasound films, both of which are obtained by technicians. Nonetheless, the ultrasound remains a highly useful initial study in patients with suspected gallstone pancreatitis.

Endoscopic Retrograde Cholangiopancreatography

ERCP allows for the direct visualization of the common bile and pancreatic ducts (Fig. 2). It may be required to determine the etiology of pancreatitis and detect gallstones or anatomical variants and tumors, but ERCP is used most commonly for therapy rather than diagnosis. ERCP is likely the most sensitive and widely available method to determine the biliary etiology of AP and may detect bile duct stones or gallstones in nearly all patients with acute gallstone pancreatitis *(38)* when the bile duct is visualized. Visualization of the bile duct can be generally

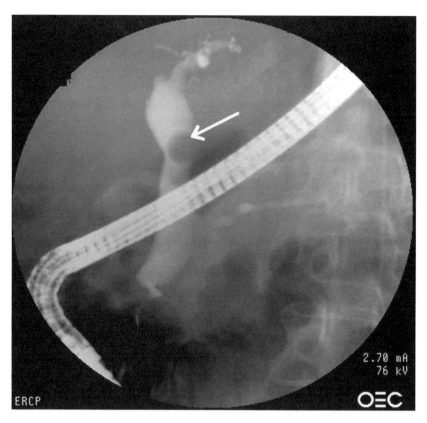

Fig. 2. An endoscopic retrograde cholangiopancreatography demonstrating a stone in the common bile duct (arrow).

accomplished in 94–98% of patients without AP but only in approximately 80–90% of patients with AP *(39,40)*. Nevertheless, the procedure is expensive, invasive, and carries risk; therefore, it is used sparingly for the diagnosis of acute gallstone pancreatitis. The role and timing of ERCP in treating (rather than diagnosing) gallstone pancreatitis has been the subject of several randomized trials. Controversies continue to exist involving the endoscopic therapy of AP, and these issues are discussed in the Treatment section. Endoscopic cannulation of the pancreatic duct in patients with pancreatitis is generally not required (unless pancreatic trauma or duct laceration is suspected), but it is also not harmful if performed inadvertently and overinjection of the duct is avoided.

Other Imaging Procedures

CT is widely used in AP and should be performed if the clinical and biochemical findings are inconclusive for pancreatitis or the patient is

suspected of having severe pancreatitis or pancreatic necrosis *(41)*.
Moreover, a CECT scan should be performed between 3 and 10 days in
patients who suffer from severe AP that do not respond to appropriate
treatment. It is the method of choice to detect pancreatic necrosis, peripancreatic or intra-abdominal fluid collections, or infected necrosis.
This last complication, which usually develops between 8 and 20 days
after admission, may require surgical intervention *(42)*. CT is actually
less sensitive than US in detecting gallstones, and patients with suspected gallstone pancreatitis often receive both an ultrasound (to assess
for gallstones as the etiology) and CT (to assess for severity). The role
of magnetic resonance cholangiopancreatography (MRCP) in the diagnosis of acute gallstone pancreatitis is not yet defined, but promising
studies have been reported from investigations pertaining to other diseases of the biliopancreatic tract *(43)*. To be useful, MRCP should be
able to visualize gallstones within the gallbladder and the bile duct.
MRCP has been shown to be a valid primary imaging alternative to
ERCP in the diagnosis of chronic pancreatitis (CP) and in patients with
malformations of the common bile duct *(44)*. More encouraging,
MRCP has been shown to be an accurate diagnostic tool for the detection of gallstones in the common bile duct with a sensitivity and positive
predictive value of 92%, along with a specificity and negative predictive
value of 96% *(45)*. This impressive accuracy is a feature relating to the
size of the stones; most patients with gallstone pancreatitis have small
stones that may limit the accuracy of MRCP.

A more accurate alternative for detecting gallstones may be endoscopic ultrasound (EUS; *46*). EUS appears to have the ability to image
common bile duct stones with an accuracy approaching (in some studies, even surpassing) that of ERCP and with less overall morbidity.
However, neither MRCP nor EUS will permit the removal of identified
gallstones. Depending on the available endoscopic expertise, EUS
might be a reasonable primary step to select patients for subsequent
ERCP. Yet, in many centers, initial ERCP may be the most practical and
cost-effective approach to patients with suspected gallstone-induced
pancreatitis *(46)* that require endoscopic therapy (discussed below).

COMPLICATIONS AND SEVERITY STRATIFICATION

In 80% of patients, AP is caused by either gallstone disease or excessive alcohol consumption. The mortality rate of acute edematous pancreatitis is below 1%, whereas patients suffering from hemorrhagic
necrotizing pancreatitis die in 10–24% of cases. The short- and long-term
complications of acute gallstone pancreatitis include parenchymal
necrosis, multiorgan failure, pancreatic pseudocyst formation, cholangitis,

Table 1
Complications of Acute Pancreatitis

	Fölsch et al., 1998		Neoptolemos et al., 1988	
Complication	Invasive treatment	Conservative treatment	Invasive treatment	Conservative treatment
Total	46	51	17	34
Pseudocyst	4	8	10.1	19.3
Necrosis	16.7	13.4	n.d.	n.d.
Abscess	2.4	0.9	n.d.	n.d.
Peritonitis	1.6	2.7	n.d.	n.d.
Respiratory insufficiency	11.9 (53)	4.5 (60)	3.4 (50)	14.0 (33)
Renal failure	7.1 (66)	3.6 (75)	None	3.3 (100)
Sepsis	10.3	14.3	n.d.	n.d.
Cardiovascular shock	4.8	3.6	1.7 (100)	8.1 (100)
DIC	3.2	1.8	1.7	1.7 (100)
Diabetes	9.5	10.7	n.d.	n.d.
Jaundice	0.8	10.7	n.d.	n.d.
Cholecystitis	10.3 (0)	17.9 (5)	n.d.	n.d.
Cholangitis	13.5	11.6	10.2	8.1
Thrombosis	0.8	0.9	n.d.	n.d.
Cerebrovascular accident	n.d.	n.d.	1.7	None

Complication rates of acute pancreatis according to two prospective controlled trials by Fölsch et al. *(40)* and Neoptolemos et al. *(39)*. n.d., not determined; DIC, disseminated intravascular coagulation; numbers in parentheses indicate percentage of death within each group of complications.

recurrence of pancreatitis, and, rarely, a transition to CP. Systemic complications include respiratory failure caused by atelectasis, pleural effusion, mediastinal abscess or acute respiratory distress syndrome, depression of the cardioavascular system (most commonly, hypotension owing to hypovolemia and hypoalbuminemia, nonspecific ST-T changes and pericardial effusion), hematological changes (e.g., disseminated intravascular coagulation), gastrointestinal bleeding, thrombosis of the portal vein and renal failure (oliguria, azotemia, renal artery or renal vein thrombosis, and acute tubular necrosis). Metabolic complications like hypocalcemia, encephalopathy, sudden blindness (Purtscher's retinopathy), and hyperglycemia and hypertriglyceridemia also occur. Complication rates in two large prospective studies of patients with gallstone pancreatitis *(39,40)* are listed in Table 1 and indicate that the previously mentioned complications mainly occur in cases of severe pancreatitis. Cardiovascular along with pulmonary and renal complications are causally related to increased mortality in the early phase of acute necrotizing pancreatitis, whereas sepsis and infected necrosis predominate after the second week of hospital care. Early identification of patients with a severe disease course is therefore important because immediate and aggressive intensive care monitoring and treatment can alter the clinical course and outcome.

Severity stratification has been shown to be useful to distinguish between groups with mild and severe AP. This is particularly important in patients with presumed gallstone pancreatitis, as the severity of the disease is often used as a significant factor to determine the need for ERCP in management. Establishment of severity can be performed by clinical assessment coupled with biochemical parameters and a CECT scan-based grading system (Table 2; 47). Multifactor scoring systems, such as the Ranson or Glasgow scoring, have been shown to accurately predict severity in 70–80% of cases (48–50). As a single parameter, CRP alone reaches an accuracy of 80% (50). The combination of the Glasgow system with CRP results in better sensitivity and specificity for those patients who develop major clinical complications (51) and is widely used in Europe. Recently, measuring hematocrit as an indicator of hemoconcentration upon hospital admission has been reported to have a good prognostic value comparable to that of the more complex Ranson and Glasgow scores, which are obtained after 48 hours (52). The major advantage of this single, easily obtainable, and cheap parameter on admission, is its high-negative predictive value. On the basis of a second study evaluating hematocrit Lankisch et al. suggest a strategy that in the absence of hemoconcentration, CECT would be unnecessary on admission and would only be necessary if the patient's condition does not improve with therapy (53).

To assess the severity of the disease and risk of complication, the Acute Physiology And Chronic Health Evaluation (APACHE II) score has also been shown to be useful. Depending on the cut-off level, it will reach a sensitivity of 95% for cases that will develop severe complications (cut-off APACHE II score of 6). When the cut-off is raised to a score of 9, the APACHE II score will indicate severe attacks with higher specificity, but a significant number of patients who later develop complications will not be detected (54). Other indicators for a systemic inflammatory response are yet to be established in routine clinical practice (29–32). If the clinical assessment and laboratory markers, as well as severity scores, predict a mild clinical course of pancreatitis, imaging studies involving CT scan and magnetic resonance imaging are generally not required, whereas patients with severe pancreatitis may require the CECT scan at some point during their clinical course to

Table 2
Contrast-Enhanced Computed Tomography Grading System

Grade	CT Morphology
A	Normal
B	Focal or diffuse gland enlargement; small intrapancreatic fluid collection
C	Any of the above plus peripancreatic inflammatory changes and less than 30–50% gland necrosis
D	Any of the above plus peripancreatic fluid collection and 30–50% gland necrosis
E	Any of the above plus extensive extrapancreatic fluid collection, pancreatic abscess, and more than 50% gland necrosis

Modified according to Balthazar (47). CT, computed tomography.

assess complications or the extent of pancreatic necrosis (47). A CT scan without an intravenous contrast agent is of little value in AP.

TREATMENT

Before the advent of interventional endoscopy, laparotomy was the only effective approach to the removal of gallstones from the biliary tract. Since the introduction of ERCP, the management of patients with AP and CP has rapidly evolved. Particularly, the introduction of EST in 1973 (55,56) has permitted much more favorable results than open laparotomy (39,57,58). It is generally accepted that ERCP is the most effective method to identify an impacted gallstone at the papilla of Vater as the triggering cause of biliary pancreatitis. ERCP should be performed in combination with EST when bile duct stones or microlithiasis are detected. One issue of debate has been when to perform an ERCP, and whether ERCP is required as an emergency procedure in all cases. Some studies suggest that all patients with pancreatitis in which clinical, laboratory, or imaging assessments indicate an involvement of gallstones in the ethiopathogenesis of pancreatitis should undergo ERCP as soon as possible (preferably within 24–72 hours after symptom onset; 59,60). Although this policy clearly reduces the morbidity and complication rate from concomitant cholangitis, it remains unclear whether the course of pancreatitis, in itself, would be directly affected (60–63). It is also uncertain if the risks of ERCP may outweigh the benefits and if the cost of ERCP was acceptable. Several randomized controlled trials have attempted to answer these questions. In a prospective single-center study by Fan et al. *(58)*, 195 patients were randomized to receive ERCP within 24 hours following admission or conservative management, irrespective of the etiology of pancreatitis. In the treatment group, EST was only performed when detectable gallstones were found; in the control group, ERCP was not carried out unless the clinical conditions deteriorated. Fan et al. found that ERCP with EST reduced the incidence of biliary sepsis when compared with the control group (0% versus 12%, $p < 0.001$), but other systemic and local complications were not reduced. The authors conclude that early ERCP and EST (if gallstones are found) are indicated in all patients presenting with AP, regardless of the expected severity of the disease, to prevent biliary sepsis. This trial has been criticized in that only about two thirds of all patients in this trial actually had gallstones as the etiology, and nearly one third of the patients randomized to conservative therapy ultimately underwent ERCP and EST. In another prospective randomized single-center trial by Neoptolemos and coworkers *(39)*, 121 patients were enrolled with suspected acute biliary pancreatitis. Patients were stratified into groups with mild and severe disease (using the modified Glasgow criteria) within 48 hours after admission. Patients randomized to ERCP underwent it within 72 hours of admission, and when bile duct stones were found, sphincterotomy was performed. Those in the conservative therapy group could receive ERCP after 5 days if necessary. No significant differences were observed in the overall mortality rate. There was a reduction in overall complication rates (17% versus 34%, $p < 0.03$), but this difference was entirely accounted for by the group of patients with predicted severe pancreatitis (complication rates of 24% versus 61%). Within the group with predicted severe disease, there was also a reduction in hospital stay and mortality (4% versus 18%) when ERCP was performed. This improvement was limited not only to the treatment or prevention of cholangitis. The authors conclude that any evidence for a biliary cause of pancreatitis should be followed by an urgent ERCP in patients with pancreatitis that is predicted to be severe. The authors also emphasize the point that ERCP in the group predicted to have mild disease, although not beneficial, does not appear to be harmful. In a recently published, prospective multicenter study by Fölsch et al. *(40)*, 235 patients were randomized to ERCP and EST within 72 hours following the onset of abdominal pain or conservative therapy. Patients were excluded if they were jaundiced (bilirubin level >5 mg/dL), and all these patients underwent ERCP and EST outside of the trial. There was no difference in local or systemic complications between the two groups and no reduction in mortality. According to these authors, ERCP in combination with EST is required as an emergency procedure only in patients with pancreatitis who have signs of bile duct obstruction and are at risk for cholangitis (the group that was excluded from this trial). A fourth randomized trial concluded that ERCP and EST is indicated in all patients with presumed biliary pancreatitis, regardless of the predicted severity of the disease *(59)*. Unfortunately, this trial has never been published and cannot be commented on further. Given that EST is a procedure associated with a significant percentage of early (5–10%) and late (5–25%) complications *(64–66)*, depending on the experience of the investigator *(67)* and institution *(68)*, a selective (rather than universal) use of ERCP seems justified. Moreover, risk factors for complications from ERCP, such as suspected sphincter of Oddi dysfunction, advanced age of the patient, and a nondilated bile duct, need to be taken into account in the decision for or against ERCP *(69,70)*. Urgent ERCP, EST, and stone extraction within 72 hours of admission should be performed in patients with acute biliary pancreatitis with evidence for bile duct obstruction or biliary sepsis, or in which clinical, imaging, or laboratory parameters predict a severe course of biliary pancreatitis *(39,40,58,71,72)*.

When multiple stones cannot be safely removed from the common bile duct after sphincterotomy, the placement of a bile duct stent has been shown to be an alternative for high-risk patients *(73)*. It might be possible to first perform endoscopic ultrasonography in such patients, whereas ERCP is reserved for those patients with visible bile duct stones as a method to minimize overall complications form ERCP. However, whether EUS before ERCP is a cost-effective approach *(74)* will have to be shown in randomized prospective trials.

Controversy also still exists concerning the subsequent clinical course of patients whose gallbladder is left *in situ* following successful endoscopic removal of stones from their common bile duct. Although the number of gallstone carriers who develop pancreatitis is small and ranges between 3 and 8% *(75)*, it is clear that stones of less than 5-mm diameter increase the risk of developing AP fourfold *(76)*. Furthermore, it has been recognized that the risk of AP in patients with gallstone disease is reduced to that of the normal population following removal of the gallbladder *(75)*. From the 1960s to 1980s, early surgical intervention was recommended for acute gallstone pancreatitis, for which reduced mortality rates were shown in a retrospective and a prospective study *(77,78)*. More recently conducted trials *(79,80)*, particularly a prospective investigation by Kelly et al. in 1988 *(57)*, which included 165 patients with acute gallstone pancreatitis, showed a decreased morbidity and mortality rate for delayed surgery and led to the recommendation that cholecystectomy should be postponed until

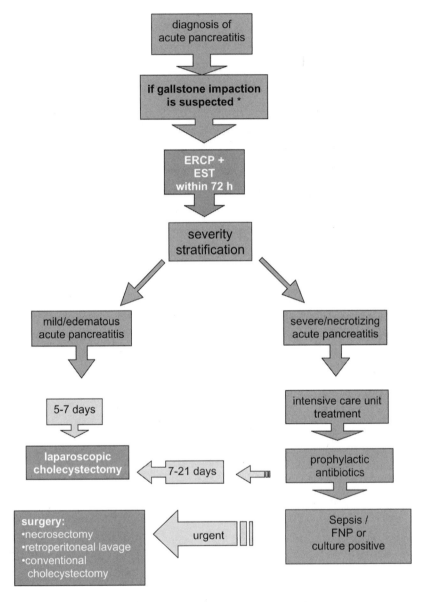

Fig. 3. Algorithm for the therapeutic approach in acute gallstone pancreatitis. Modified according to Uhl et al. *(83)*. *Based on jaundice, persistently elevated liver chemistries, a dilated common bile duct, suspected cholangitis, or predicted severe pancreatitis.

pancreatitis has subsided. According to the British Society of Gastroenterology guidelines, patients with mild gallstone pancreatitis should have definitive management of their gallstone disease ideally within 2–4 weeks after recovery from an episode of AP *(81,82)*. Another publication by Uhl et al. *(83)* recommends laparoscopic cholecystectomy 5–7 days after the onset of mild/edematous AP. These data are in line with a National Institutes of Health consensus conference, recommending cholecystectomy in acute gallstone pancreatitis 5–6 days after the onset of the disease. One reason to postpone surgical cholecystectomy in acute gallstone pancreatitis until day 4–5 is that the development of severe disease with necrosis usually takes approximately 4 days to develop *(84)*. Cholecystectomy before day 4, even in mild or edematous pancreatitis, is therefore not recommended, as the rate of complications may rise. A recently published study by Sargen et al. *(82)* analyzed the effect of deviation from these clinical guidelines and concluded that this will result in high rates of re-admission to the hospital.

In cases of severe/necrotizing AP, cholecystectomy should be performed after 7–21 days, provided that the episode of pancreatitis has subsided. In elderly high-risk patients with gallstone-induced pancreatitis, biliary sphincterotomy and removal of stones from the common bile duct may be sufficient *(85)*. Whether the placement of a pancreatic duct stent in combination with sphincterotomy, which has been reported to lower post-ERCP pancreatitis rates *(86,87)*, is of any benefit for patients undergoing sphincterotomy for biliary pancreatitis needs further evaluation. An algorithm for the treatment of acute gallstone pancreatitis is given in Fig. 3.

PROGNOSIS AND PREVENTION

Because of the high incidence of up to 45% of recurrent pancreatitis *(88)*, when the gallbladder is left *in situ*, cholecystectomy has been advocated after gallstone pancreatitis. Very low rates (4–8%) of recurrent pancreatitis in patients who underwent cholecystectomy have been noted during long-term follow-up *(89–91)*. Recurrent bile duct calculi have been reported in 2–6% of patients after EST *(92–94)*. The overall mortality of patients with gallstone pancreatitis is 6% in the first 28 days with a median age at death of 80.5 years *(95)*. In severe pancreatitis, which accounts for about 20% of cases, the mortality rate reaches 20% *(96)*. Unlike alcohol consumption, gallstones are not an established risk factor for the development of chronic pancreatitis if cholecystectomy is performed after the first episode of pancreatitis.

SUMMARY

- The diagnosis of AP should be established within 48 hours after onset of symptoms and/or hospital admission.
- Early identification of a biliary etiology is recommended using clinical, laboratory, and imaging studies.
- In patients with severe pancreatitis a CECT scan or MRCP may be required to detect complications and the extent of pancreatic necrosis.
- Signs of biliary obstruction, sepsis, and severe gallstone pancreatitis should prompt an urgent ERCP.
- EST is the treatment of choice in patients with bile duct or papillary stones.
- For patients with gallstones, cholecystectomy should be performed within 5–7 days after mild pancreatitis and within 3–4 weeks in patients with severe pancreatitis.

REFERENCES

1. Bernard C. Lecons de physiologie experimentale. Paris Bailliere 1856; 2: 758.
2. Opie E. The relation of cholelithiasis to disease of the pancreas and to fat necrosis. Johns Hopkins Hosp Bull 1901; 12: 19–21.
3. Opie E. The etiology of acute hemorrhagic pancreatitis. John Hopkins Hosp Bull 1901; 12: 182–188.
4. Neoptolemos JP. The theory of 'persisting' common bile duct stones in severe gallstone pancreatitis. Ann R Coll Surg Engl 1989; 71: 326–331.
5. Lerch MM, Saluja AK, Runzi M. Pancreatic duct obstruction triggers acute necrotizing pancreatitis in the opossum. Gastroenterology 1993; 104: 853–861.
6. DiMagno EP, Shorter RG, Taylor WF, et al. Relationships between pancreaticobiliary ductal anatomy and pancreatic ductal and parenchymal histology. Cancer 1982; 49: 361–368.
7. Mann FC, Giordano AS. The bile factor in pancreatitis. Arch Surg 1923; 6: 1–30.
8. Carr-Locke DL, Gregg JA. Endoscopic manometry of pancreatic and biliary sphincter zones in man. Basal results in healthy volunteers. Dig Dis Sci 1981; 26: 7–15.
9. Menguy RB, Hallenback GA, Bollmann JL, et al. Intradcutal pressures and sphincteric resistance in canine pancreatic and biliary ducts after various stimuli. Surg Gynecol Obstet 1958; 26: 306–320.
10. Kim JY, Kim KH, Lee JA, et al. Transporter-mediated bile acid uptake causes Ca2+-dependent cell death in rat pancreatic acinar cells. Gastroenterology 2002; 122: 1941–1953.
11. Schleicher C, Baas JC, Elser H, et al. Reticuloendothelial system blockade promotes progression from mild to severe acute pancreatitis in the opossum. Ann Surg 2001; 233: 528–536.
12. Cuschieri A, Cumming JG, Wood RA, et al. Evidence for sphincter dysfunction in patients with gallstone associated pancreatitis: effect of ceruletide in patients undergoing cholecystectomy for gallbladder disease and gallstone associated pancreatitis. Br J Surg 1984; 71: 885–888.
13. Guelrud M, Mendoza S, Vicent S, et al. Pressures in the sphincter of Oddi in patients with gallstones, common duct stones, and recurrent pancreatitis. J Clin Gastroenterol 1983; 5: 37–41.

14. Eversman D, Fogel EL, Rusche M, et al. Frequency of abnormal pancreatic and biliary sphincter manometry compared with clinical suspicion of sphincter of Oddi dysfunction. Gastrointest Endosc 1999; 50: 637–641.

15. Hernandez CA, Lerch MM. Sphincter stenosis and gallstone migration through the biliary tract. Lancet 1993; 341: 1371–1373.

16. Arendt T, Nizze H, Liebe S, et al. Does bile of patients with acute gallstone pancreatitis cause pancreatic inflammatory lesions? A study of the pancreatic toxicity of choledochal secretions collected at ERCP. Gastrointest Endosc 1999; 50: 209–213.

17. Arendt T, Nizze H, Monig H, et al. Biliary pancreatic reflux-induced AP—myth or possibility? Eur J Gastroenterol Hepatol 1999; 11: 329–335.

18. Csendes A, Sepulveda A, Burdilles P, et al. Common bile duct pressure in patients with common bile duct stones with or without acute suppurative cholangitis. Arch Surg 1988; 123: 697–699.

19. Lerch MM, Saluja AK, Dawra R, et al. Acute necrotizing pancreatitis in the opossum: earliest morphological changes involve acinar cells. Gastroenterology 1992; 103: 205–213.

20. Lerch MM, Weidenbach H, Hernandez CA, et al. Pancreatic outflow obstruction as the critical event for human gall stone induced pancreatitis. Gut 1994; 35: 1501–1503.

21. Dickson AP, Imrie CW. The incidence and prognosis of body wall ecchymosis in acute pancreatis. Surg Gynecol Obstet 1984; 159: 343–347.

22. Imrie CW, McKay AJ, Benjamin IS, et al. Secondary acute pancreatis: aetiology, prevention, diagnosis and management. Br J Surg 1978; 65: 399–402.

23. Whitcomb DC, Gorry MC, Preston RA, et al. Hereditary pancreatitis is caused by a mutation in the cationic trypsinogen gene. Nat Genet 1996; 14: 141–145.

24. Simon P, Weiss FU, Shahin-Tooth M, et al. Hereditary pancreatitis caused by a novel PRSS1 mutation (Arg-122 —> Cys) that alters autoactivation and autodegradation of cationic trypsinogen. J Biol Chem 2002; 277: 5404–5410.

25. Simon P, Weiss FU, Zimmer KP, et al. Spontaneous and sporadic trypsinogen mutations in patients with idiopathic pancreatitis. JAMA 2002, 288: 2122.

26. Steinberg WM, Goldstein SS, Davis ND, et al. Diagnostic assays in acute pancreatitis. A study of sensitivity and specificity. Ann Intern Med 1985; 102: 576–580.

27. Kolars JC, Ellis CJ, Levitt MD. Comparison of serum amylase pancreatic isoamylase and lipase in patients with hyperamylasemia. Dig Dis Sci 1984; 29: 289–293.

28. Ventrucci M, Pezzilli R, Gullo L, et al. Role of serum pancreatic enzyme assays in diagnosis of pancreatic disease. Dig Dis Sci 1989; 34: 39–45.

29. Yadav D, Agarwal N, Pitchumoni CS. A critical evaluation of laboratory tests in acute pancreatitis. Am J Gastroenterol 2002; 97: 1309–1318.

30. Bidarkundi GK, Wig JD, Bhatnagar A, et al. Clinical relevance of intracellular cytokines IL-6 and IL-12 in acute pancreatitis, and correlation with APACHE III score. Br J Biomed Sci 2002; 59: 85–89.

31. Mayer J, Rau B, Gansauge F, et al. Inflammatory mediators in human acute pancreatitis: clinical and pathophysiological implications. Gut 2000; 47: 546–552.

32. Rau B, Steinbach G, Baumgart K, et al. Serum amyloid A versus C-reactive protein in acute pancreatitis: clinical value of an alternative acute-phase reactant. Crit Care Med 2000; 28: 736–742.

33. Neoptolemos JP, Kemppainen EA, Mayer JM, et al. Early prediction of severity in acute pancreatitis by urinary trypsinogen activation peptide: a multicentre study. Lancet 2000; 355: 1955–1960.

34. Silverstein W, Isikoff MB, Hill MC, et al. Diagnostic imaging of acute pancreatitis: prospective study using CT and sonography. AJR Am J Roentgenol 1981; 137: 497–502.

35. McKay AJ, Imrie CW, O'Neill J, et al. Is an early ultrasound scan of value in acute pancreatitis? Br J Surg 1982; 69: 369–372.
36. Block S, Maier W, Bittner R, et al. Identification of pancreas necrosis in severe acute pancreatitis: imaging procedures versus clinical staging. Gut 1986; 27: 1035–1042.
37. Lerch MM, Riehl J, Buechsel R, et al. Bedside ultrasound in decision making for emergency surgery: its role in medical intensive care patients. Am J Emerg Med 1992; 10: 35–38.
38. Scholmerich J, Lausen M, Lay L, et al. Value of endoscopic retrograde cholangiopancreatography in determining the cause but not course of acute pancreatitis. Endoscopy 1992; 24: 244–247.
39. Neoptolemos JP, Carl-Locke DL. London LJ, et al. Controlled trial of urgent endoscopic retrograde cholangiopancreatography and endoscopic sphincterotomy versus conservative treatment for acute pancreatitis due to gallstones. Lancet 1988; 2: 979–983.
40. Folsch UR, Nitsche R, Ludtke R, et al. Early ERCP and papillotomy compared with conservative treatment for acute biliary pancreatitis. The German Study Group on Acute Biliary Pancreatitis. N Engl J Med 1997; 336: 237–242.
41. Hill MC, Huntington DK. Computed tomography and acute pancreatitis. Gastroenterol Clin North Am 1990; 19: 811–842.
42. Balthazar EJ, Robinson DL, Mebigow AJ, et al. Acute pancreatitis: value of CT in establishing prognosis. Radiology 1990; 174: 331–336.
43. Albert JG, Riemann JF. ERCP and MRCP—when and why. Best Pract Res Clin Gastroenterol 2002; 16: 399–419.
44. Del Frate C, Zanardi R, Mortele K, et al. Advances in imaging for pancreatic disease. Curr Gastroenterol Rep 2002; 4: 140–148.
45. Brisbois D, Blomteux O, Nehimi A, et al. Value of MRCP for detection of choledocholithiasis in symptomatic patients: one-year experience with a standardized high resolution breath-hold technique. Jbr-Btr 2001; 84: 258–261.
46. Arguedas MR, Dupont AW, Wilcox CM. Where do ERCP, endoscopic ultrasound, magnetic resonance cholangiopancreatography, and intraoperative cholangiography fit in the management of acute biliary pancreatitis? A decision analysis model. Am J Gastroenterol 2001; 96: 2892–2899.
47. Balthazar EJ. Acute pancreatitis: assessment of severity with clinical and CT evaluation. Radiology 2002; 223: 603–613.
48. Ranson JH, Rifkind KM, Roses RF, et al. Prognostic signs and the role of operative management in acute pancreatitis. Surg Gynecol Obstet 1974; 139: 69–81.
49. Blamey SL, Imrie CW, O'Neill J, et al. Prognostic factors in acute pancreatitis. Gut 1984; 25: 1340–1346.
50. Wilson C, Heads A, Shankin A, et al. C-reactive protein, antiproteases and complement factors as objective markers of severity in acute pancreatitis. Br J Surg 1989; 76: 177–181.
51. Imrie CW. Prognosis of acute pancreatitis. Ann Ital Chir 1995; 66: 187–189.
52. Brown A, Orav J, Banks PA. Hemoconcentration is an early marker for organ failure and necrotizing pancreatitis. Pancreas 2000; 20: 367–372.
53. Lankisch PG, Mahlke R, Blum T, et al. Hemoconcentration: an early marker of severe and/or necrotizing pancreatitis? A critical appraisal. Am J Gastroenterol 2001; 96: 2081–2085.
54. Wilson C, Heath DI, Imrie CW. Prediction of outcome in acute pancreatitis: a comparative study of APACHE II, clinical assessment and multiple factor scoring systems. Br J Surg 1990; 77: 1260–1264.

55. Demling L, Koch H, Classen M, et al. [Endoscopic papillotomy and removal of gall-stones: animal experiments and first clinical results (author's transl)]. Dtsch Med Wochenschr 1974; 99: 2255–2257.

56. Classen M, Demling L. Endoscopic sphincterotomy of the papilla of vater and extraction of stones from the choledochal duct (author's transl). Dtsch Med Wochenschr 1974; 99: 496–497.

57. Kelly TR, Wagner DS. Gallstone pancreatitis: a prospective randomized trial of the timing of surgery. Surgery 1988; 104: 600–605.

58. Fan ST, Lay EC, Mock MP, et al. Early treatment of acute biliary pancreatitis by endoscopic papillotomy. N Engl J Med 1993; 328: 228–232.

59. Nowak A, Nowakowska-Dulawa E, Marek TA, et al. Final results of the prospective, randomized, controlled study of endoscopic versus conventional management in acute biliary pancreatitis. Gastroenterology 1995; 108: A380.

60. Ricci F, Castaldini G, de Manzoni G, et al. Minimally invasive treatment of acute biliary pancreatitis. Surg Endosc 1997; 11: 1179–1182.

61. Moreira VF, Sanroman AL. Endoscopic sphincterotomy and gallstone pancreatitis: some answers and more fuel for the flames. J Clin Gastroenterol 1992; 14: 85–87.

62. Ricci F, Castaldini G, de Manzoni G, et al. Treatment of gallstone pancreatitis: six-year experience in a single center. World J Surg 2002; 26: 85–90.

63. Uomo G, Galloro V, Rabitti PG, et al. Early endoscopic cholangiopancreatography and sphincterotomy in acute biliary pancreatitis: report of 50 cases. Ital J Gastroenterol 1991; 23: 564–566.

64. Freeman ML, Nelson DB, Sherman S, et al. Complications of endoscopic biliary sphincterotomy. N Engl J Med 1996; 335: 909–918.

65. Freeman ML. Complications of endoscopic biliary sphincterotomy: a review. Endoscopy 1997; 29: 288–297.

66. Leese T, Neoptolemos JP, Carr-Locke DL. Successes, failures, early complications and their management following endoscopic sphincterotomy: results in 394 consecutive patients from a single centre. Br J Surg 1985; 72: 215–219.

67. Ell C, Rabenstein T, Ruppert T, et al. [20 years of endoscopic papillotomy. Analysis of 2752 patients at Erlangen Hospital]. Dtsch Med Wochenschr 1995; 120: 163–167.

68. Ell C, Rabenstein T, Schneider HT, et al. Safety and efficacy of pancreatic sphincterotomy in chronic pancreatitis. Gastrointest Endosc 1998; 48: 244–249.

69. Enns R, Eloubaidi ML, Mergener K, et al. ERCP-related perforations: risk factors and management. Endoscopy 2002; 34: 293–298.

70. Freeman ML, DiSario JA, Nelson DB, et al. Risk factors for post-ERCP pancreatitis: a prospective, multicenter study. Gastrointest Endosc 2001; 54: 425–434.

71. Forssmann K, Singer MV. How to proceed? ERCP in acute pancreatitis? Schweiz Rundsch Med Prax, 1999; 88: 13–17.

72. Nitsche R, Folsch UR. Endoscopic sphincterotomy for acute pancreatitis: arguments against. Ital J Gastroenterol Hepatol 1998; 30: 562–565.

73. Chopra KB, Peters RA, O'Toole PA, et al. Randomised study of endoscopic biliary endoprosthesis versus duct clearance for bileduct stones in high-risk patients. Lancet 1996; 348: 791–793.

74. Prat F, Ederi J, Meduri B, et al. Early EUS of the bile duct before endoscopic sphincterotomy for acute biliary pancreatitis. Gastrointest Endosc 2001; 54: 724–729.

75. Moreau JA, Zinsmeister RA, Melton 3rd LJ, et al. Gallstone pancreatitis and the effect of cholecystectomy: a population-based cohort study. Mayo Clin Proc 1988; 63: 466–473.

76. Diehl AK, Hollemann DR Jr, Chapman JB, et al. Gallstone size and risk of pancreatitis. Arch Intern Med 1997; 157: 1674–1678.
77. Acosta JM, Rossi R, Galli OM, et al. Early surgery for acute gallstone pancreatitis: evaluation of a systematic approach. Surgery 1978; 83: 367–370.
78. Stone HH, Fabian TC, Dunlop WE. Gallstone pancreatitis: biliary tract pathology in relation to time of operation. Ann Surg 1981; 194: 305–312.
79. Runkel NS, Buhr HJ, Herfarth C. Outcome after surgery for biliary pancreatitis. Eur J Surg 1996; 162: 307–313.
80. Frei GJ, Frei VT, Thirlby RC, et al. Biliary pancreatitis: clinical presentation and surgical management. Am J Surg 1986; 151: 170–175.
81. Glazer G, Mann MV. United kingdom guidlines for the management of acute pancreatitis. British society of Gastreoenterology. Gut 1998; 42: S1–13.
82. Sargen K, Kingsnorth AN. Management of gallstone pancreatitis: effects of deviation from clinical guidelines. JOP 2001; 2: 317–322.
83. Uhl W, Mueller CA, Krahenbuhl L, et al. Acute gallstone pancreatitis: timing of laparoscopic cholecystectomy in mild and severe disease. Surg Endosc 1999; 13: 1070–1076.
84. Isenmann R, Buchler M, Uhl W, et al. Pancreatic necrosis: an early finding in severe acute pancreatitis. Pancreas 1993; 8: 358–361.
85. Boytchev I, Pelletier G, Prat F, et al. Late biliary complications after endoscopic sphincterotomy for common bile duct stones in patients older than 65 years of age with gallbladder in situ. Gastroenterol Clin Biol 2000; 24: 995–1000.
86. Fogel EL, Eversmann D, Jamidar P, et al. Sphincter of Oddi dysfunction: pancreaticobiliary sphincterotomy with pancreatic stent placement has a lower rate of pancreatitis than biliary sphincterotomy alone. Endoscopy 2002; 34: 280–285.
87. Devereaux BM, Sherman S, Lehman GA. Sphincter of Oddi (pancreatic) hypertension and recurrent pancreatitis. Curr Gastroenterol Rep 2002; 4: 153–159.
88. DeIorio AV Jr, Vitals GC, Reynolds M, et al. Acute biliary pancreatitis. The roles of laparoscopic cholecystectomy and endoscopic retrograde cholangiopancreatography. Surg Endosc 1995; 9: 392–396.
89. Freund H, Pfeffermann R, Durst AL, et al. Gallstone pancreatitis. Exploration of the biliary system in acute and recurrent pancreatitis. Arch Surg 1976; 111: 1106–1107.
90. Kelly TR. Gallsonte pancreatitis. Arch Surg 1974; 109: 294–297.
91. Dixon JA, Hillam JD. Surgical treatment of biliary tract disease associated with acute pancreatitis. Am J Surg 1970; 120: 371–375.
92. Riemann JF, Lux G, Forster P, et al. Long-term results after endoscopic papillotomy. Endoscopy 1983; 15 (Suppl 1): 165–168.
93. Hammarstrom LE, Holmin T, Stridbeck H. Endoscopic treatment of bile duct calculi in patients with gallbladder in situ: long-term outcome and factors. Scand J Gastroenterol 1996; 31: 294–301.
94. Seifert E, Gail K, Weismuller J. Long term results after endoscopic sphincterotomy. Dtsch Med Wochenschr 1982; 107: 610–614.
95. Norton SA, Cheruvu CV, Collins J, et al. An assessment of clinical guidelines for the management of acute pancreatitis. Ann R Coll Surg Engl 2001; 83: 399–405.
96. Lichtenstein DR. Gallstone Pancreatitis. Curr Treat Options Gastroenterol 2002; 5: 355–363.
97. Lerch MM, Adler G. Experimental pancreatitis. Current Opin Gastroenterol 1993; 9: 752–759.

4 Other Causes of Acute Pancreatitis

Charles D. Ulrich, II, MD, FACP, FACG

INTRODUCTION

Proven and potential causes of acute pancreatitis (AP) are legion. In most epidemiological studies, alcohol abuse and gallstones are the most common causes of AP. In most series, the third most common etiology is idiopathic. Several other etiologies are also described, all of which are rare. However, studies of these rare forms of AP have provided impressive insight into the pathophysiology of AP and have begun to allow investigators to study idiopathic acute pancreatitis (IAP) with progressively more sophisticated scientific tools. Two causes of AP are described in other chapters and are only briefly discussed here. Endoscopic retrograde cholangiopancreatography (ERCP)-induced pancreatitis is discussed in Chapter 5. Gallstones and microlithiasis are reviewed in Chapter 3 of this volume. This chapter reviews other causes

From: *Pancreatitis and Its Complications*
Edited by: C. E. Forsmark © Humana Press Inc., Totowa, NJ

of AP with a particular emphasis on genetic predisposition and autoimmune pancreatitis (AIP).

CATEGORIZATION

Causes of AP can be categorized as toxic-metabolic, mechanical, genetic, autoimmune, and miscellaneous. Items within certain categories are then characterized as established or suspected based on available data.

TOXIC–METABOLIC CAUSES

Alcohol, hypertriglyceridemia, hypercalcemia, medications, organophosphates, Scorpion toxin, certain infections, and methylene chloride fall into the category of toxic–metabolic causes. Alcohol is clearly the most common of these causes and attributes to approximately 30% of cases of AP in the United States.

The long-standing belief has been that dedicated ethanol ingestion over a 3- to 5-year period was necessary to "prime" the pancreas before AP becomes clinically apparent. Although this is true in most cases, most experts in the field now agree that a single episode of binge drinking may be sufficient to cause AP *(1,2)*. Most patients fit into the former category, and the pathophysiological mechanisms differentiating the two phenotypes have yet to be ascertained. In most patients, it has been thought that histologic chronic pancreatitis (CP) has already developed at the time of the initial attack of pancreatitis, which may not be apparent because histological material is rarely available. If not already apparent at the time of the initial attack, radiological evidence of CP usually develops within a few years of the initial attack. A rare number of patients may have multiple acute attacks of pancreatitis over several years before developing obvious CP. Yet, a small group of patients will not progress to CP despite continued alcohol abuse. Once CP develops, however, abstinence from alcohol may slow but will not stop the subsequent continued deterioration of pancreatic function. The mechanism by which alcohol causes AP and CP remains unknown. Hypotheses include direct acinar or ductal cell damage by alcohol or one of its metabolites, changes in acinar cell synthesis or secretion, and other theories.

Sustained serum triglycerides 1000 or greater are generally required to induce AP *(3)*. Most adults who develop triglyceride elevations of this magnitude suffer from hyperchylomicronemia owing to type I or IV hyperlipoproteinemia. Many have a secondary condition that further increases serum lipids. Diabetes mellitus is the most common condition, although obesity, pregnancy, estrogen therapy, or glucocorticoid therapy may also contribute. Estrogens cause AP via hypertriglyceridemia *(2)*. A normal triglyceride level effectively excludes estrogen supplements as causative. The mechanism by which triglyceride elevations to this level cause pancreatitis is thought to be the release of toxic-free fatty acids that could directly injure pancreatic acinar cells. Notably, elevations in serum triglycerides might be seen as a consequence of AP as well as a cause. In this situation, elevations of triglycerides are usually mild (< 300 mg/dL). The diagnosis of hyperlipidemic pancreatitis may be difficult in that very high triglyceride levels interfere with the laboratory assay for amylase. Triglyceride levels usually fall rapidly when these patients are fasted; occasional patients require plasmapheresis for persistent high-level elevations. Control of serum lipids after recovery by dietary and drug therapy prevents recurrent pancreatitis.

Numerous medications have been implicated in AP (2), overall, medications are an uncommon cause of AP. More than 50 drugs have been implicated. The strongest evidence of causation derives from cases where pancreatitis repeatedly developed with reexposure. Rechallenge data exist for α-methyldopa, 5-aminosalicylate, azathioprine and 6-mercaptopurine, cimetidine, cytosine arabinoside, dexamethasone, ethinylestradiol/lynestrenol, furosemide, isoniazid, metronidazole, norethindrone/mestranol, pentamidine, procainamide, stibogluconate, sulfamethazole, sulfamethoxazole, sulindac, tetracycline, trimethorpim/sulfamethoxazole, and valproic acid. There is general agreement that asparaginase, other corticosteroids, didanosine, other estrogens, other salicylates, and thiazides are also capable of causing acute pancreatitis. The highest attack rate is with 6-mercaptopurine and azathioprine, where up to 3% of patients taking these drugs will develop AP. The prognosis of drug-induced pancreatitis is usually quite good if the offending agent is removed.

Pancreatitis owing to hypercalcemia is a very rare event. Untreated hyperparathyroidism, vitamin D toxicity, sarcoidosis, and iatrogenic hypercalcemia are the most common explanations.

Certain toxins may cause AP. In the Caribbean, a particular scorpion sting can inject a toxin, which releases acetylcholine from pancreatic nerves, leading to a hyperstimulation of the pancreatic acinar cells. This causes AP by the same mechanism used in animal models to precipitate AP—hyperstimulation by the cholecystokinin analog caerulein. Organophosphate insecticides also cause AP via a cholinergic hyperstimulation mechanism.

MECHANICAL CAUSES

Mechanical causes of AP are believed to induce pancreatitis by transiently or chronically obstructing the pancreatic duct or by direct trauma to the pancreas. The mechanism by which pancreatic ductal obstruction leads to AP is not defined. The slow ductal obstruction of pancreatic cancer rarely leads to AP, whereas the more rapid and transient passage of a gallstone does. Similarly, pancreas divisum is quite common in the population, but very few of these patients develop pancreatitis. The nature, severity, and rapidity of the ductal obstruction appear to influence the risk of AP.

Gallstones are certainly the most common of these mechanical causes, accounting for at least 35% of all cases of acute pancreatitis, which is discussed in detail in Chapter 3. It is worth noting that tiny stones and biliary crystals (biliary sludge or microlithiasis) are common explanations for IAP, making gallstones an even more common cause of AP.

Obstruction of the pancreatic duct at the ampulla or periampullary region may result from a diverticulum, cyst, polyp, tumors, strictures, Crohn's disease of the duodenum, congenital malformations, or a blind loop. Villous adenomas of the ampulla and periampullary malignancies may present as AP, leading to a recommendation for a complete diagnostic evaluation (including ERCP) in patients more than 45 years of age with unexplained pancreatitis. Pancreatic adenocarcinoma may also cause AP, as can other more rare forms of pancreatic neoplasia (e.g., intraductal papillary mucinous tumors, and islet cell tumors). Blunt or penetrating trauma to the pancreas may directly cause pancreatitis by a crush injury, transect the pancreas, or result in ductal strictures. The diagnosis is usually suspected based on the clinical circumstances, although sometimes mild blunt trauma may contuse the pancreas where it crosses the spine. Diagnosis is commonly made with a high-quality computed tomography (CT), although ERCP may be needed to define ductal anatomy and plan therapy. ERCP-induced pancreatitis is thought to be caused, at least in part, by the obstruction of the pancreatic duct at the time of the procedure (discussed in more detail in Chapter 5).

Two additional conditions may cause AP by obstructing the pancreatic duct: sphincter of Oddi dysfunction (SOD) and pancreas divisum, both are controversial putative causes. SOD may occur via fibrosis of the sphincter (likely better termed "ampullary stenosis" than SOD) and, perhaps, only because of dyskinesia (spasm or other motility disturbance in the absence of fixed stenosis). SOD is defined by manometry of the sphincter performed at the time of ERCP. It is possible to measure pressures in both the pancreatic and biliary portion of the sphincter of Oddi. There are syndromes attributed to biliary sphincter dysfunction (biliary pain, elevated liver chemistries, or a dilated common bile duct) and syndromes thought to be caused by dysfunction of the pancreatic portion of the sphincter (pancreatic pain, recurrent pancreatitis, a dilated pancreatic duct). Pancreatic SOD is usually classified as type I, documented recurrent attacks of AP with a dilated pancreatic duct and slow drainage of contrast after ERCP, associated with fixed stenosis of the pancreatic duct at the sphincter of Oddi; and type II, recurrent AP or pancreatic pain with elevated basal sphincter pressures more than 40 mmHg in the absence of stenosis *(2)*. Most clinicians agree that stenosis of the ampulla is a cause of recurrent pancreatitis, but controversy exists as to whether dyskinesia alone is a cause of recurrent pancreatitis. The pancreatic and biliary sphincters are conjoined for much of their length; it is unknown whether biliary SOD in the absence of pancreatic SOD is causative of AP. Some studies claim that relief of symptoms is potentially attributable to SOD following biliary sphincterotomy alone in up to 50% of cases. However, performance of manometry in both sphincters with subsequent biliary and pancreatic sphincterotomy, the latter if pancreatic pressures are elevated, has been advocated as more beneficial than pancreatic sphincterotomy alone *(7)*. Data supporting pancreatic SOD as causative of AP come from studies with a small number of patients and all are essentially uncontrolled *(4–7)*. Cumulatively, this data is supportive and leads many clinicians to pursue pancreatic sphincter of Oddi manometry in patients with recurrent AP once all other potential etiologies have been excluded. It should be noted that the data for symptom improvement after biliary or pancreatic sphincterotomy for SOD is strongest in patients with discrete episodes of relapsing AP, in whom there is confirmation of attacks by either amylase greater than three times normal or imaging evidence of AP. Those patients with pain only, particularly chronic abdominal pain considered of pancreatic origin, but without discrete episodes of confirmed pancreatitis, respond poorly to sphincterotomy. This patient group often has associated intestinal motility disorders and visceral hyperalgesia with high levels of somatization and depression.

Documenting SOD with pancreatic or biliary manometry is not without risk, where rates of ERCP-induced pancreatitis average 20%. A recent report from Freeman and colleagues suggest sphincterotomy as the risk factor for ERCP-induced AP in SOD, not the actual manometry *(8)*. Sherman et al. claim a substantial reduction in the risk of sphincterotomy-induced AP in this cohort through placement of a small (3 cm, 5 Fr) temporary pancreatic duct stent *(9)*. Therefore, it may be possible to mitigate the risk to an extent, but a substantial risk remains that requires careful informed consent. Randomized trials in this condition are sorely needed.

Pancreas divisum is a congenital variant that occurs in up to 7% of the general population. In this condition, the dorsal and ventral pancreatic buds fail to fuse during embryogenesis, leaving the larger dorsal pancreas to drain through the smaller minor papilla. The vast majority of these patients do not suffer from any form of pancreatic disease. In some patients with pancreas divisum, AP is believed to occur through pancreatic ductal hypertension caused by an inadequately patent or stenosed minor papilla or by some excessive stimuli for pancreatic secretion, which cannot be accommodated through the minor papilla. Most but not all numerous studies have reported a significantly higher prevalence of pancreas divisum in patients with recurrent AP when compared to controls (10–14). Data supporting pancreas divisum as causative of AP derive from small studies reporting success of either transpapillary stent placement across or sphincterotomy of the minor papilla in preventing recurrent episodes of pancreatitis and relieving symptoms (15–17). Although these studies are not properly controlled, the combined data are compelling. Minor papilla sphincterotomy with short-term stent placement is favored over long-term stent placement owing to valid concerns that the stents themselves may cause ductal changes with the potential to contribute to the pathology. As in the case of SOD, those patients with pancreatic pain only, particularly chronic pain, do not appear to respond to endoscopic minor papilla therapy.

GENETIC CAUSES

Technological advances in conjunction with the human genome project have facilitated the identification of several gene mutations that may either directly cause, predispose, or enhance the risk of other factors causing AP.

Cationic Trypsinogen

Hereditary pancreatitis is an autosomal dominant genetic disorder that consists of recurrent episodes of AP, frequent progression to CP with a substantially enhanced risk of pancreatic cancer (18). In the majority of hereditary pancreatitis kindreds, the phenotype is caused by mutations in the gene encoding cationic trypsinogen (PRSS1), the inactive precursor of a serine protease. Those carrying R122H, R122C, N29I, or N29T mutations in this gene express the phenotype in 80% of cases (18,19). Kindreds with K23R, D22G, and A16V mutations in the same gene have also been described (18). Owing to small numbers, the true phenotypic significance of the latter mutations has yet to be ascertained.

Heated debate exists within the scientific community as to whether or not these mutations in cationic trypsinogen cause a gain-of-function, resulting in excessive levels of protease activation within pancreatic acini or a loss of function that somehow leads to the creation of a milieu conducive to pancreatitis. Individuals with (1) AP and a family history of pancreatitis of unclear etiology or (2) otherwise idiopathic recurrent AP in the absence of a family history should undergo testing for R122H, R122C, N29I, and N29T mutations in the PRSS1 gene (20). Testing for other mutations in this gene is controversial outside of research protocols. All patients undergoing testing should be appropriately counseled before and after testing regarding the potential risks (e.g., impact on insurability) and benefits (e.g., risk factor reduction, enrollment in pancreatic cancer screening protocols, and family planning).

Cystic Fibrosis Transmembrane Conductance Regulator

Mutations in the cystic fibrosis (*CFTR*) gene, which encodes the cystic fibrosis transmembrane conductance regulator (*CFTR*) chloride channel, may enhance the risk of pancreatitis *(18,21)*. Several studies have documented that patients with otherwise idiopathic recurrent AP lacking a family history of pancreatitis have a much higher prevalence of *CFTR* mutations than *PRSS1* gene mutations *(22)*. The majority of patients with recurrent AP or CP attributable to *CFTR* gene mutations are compound heterozygotes (i.e., they have one dominant CF-causing gene mutation and one mild/variable mutation; *22*). This results in a phenotype lacking the overt pulmonary manifestations of CF, yet capable of causing pancreatitis. Indeed, most of the patients exhibit normal sweat chloride and baseline nasal potential difference (PD) with a ΔPD less abnormal than that seen in overt CF.

Not all *CFTR* compound heterozygotes develop pancreatitis. In fact, the exact risk of developing pancreatitis for a compound heterozygote has yet to be defined. The natural history of the disease and risk of developing pancreatic cancer is not well-described and likely varies depending on which mutations are present and what other risk factors (e.g., environmental or genetic) are present. Counseling of these patients is consequently problematic. Most investigators in the field advocate testing for *CFTR* gene mutations only within research protocols. If genetic testing is to be performed outside of Institutional Review Board-approved protocols, it should be driven by abnormal nasal ΔPD testing. An initial search for dominant CF-causing mutations should be undertaken prior to the consideration of complete sequencing of the *CFTR* gene for mild/variable mutations.

Pancreatic Secretory Trypsin Inhibitor

Pancreatic secretory trypsin inhibitor (*PSTI*), otherwise known as *SPINK1*, is an inhibitor of trypsin. Patients with AP have an increased prevalence of N34S *SPINK1* mutations when compared to the general population *(23)*. Families with a history of pancreatitis but no known cause, including no detectable mutations in *PRSS1*, have an increased prevalence of the N34S *SPINK1* mutation *(24)*. Concomitance of *CFTR* and *SPINK1* mutations enhances the risk of pancreatitis above that of *CFTR* mutations alone (600-fold versus 40-fold; *22*). *SPINK1* mutations are also associated with tropical pancreatitis and type II diabetes mellitus in Bangladesh *(25)*. However, the vast majority of patients with *SPINK1* mutations never develop pancreatitis *(23)*. The spectrum of pancreatic manifestations attributable to mutations in *SPINK1*, or lack thereof, is likely the result of variations in concomitant genetic and/or environmental factors.

AUTOIMMUNE PANCREATITIS

In 1965, Sarles and colleagues reported a case of pancreatitis associated with hypergammaglobulinemia *(26)*. Only in the past few years has "autoimmune pancreatitis" (AIP) become recognized as a distinct entity of clinical relevance. In a recent review of the topic *(27)*, Okazaki and Chiba summarized the features characterizing AIP as:

1. Increased levels of serum γ-globulins or immunoglobulin G (IgG).
2. Presence of autoantibodies.
3. Diffuse enlargement of the pancreas.
4. Diffusely irregular narrowing of the main pancreatic duct and occasional stenosis of the intrapancreatic bile duct.
5. Fibrotic changes with lymphocytic infiltration.
6. No symptoms or only mild symptoms, usually without acute attacks of pancreatitis.
7. Rare pancreatic calcification or cysts.
8. Occasional association with other autoimmune diseases.
9. Effective steroid therapy.

Primary AIP occurs in the absence of an established autoimmune syndrome outside of the pancreas. Serologic markers may include antinuclear antibody, antilactoferrin antibody, anticarbonic anyhydrase II antibody, and rheumatoid factor. Serum levels of IgG4 are frequently elevated. Unfortunately, none of these markers are adequately specific to make the diagnosis independent of other clinical, radiological, or histological features. The presence of such features in the setting of another autoimmune disease process (e.g., Sjogren's syndrome, systemic lupus erythematosis, primary sclerosing cholangitis, or ulcerative colitis) suggests a diagnosis of secondary AIP. Diabetes mellitus is frequently shown in patients with AIP (43–68%).

Most experts in the field agree that AIP should be considered a diagnosis of exclusion in the setting of suggestive serologic markers and typical clinical, radiological and histological features. An extensive evaluation leading to the identification and elimination of other causative factors of AP or CP should precede any consideration of a trial of steroid therapy. In a subset of these patients, glucose intolerance improves with steroid therapy. The appropriate duration of therapy and possible need for chronic immunosuppression has yet to be defined.

Therefore, physicians managing a patient with suspected AIP should involve a pancreatic specialist prior to the initiation of steroids.

MISCELLANEOUS CAUSES

Hypotension, vasculitis, hypercoagulable states, and embolic disease may lead to vascular insufficiency and ischemic pancreatitis *(2)*. Infectious agents, such as cytomegalovirus, *Myocardium tuberculosis,* Coxsackie virus, mumps, human immunodeficiency virus, and parasites, are also capable of inducing an episode of pancreatitis *(2)*. Tropical pancreatitis is generally classified as chronic *(25)*.

IDIOPATHIC ACUTE PANCREATITIS

No obvious cause of AP is found in 25–30% of patients. Some patients are alcohol users, but this cause is not elucidated in the medical history. Many of these patients suffer from microlithiasis, and certainly some have genetic mutations as delineated previously. As the understanding of AP causes expands, the percentage of patients with true IAP will continue to decrease. In one study, only 1 of 31 patients with IAP had a second attack within the following 36 months *(28)*, leading to the recommendation that extensive evaluation of unexplained AP be delayed until after the second attack. This approach is usually modified in those patients with a higher risk for malignancy causing AP (age >40–45 years).

SUMMARY

The differential diagnosis in patients with AP is broad. Identification and elimination of factors inciting AP is of paramount importance in reducing the risk of recurrent episodes and progression to CP. Toxic–metabolic causes of AP are both common and can be eliminated. Knowledge of the mechanisms through which ethanol may cause AP is still evolving. Risk factors for and the prevention of ERCP-induced pancreatitis, as well as the diagnosis and management of patients with gallstone pancreatitis, are discussed in other chapters of this volume. Although evidence is mounting that SOD and pancreas divisum may play an important role in patients with AP of otherwise unclear etiology, endoscopic intervention remains controversial.

Recent advances have led to the identification of genetic mutations that are either directly causative (R122H, R122C, N29I, or N29T mutations in cationic trypsinogen), presumably causative (compound heterozygous mutations in *CFTR*), or enhance the risk of AP (N34S mutations in *SPINK1*). Testing for such mutations must be undertaken only in an appropriate clinical setting and with prospective counseling regarding the potential ramifications of a positive test. Autoimmune pancreatitis is an accepted entity that should be treated only following the exclusion of other potential etiologies of pancreatitis and in collaboration with a pancreatic specialist.

REFERENCES

1. Bank S, Indaram A. Causes of acute and recurrent pancreatitis. *Gastroenterol Clin North Am* 1998; 28: 571–589.
2. Somogyi L, Martin SP, Venkatesan T, Ulrich CD. Recurrent acute pancreatitis: an algorithmic approach to identification and elimination of inciting factors. *Gastroenterology* 2001; 120: 708–717.
3. Yadav D, Pitchumoni CS. Issues in hypertriglyceridemic pancreatitis. *J Clin Gastroenterol* 2003; 36: 54–62.
4. Catalano MF, Sivak MV, Falk GW, et al. Idiopathic pancreatitis: diagnostic role of sphincter of Oddi manometry (SOM) and response to endoscopic sphincterotomy (ES). *Gastrointest Endosc* 1993; 39 (Abstract): 310A.
5. Sherman S. Idiopathic acute recurrent pancreatitis: endoscopic approach to diagnosis and therapy. *Gastrointest. Endosc* 1992; 38 (Abstract): 261A.
6. Venu RP, Geenen JE, Hogan W, et al. Idiopathic recurrent pancreatitis: an approach to diagnosis and treatment. *Dig Dis Sci* 1989; 34: 56–60.
7. Eversman D, Fogel EL, Rusche M, et al. Frequency of abnormal pancreatic and biliary sphincter manometry compared with clinical suspicion of sphincter of Oddi dysfunction. *Gastrointest Endosc* 1999; 50: 637–641.
8. Freeman ML, DiSario, JA, Nelson DB, et al. Risk factors for post-ERCP pancreatitis: a prospective, multicenter study. *Gastrointest Endosc* 2001; 54: 425–434.
9. Sherman S, Eversman D, Fogel E, et al. Sphincter of Oddi dysfunction (SOD): needle-knife pancreato-biliary sphincterotomy over pancreatic stent (NKOPS) has a lower post-procedure pancreatitis rate than pull-type biliary sphincterotomy (BES). *Gastrointest Endosc* 1997; 45 (Abstract): 148A.
10. Delhaye M, Engelholm L, Cremer M. Pancreas divisum: congenital anatomic variant or anomaly? Contribution of endoscopic retrograde dorsal pancreatography. *Gastroenterology* 1985; 89: 951–958.
11. Morgan D, Logan K, Baron T, et al. Pancreas divisum: implications for diagnostic and therapeutic pancreatography. *Am J Roentgenol* 1999; 173: 193–198.
12. Bernard JP, Sahel J, Giovannini M, et al. Pancreas divisum is a probable cause of pancreatitis: a report of 137 cases. *Pancreas* 1990; 5: 248–254.
13. Brenner P, Duncombe V, Ham JM. Pancreatitis and pancreas divisum: aetiological and surgical considerations. *Aust NZ J Surg* 1990; 60: 899–903.
14. Richter JM, Schapiro RH, Mulley AG, et al. Association of pancreas divisum and pancreatitis, and its treatment by sphincteroplasty of the accessory ampulla. *Gastroenterology* 1981; 81: 1104–1110.
15. Lans J, Geenen J, Johanson J, et al. Endoscopic therapy in patients with pancreas divisum and acute pancreatitis: a prospective, randomized, controlled clinical trail. *Gastrointest Endosc* 1992; 38: 430–434.
16. Lehman GA, Sherman S, Nisi R, et al. Pancreas divisum: results of minor papilla sphincterotomy. *Gastrointest Endosc* 1993; 39: 1–8.
17. Ertan A. Long-term results after endoscopic pancreatic stent placement without pancreatic papillotomy in acute recurrent pancreatitis due to pancreas divisum. *Gastrointest. Endosc* 2000; 52: 9–14.

18. Sweeney J, Ulrich CD. Genetics of pancreatic disease. *Clin Perspect Gastroenterol* 2002; 5: 110–116.
19. Pfutzer R, Myers E, Applebaum-Shapiro S, et al. Novel cationic trypsinogen (*PRSS1*) N29T and R122C mutations cause autosomal dominant hereditary pancreatitis. *Gut* 2002; 50: 271–272.
20. Ellis I, Lerch MM, Whitcomb DC, et al. Genetic testing for hereditary pancreatitis: guidelines for indications, counseling, consent, and privacy issues. *Pancreatology* 2001; 1: 405–415.
21. Noone PG, Zhou Z, Silverman LM, et al. Cystic fibrosis gene mutations and pancreatitis risk: relation to epithelial ion transport and trypsin inhibitor gene mutations. *Gastroenterology* 2001; 121: 1508–1512.
22. Cohn JA, Noone PG, Jowell PS. Idiopathic pancreatitis related to *CFTR*: complex inheritance and identification of a modifier gene. *J Invest Med* 2002; 50: 247S–255S.
23. Pfutzer RH, Whitcomb DC. *SPINK1* mutations are associated with multiple phenotypes. *Pancreatology* 2001; 1: 457–460.
24. Threadgold J, Greenhalf W, Ellis I, et al. The N34S mutation of *SPINK1* (*PSTI*) is associated with a familial pattern of idiopathic chronic pancreatitis but does not cause the disease. *Gut* 50: 675–681.
25. Schneider A, Suman A, Rossi L, et al. *SPINK1/PSTI* mutations are associated with tropical pancreatitis in Bangladesh. *Gastroenterology* 2002; 123: 1026–1030.
26. Sarles H, Sarles JC, Camatte R, et al. Observation on 205 confirmed cases of acute pancreatitis, recurring pancreatitis, and chronic pancreatitis. *Gut* 1965; 6: 545–559.
27. Okazaki K, Chiba T. Autoimmune related pancreatitis. *Gut* 2002; 51: 1–4.
28. Ballinger AB, Barnes E, Alstead EM, et al. Is intervention necessary after a first episode of idiopathic acute pancreatitis? *Gut* 1996; 28: 293–295.

5 Treatment of Mild Acute Pancreatitis and Prevention of Post-Endoscopic Retrograde Cholangiopancreatography Pancreatitis

Michael Morelli, MD
and Lehel Somogyi, MD

CONTENTS

INTRODUCTION
TREATMENT OF MILD ACUTE PANCREATITIS
SUMMARY: TREATMENT OF MILD ACUTE PANCREATITIS
PHARMACOLOGICAL PREVENTION OF POST-ERCP PANCREATITIS
SUMMARY: PHARMACOLOGICAL PREVENTION OF PANCREATITIS AFTER ERCP
TECHNIQUE-RELATED PREVENTION OF POST-ERCP PANCREATITIS
SUMMARY: TECHNIQUE-RELATED PREVENTION OF POST-ERCP PANCREATITIS
REFERENCES

INTRODUCTION

The treatment of mild acute pancreatitis (AP) is largely supportive and includes the administration of fluids intravenously, pain medications, antiemetics, and bowel rest until nausea and vomiting have resolved and

From: *Pancreatitis and Its Complications*
Edited by: C. E. Forsmark © Humana Press Inc., Totowa, NJ

narcotics are not required for pain control. Several medications have been studied with the goal to improve patient outcomes, avoid complications associated with pancreatitis, and reduce the time needed for recovery. However, to date, there is no medication proven to alter the course of the disease. This data, as well as the limited data available for the initiation of analgesics and feeding, are reviewed in this chapter. Additionally, the literature on prophylaxis of post-endoscopic retrograde cholangiopancreatography (ERCP) pancreatitis is reviewed.

TREATMENT OF MILD ACUTE PANCREATITIS

Fluids

Patients with mild AP are frequently dehydrated but rarely exhibit signs of severe hypotension or third spacing of fluid, which is much more common with severe acute pancreatitis (SAP). Normal saline should be administered intravenously to prevent dehydration, as possibly manifested by tachycardia, hypotension, the presence of orthostasis, an elevated blood urea netrogen (BUN) or creatinine, or elevated serum sodium. Hemoconcentration is another marker of third-space fluid loss and is also a predictor of more severe pancreatitis. A case-control study showed that an admission hematocrit of 47% or greater or a failure of admission hematocrit to decrease at 24 hours were strong risk factors for the development of pancreatic necrosis (1). The rate of administration varies based on other possible coexisting conditions, such as end-stage renal disease or congestive heart failure, and also based on the degree of dehydration. There are no published studies in humans that provide an evidence-based approach to the administration of fluids in the AP setting, but adequate fluid resuscitation is generally thought to be a key component of medical management.

Analgesia

Pain control is an important part of the management of patients with AP. The preferred route of analgesic administration is intravenous. There has been much debate about the choice of narcotic in this patient population. Traditional teaching states that morphine sulphate is contraindicated in patients with pancreatitis as this can lead to sphincter of Oddi spasm, which could worsen pancreatitis and pain. Meperidine has historically been the preferred narcotic for the treatment of pain associated with pancreatitis because of a widely held belief that this medication does not affect the sphincter of Oddi in the manner morphine does. During direct measurements, sphincter of Oddi mean basal pressure was not affected by meperidine, whereas morphine, at doses of 10–20 μg/kg, resulted in an average increase from 12 to 30 mmHg (2). This result is still below the threshold used to diagnose sphincter of Oddi dysfunction (SOD). The clinical significance of these findings is unknown. No studies have directly compared the effects of meperidine and morphine on sphincter of Oddi manometry, and there have been no clinical studies that compares the use of the two drugs in patients with AP. No direct evidence exists that indicates morphine is contraindicated or should not be used in the treatment of AP-induced pain. In fact, morphine may offer longer pain relief with less risk of seizures in comparison to meperidine. Hydromorphone is also an alternative drug.

Typically, patients with mild AP will have adequate pain relief with the aforementioned intravenous or intramuscular narcotics. Additional benefit may be obtained with the use of patient-controlled analgesia. Segmental epidural blocks have been reported to control pain successfully in those cases where traditional methods of pain management fail *(3)*.

Nutrition

Because of pain, nausea, and vomiting, oral intake is usually withheld in the early phases of the disease. Important considerations in patient care with pancreatitis are when and how to initiate nutrition. Decreased oral intake in the setting of a hypermetabolic condition leads to a negative energy and nitrogen balance. In mild cases of pancreatitis, this is of little clinical importance as most patients are able to eat within 5 days. Insufficient nutrition in this brief time does not seem to negatively influence outcome *(4)*. There is considerable variation to the approaches of when and by what means these patients should be fed. Most patients are not fed orally until their pain and appetite are considerably improved. Although there is no data to support this approach, some advocate awaiting a normalization of the amylase level. A randomized trial compared early initiation (within 24 hours) of total parenteral nutrition (TPN) with management that included intravenous fluids, analgesics, nasogastric (NG) suction, and cimetidine in patients with mild pancreatitis. The TPN group was found to have a higher rate of catheter-related sepsis (10.5 versus 1.5%). No advantage was found in using early TPN with respect to the length of days to oral intake, total hospital stay, or number of complications of pancreatitis *(5)*. A more recent study of TPN versus enteral feeding in patients with mild AP to SAP showed that enteral feeding improved the acute phase response and indicated a trend toward improvement in clinical disease severity over TPN. How clinically applicable this data is remains unclear owing to the small number of patients included in the study *(6)*.

There have been several studies that evaluated enteral versus parenteral nutrition in mild AP. A recent review of these studies concluded that enteral nutrition via nasojejunal tubes is substantially less costly than TPN and is associated with similar outcomes, including length of stay, time to oral feeding, and complications *(7)*. Thus, enteral nutrition beyond the ligament of Treitz should be given to those patients with pancreatitis who are unable to tolerate oral feeding within 48–72 hours of admission, as long as they do not have an ileus severe enough to preclude this approach.

Nasogastric Suction

NG suction is often used in the treatment of AP, especially if associated with vomiting. In addition, NG suction has been used with the rationale that it will prevent hormone-stimulated pancreatic secretion by removing acid from the stomach before it reaches the duodenum and therefore beneficially alter the course of the disease. This practice has been studied comparing NG suction to fasting in patients with mild to moderately severe pancreatitis and did not demonstrate a difference between NG suction and fasting regarding the duration or intensity of abdominal pain, the necessity for narcotic administration, or the incidence of complications associated with pancreatitis *(8)*. Another study that compares NG suction with fasting and cimetidine actually showed a prolonged duration of pain and hospitalization and increased analgesic needs in the NG suction group *(9)*. These findings have been consistent regardless of the etiology of pancreatitis *(10)*. Consequently, NG suction should be reserved for those patients who meet other indications for its use, such as bowel obstruction, ileus, or intractable vomiting.

Acid Suppression

Antacids, antihistamines, and more recently, proton pump inhibitors, have been used in the treatment of AP with similar reasoning as NG suction, i.e., to decrease acid-induced pancreatic secretions. Randomized studies of this practice have demonstrated that antacids or cimetidine are not superior to fasting in any measured variable, including duration of abdominal pain, length of hospital stay, and time taken for patients to resume an oral diet *(11,12)*. There have been no randomized studies of proton pump inhibitors in the AP setting, but substantial beneficial effects in the absence of other indications seem unlikely.

Somatostatin/Octreotide

Somatostatin is a hormone that suppresses pancreatic exocrine function directly by depressing pancreatic exocrine secretion and indirectly by suppressing gastrointestinal hormone secretion. Octreotide is a long-acting analog of somatostatin that can be given subcutaneously. Theoretical benefit from the use of these medications to suppress pancreatic secretions in the AP setting has never materialized. An early study showed statistically significant benefits with somatostatin use in the surrogate endpoints of laboratory values e.g., white blood count and lactate dehydrogenase, along with trend toward fewer complications *(13)*. One study showed a statistically significant difference between those given 0.5 μg/kg/hour octreotide versus the control group in earlier intake of oral feedings, but the effect was small (3.76 days versus 4.9 days; *14*). A study of octreotide in moderate-to-severe pancreatitis failed to show any benefit of therapy over placebo in mortality or complications of pancreatitis *(15)*. Overall, the results of these studies have not shown consistent benefits, and, thus, somatostatin or its analogs are not routinely recommended.

Gabexate Mesilate

Gabexate mesilate is a low-molecular-weight protease inhibitor. As intracellular activation of proteolytic enzymes is believed to play an important role in the development of AP *(16)*, blockade of this process appears to be a logical therapeutic and prophylactic target. An early controlled study demonstrated a trend toward lower morbidity and mortality in the gabexate group versus the control group *(17)*. A retrospective study of 88 patients with mild AP to moderately SAP showed that gabexate administration within 24 hours of admission resulted in significantly earlier recovery from abdominal pain, hyperamylasemia, and leukocytosis when compared to late administration of the drug *(18)*. However, a subsequent prospective, double-blinded, randomized study failed to show any benefit with the administration of gabexate over placebo in patients with mostly mild AP *(19)*. These conflicting results were addressed in a meta-analysis of five randomized trials evaluating the three endpoints of mortality, complications, and complications that require surgery. This analysis showed no mortality benefit of gabexate but did demonstrate a significant reduction in the incidence of complications needing surgery with an odds ratio (OR) of 0.61 and of general complications with OR of 0.69. However, the overall clinical impact seemed small, and the use of this expensive medication may not be cost-effective, particularly in mild pancreatitis expected to follow a benign course *(20)*. Furthermore, a multicenter, double-blind, randomized, controlled trial of gabexate mesilate failed to show benefit in patients with moderate AP to SAP *(21)*. This medication is not currently available in the United States.

Other Interventions and Treatments

Continuous peritoneal lavage with crystalloid solution has been evaluated in numerous studies in patients with varying degrees of severity of pancreatitis. Eight randomized, prospective trials were evaluated in one recent meta-analysis which found effect on morbidity and mortality when compared to control patients *(22)*.

Pirenzepine, an anticholinergic drug with specific antagonistic action on cholinergic receptors in the acinar cells of the pancreas, was studied in one prospective randomized trial of 115 patients with mild AP to SAP. Patients received either 10 or 20 mg intravenously of pirenzepine every 12 hours. This study showed a statistically significant benefit in the surrogate duration endpoint of hyperamalyasemia and the duration of pain with no major side effects *(23)*. For reasons that are unclear, there have been no other published clinical studies that evaluate the utility of pirenzepine in AP.

Calcitonin has been shown to depress the basal- and pentagastrin-stimulated secretion of gastric acid, pepsin, and gastrin release. Because of this, it was considered to be of potential benefit in patients with AP. Synthetic salmon calcitonin was evaluated in a randomized double-blind placebo-controlled trial of 99 patients with AP. Most patients had mild-to-moderate disease. Salmon calcitonin was given three times per day at a dose of 20 μg intravenously for 6 days. The number of patients without pain and with normalized serum amylase was significantly higher in the group treated with salmon calcitonin *(24)*. This data has not been confirmed in other studies but raises interesting questions about the potential utility of calcitonin.

SUMMARY: TREATMENT OF MILD ACUTE PANCREATITIS

Patients who present with mild AP should be hydrated aggressively based on body weight, degree of dehydration, and on the presence of comorbid conditions that may affect fluid tolerance. Pain control is important in symptomatic management, and it is usually accomplished by narcotics as needed. There is no convincing evidence to suggest that morphine is contraindicated. Patients should be kept *null per os* and the use of NG tubes should be reserved for those with ileus or intractable vomiting. If patients are not able to resume oral intake within several days of admission, nutrition should be administered, preferably via nasojejunal feeding tubes, which have proven to be less expensive and safer than TPN. There is no data to support the use of acid suppression in mild AP. Strategies that have been evaluated, but appear to have no proven role in the management of these patients, include peritoneal lavage, octreotide, somatostatin, and gabexate. Further studies are needed before the use of calcitonin or pirenzepine can be recommended. Table 1 summarizes the proposed mechanism of action and efficacy for some agents evaluated in the treatment of pancreatitis.

Table 1
Pharmacological Treatment of Mild Acute Pancreatitis

Agent	Mechanism of action	Efficacy
Antacids/cimetidine	Decreased acid-induced pancreatic secretion	Proven to be of no benefit
Somatostatin/ octreotide	Inhibition of pancreatic secretion	Proven to be of little to no benefit especially in mild acute pancreatitis
Gabexate mesilate	Blocks intracellular activation of proteolytic enzymes	Proven to be of no benefit, expensive, and unavailable in United States
Pirenzipine	Antagonizes cholinergic receptors on pancreatic acinar cells	Shown to be beneficial in one RCT. No confirmatory studies have been performed
Salmon calcitonin	Decreases pentagastrin-stimulated secretion of gastric acid, pepsin, and release of gastrin	Demonstrated to be useful in one RCT. No confirmatory studies have been performed

RCT, randomized controlled trial.

PHARMACOLOGICAL PREVENTION OF POST-ERCP PANCREATITIS

Pancreatitis is a known complication of ERCP, occurring in approximately 5–7% of all patients who undergo the procedure. Independent risk factors found on multivariate analysis for the development of post-ERCP pancreatitis included a prior history of pancreatitis after ERCP, suspected SOD, female gender, difficulty with cannulation, pancreatic sphincterotomy, biliary sphincter balloon dilation, more than one injection into the pancreatic duct, absence of chronic pancreatitis, and a normal serum bilirubin (25). To decrease the frequency of post-ERCP pancreatitis, many trials have been performed using various medications prior to ERCP. Research has focused on gabexate, corticosteroids, somatostatin and its analog octreotide, glyceryl trinitrate, heparin, interleukin (IL)-10, and diclofenac.

Gabexate Mesilate

Two small, nonrandomized studies showed a reduction in post-ERCP pancreatitis with the use of gabexate mesilate (26,27). These findings were confirmed via a prospective, double-blinded, randomized, placebo-controlled study of gabexate that indicated statistically significant benefits in favor of gabexate over placebo in the development of pancreatitis after ERCP (2.4 versus 7.6%). The benefit was seen using 1 g of intravenous gabexate by continuous infusion starting 30–90 minutes prior to the procedure and continuing for 12 hours following. No significant differences between the two groups regarding side effects were noted *(28)*, despite that rare cases of anaphylaxis have been reported with gabexate. A meta-analysis of these trials concluded that gabexate lowers the risk of post-ERCP pancreatitis with a number needed to treat (NNT) of 27 to prevent one case of post-ERCP pancreatitis *(29)*. One recent study using a shorter infusion that began 30 minutes before ERCP and continued for 2 hours afterward showed no benefit, suggesting a longer infusion is required *(30)*. Gabexate is unavailable in the United States.

Corticosteroids

Hydrocortisone at a dose of 100 mg intravenously given immediately before ERCP was compared to placebo in a randomized, double-blinded, placebo-controlled trial and was found to be no different from placebo in the prevention of post-ERCP pancreatitis *(31)*. Another prospective randomized trial involving 40 mg prednisone in comparison with 200 mg allopurinol and placebo given 3 and 15 hours prior to ERCP showed no statistically significant difference between groups in the development of pancreatitis *(32)*. These studies indicate that corticosteroids have no benefit for prophylaxis of post-ERCP pancreatitis.

Somatostatin/Octreotide

The studies using somatostatin as prophylaxis for ERCP-induced pancreatitis have yielded conflicting results. Several small randomized studies of 20–60 patients showed no benefit from somatostatin in the prevention of post-ERCP pancreatitis *(33–35)*. A larger prospective, randomized, double-blind study of 230 patients using somatostatin infusion versus placebo infusion that started 30 minutes prior to ERCP and continued for 12 hours postprocedure, however, showed that clinical post-ERCP pancreatitis was significantly higher in the placebo group than in the somatostatin group (10% versus 3%). No difference existed between groups pertaining to factors that may predispose patients to developing post-ERCP pancreatitis, including pancreatic duct injection, difficulty of bile duct cannulation, sphincterotomy, and stenting. No difference in side effects was noted *(36)*. This expensive and time-consuming intervention to prevent a typically mild disease is unlikely to be cost-effective.

The use of bolus somatostatin given at the time of papilla identification versus placebo to prevent pancreatitis after ERCP has also been addressed in a double-blind randomized study of 160 patients, which showed a statistically significant difference in favor of somatostatin in the development of post-ERCP pancreatitis (2.5% versus 10%). Subgroup analysis revealed that the difference was in those patients undergoing sphincterotomy rather than routine ERCP *(37)*. The results of this study were in direct contrast to an earlier, but smaller study, of 33 patients by the same authors that showed no difference in the rate of post-ERCP pancreatitis with the use of bolus somatostatin *(38)*.

Multiple randomized studies of octreotide for the prevention of post-ERCP pancreatitis have failed to demonstrate any significant benefit over placebo, and it is therefore not currently recommended *(39–42)*.

Glyceryl Trinitrate

Glyceryl trinitrate, a nitric oxide donor, lowers basal pressure and contraction amplitude of the sphincter of Oddi *(43)*. Difficult cannulation is a known risk factor for post-ERCP pancreatitis. It is conceivable that glyceryl trinitrate administration will result in decreased sphincter of Oddi tone and might either make cannulation easier or reduce the chance of postmanipulation spasm, which could reduce the incidence of post-ERCP pancreatitis. A randomized double-blinded placebo-controlled trial was conducted in 186 patients using glyceryl trinitrate in the prevention of post-ERCP pancreatitis. Glyceryl trinitrate was given in a dose of 2 mg sublingual 5 minutes before the procedure. This study documented a statistically significant difference between groups in the development of pancreatitis after ERCP in favor of glyceryl trinitrate (7% versus 18%). Subgoup analysis showed that results were greatest in patients having cholangiography only without delineation of the pancreatic duct and in those undergoing diagnostic rather than therapeutic ERCP *(44)*. It should be noted that the rate of post-ERCP pancreatitis in the glyceryl trinitrate group was similar to the usually reported rate of pancreatitis in those patients who do not receive prophylactic medication. Interestingly, the rate was unusually high in the control group, which may have resulted in statistical differences, and the significance of this study is therefore unclear. A letter to the editor reported preliminary results of another double-blind study using a 15 mg glyceryl trinitrate patch applied 30–40 minutes before the procedure that showed a reduction in post-ERCP pancreatitis *(45)*. More confirmatory studies are needed before this medication to be recommended for routine use.

Heparin

Heparin has been shown to have a direct inhibitory effect on pancreatic proteases and improve pancreatic microcirculation in studies of experimentally induced pancreatitis in animals *(46,47)*. Based on this evidence, heparin has been postulated to have a role in the prevention of post-ERCP pancreatitis. An exploratory analysis of the effect of heparin on post-ERCP pancreatitis in 815 patients who underwent ERCP with sphincterotomy demonstrated possible beneficial effects of heparin versus control group. Patients received heparin for reasons unrelated to the procedure, and the review was made on patients who were prospectively studied to evaluate risk factors using multivariate analysis for complications that arise from endoscopic sphincterotomy (EST). The overall rate of pancreatitis was 6.4%, the heparin group rate was 3.4% (9 of 268), and the control group (no heparin) rate was 7.9% (43 of 547), a difference that reached statistical significance. No increase in bleeding complications between the two groups was noted. Although interesting, this study was not originally designed to assess the effect of heparin on the development of post-ERCP pancreatitis, and other confounding variables may therefore have contributed to the observed outcomes *(48)*. More studies are needed before heparin can be recommended for routine use.

Interleukin-10

Two randomized studies on the use of IL-10 for the prevention of pancreatitis after ERCP have yielded conflicting results. One prospective randomized study of 144 patients displayed a decrease in the incidence of pancreatitis with the use of IL-10 given as a single injection 30 minutes prior to the procedure versus placebo *(49)*. It should be noted that the rate of pancreatitis in the placebo group was unusually high at 24%. The other study was also prospective, randomized, and double-blind and included 200 patients but failed to show a decrease in the incidence of post-procedure pancreatitis *(50)*. Therefore, IL-10 use should be limited at this point to further randomized trials.

Diclofenac

A prospective double-blind, randomized, placebo-controlled trial was recently performed reviewing the use of 100 mg rectal suppository diclofenac given immediately after endoscopy for the prevention of post-ERCP pancreatitis. This study was limited to patients undergoing ERP and to patients with manometrically confirmed sphincter of Oddi hypertension. A total of 7 of 110 patients (6.4%) who received rectal diclofenac and 17 of 110 patients (15.5%) who receiving placebo suffered from post-ERCP pancreatitis ($p < 0.05$), yielding an absolute risk reduction (ARR) of 9% and a NNT of 11. Subgroup analysis suggested that the benefit was limited to those patients who underwent EST (116 patients) and did not extend to those who had sphincter of Oddi hypertension (53 patients), although the study was not focused specifically at this subgroup. The benefit is thought to occur via an inhibition of phospholipase 2 and the inflammatory cascade that results *(51)*. Even if a single study, it was well-designed and represents a practical and inexpensive method to prevent post-ERCP pancreatitis in a group of patients at the highest risk for this complication.

SUMMARY: PHARMACOLOGICAL PREVENTION OF PANCREATITIS AFTER ERCP

Given the relatively low incidence of pancreatitis post-ERCP, large studies are needed to show significant differences with the administration of medications prior to procedure. Additionally, the NNT to prevent one episode of severe pancreatitis are high and nay not be worth the associated costs, especially if medication administration requires hospitalization in patients that would otherwise be managed in an outpatient setting. The available data do not support the routine use of somatostatin, gabexate, corticosteroids, allopurinol, octreotide, and IL-10. Prophylactic glyceryl trinitrate and heparin are promising, but more confirmatory studies are needed before they can be recommended. Rectal diclofenac may represent a practical and inexpensive intervention in high-risk patients undergoing EST. Table 2 summarizes the proposed mechanism of action and efficacy of these agents in the prevention of post-ERCP pancreatitis.

TECHNIQUE-RELATED PREVENTION OF POST-ERCP PANCREATITIS

The precise mechanism of pancreatitis post ERCP is not clear, but is felt to be secondary to papillary edema/spasm and pancreatic sphincter hypertension in the setting of sphincterotomy or repeated injection of the pancreatic duct. Based on this theory, five studies have been performed analyzing the effect of the placement of pancreatic duct stents to relieve ductal hypertension during ERCP on the incidence of post-ERCP pancreatitis.

The first analysis was a prospective randomized study that reviewed the effect of stenting of the main pancreatic duct on the incidence of post-ERCP pancreatitis in high-risk patients undergoing biliary sphincterotomy. High-risk patients were defined as those with SOD, a common bile duct less than 10 mm or those requiring precut sphincterotomy. Patients were randomized to stent (48 patients with stent removal 10–14 days after placement) or no stent (50 patients). The incidence of post-ERCP pancreatitis was 18% in the no-stent group and 14% in the stent group ($p = 0.6$). Trends in favor of the stent group were noted with respect to hospital days required to treat pancreatitis (2.5 days versus 9.5 days) and regarding frequency of

Table 2
Pharmacological Prevention of Post-ERCP Pancreatitis

Agent	Mechanism of action	Efficacy
Gabexate mesilate	Blocks intracellular activation of proteolytic enzymes	Efficacious but expensive, must be given for 12 hours postprocedure and not available in Unites States
Corticosteroids	Inhibition of pancreatic inflammation	Proven to be of no benefit
Somatostatin	Inhibition of pancreatic secretion	Conflicting results but appears to be effective. Requires prolonged postprocedure infusion
Octreotide	Inhibition of pancreatic secretion	Proven to be of no benefit
Glyceryl trinitrate	Lowers basal pressure of SO and decreases SO contraction pressure	Proven to be useful in two studies: inexpensive and easy to administer; should be considered for use pending further trials
Heparin	Improved pancreatic-micro circulation and acts as protease inhibitor	Post-hoc analysis suggested benefit, but more valid studies are needed before further recommendations can be made
Interleukin-10	Decrease inflammatory cytokines released during pancreatitis that may cause parenchymal edema and necrosis	Conflicting results in trials but does not appear to be effective
Diclofenac suppository	Inhibits phospholipase A_2 and resulting inflammatory cascade	Found useful in one randomized controlled study

ERCP, endoscopic retrograde cholangiopancreatography; SO, Sphincter of Oddi.

moderate-to-severe pancreatitis (2% versus 8%). Small common bile duct diameter of less than 6 mm was found to be an independent risk factor for pancreatitis after EST *(52)*.

Another prospective randomized study of 93 patients was performed reviewing the incidence of post-procedure pancreatitis in patients who underwent pancreatic duct stenting as a guide to precut biliary sphincterotomy in those patients where free cannulation of the bile duct was not able to be performed. This demonstrated that maintaining the pancreatic duct stent in place for 7–10 days reduced the frequency of post-ERCP pancreatitis from 21% to 2% when compared to patients who had immediate removal of the pancreatic stent after successful precut sphincterotomy. The rate of pancreatitis following precut sphincterotmy in 58 patients who did not have pancreatic duct stent placement as a guidance to precut sphincterotomy was 13%. The results of this study were published in abstract form, only making it difficult to determine the validity of the study and consequently to generalize the results to clinical practice *(53)*.

The next study involved 80 patients with unexplained pancreatico-biliary pain or prior AP who had manometrically confirmed pancreatic sphincter hypertension. Patients were randomized to the placement of pancreatic duct stent (41 patients) or no stent (39 patients) after biliary sphincterotomy. The incidence of post-ERCP pancreatitis in the stent group was 2% versus 26% in the no-stent group ($p = 0.003$, ARR of 24% with an NNT of 4). Of note, the no-stent group had a significantly greater difficulty of cannulation and a significantly longer time to repeat pancreatic access after biliary sphincterotomy. After the correction for these differences by logistic regression analysis, the risk of post-ERCP pancreatitis after biliary sphincterotomy remained significantly higher in the no-stent group (OR 14.4; 95% confidence interval (CI) 1.7–125; $p = 0.002$). Subgroup analysis revealed that the incidence of post-ERCP pancreatitis was much greater in those without a patent accessory papilla (23% versus 0%), and that all of the patients in the no-stent group who developed post-ERCP pancreatitis (43%) had a nonpatent accessory papilla. Criticisms of this study include unblinded investigators who were analyzing the primary outcome and the fact that patients in both study groups underwent repeat pancreatic manometry and, if not done already, pancreatography after biliary sphincterotomy. This may have contributed to the development of post-ERCP pancreatitis and confounded the results of the study *(54)*.

Another study was performed that analyzed the effect of pancreatic duct stent placement in patients undergoing endoscopic sphincter dilation for removal of bile duct stones. In this analysis, 38 of 40 patients who had successful placement of a pancreatic duct stent during ERCP were compared to 92 controls undergoing the same procedure that did not have a stent placed. No randomization was done, but there were no significant difference between the stated group characteristics. There was a nonsignificant ($p = 0.11$) trend toward a decreased rate of pancreatitis in the stent group (0%) versus the no-stent control group (6%). However, the study, may not have been powered enough to demonstrate a significant difference. A significant difference in favor of the stent group between levels of postprocedure hyperamylasemia was seen, but the clinical importance is likely negligible *(55)*.

A recent prospective, randomized controlled trial was performed analyzing the effect of pancreatic duct stent placement versus no-stent placement on the incidence of post-ERCP pancreatitis in 76 patients considered at high risk for the complication, including those with difficult ductal cannulation (defined as >30 minutes required to cannulate) or the performance of sphincter Oddi manometry and/or EST. Twenty-eight percent of the no-stent group versus 5% ($p < 0.05$) of the stent group developed post-ERCP pancreatitis. Pancreatitis tended to be less severe in patients who had a pancreatic duct stent placed. No CIs were mentioned in this unblinded study *(56)*.

A meta-analysis published in abstract form only compiled data on 371 patients at higher than average risk for post-ERCP pancreatitis, including the presence of SOD, performance of precut sphincterotomy, or a common bile duct less than 10 mm. Pancreatic duct stents were placed in 158 patients and not placed in 213 patients. A significantly lower incidence of postprocedure pancreatitis was observed in the stent group vs. no stent group (9% versus 18%; OR = 0.3. 95% CI, 0.18–0.7; $p = 0.003$; NNT 11; *57*).

SUMMARY: TECHNIQUE-RELATED PREVENTION OF POST-ERCP PANCREATITIS

Although small in numbers and variable in patient characteristics, the studies to date, report an overall reduction in post-ERCP pancreatitis in those patients at a high risk for this complication, including those patients undergoing precut sphincterotomy, those with SOD, and those with a common bile duct diameter of less than 10 mm. It is estimated that 11 main pancreatic duct stents would have to be placed to prevent one case of post-ERCP pancreatitis, which appears to be a cost-effective measure and should be considered by experienced endoscopists. Use of stents without internal barbs would prevent inward migration and reduce the need for a repeat procedure to remove the stents.

REFERENCES

1. Baillargeon, JD, Orav J, Vinodhini R, et al. Hemoconcentration as an early risk factor for necrotizing pancreatitis. Am J Gastroenterol 1998; 93: 2130–2134.
2. Thompson DR. Narcotic analgesic effects on the sphincter of Oddi: A review of the data and therapeutic implications in treating pancreatitis. Am J Gastroenterol 2001; 96: 1266–1272.
3. Rykowski JJ, Hilgier M. Continuous celiac plexus block in acute pancreatitis. Reg Anesth 1995; 20: 528–532.
4. Archer SB, Burnett RJ, Fischer JE. Current uses and abuses of total parental nutrition. Adv Surg 1996; 29: 165–189.

5. Sax HC, Warner BW, Talamini MA, et al. Early total parenteral nutrition in acute pancreatitis: Lack of beneficial effects. Am J Surg 1987; 153: 117–122.

6. Windsor ACJ, Kanwar S, Li AGK, et al. Compared with parenteral nutrition, enteral feeding attenuates the acute phase response and improves disease severity in acute pancreatitis. Gut 1998; 42: 431–435.

7. Erstad BL. Enteral nutrition support in acute pancreatitis. Ann Pharmacother 2000; 34: 514–521.

8. Sarr MG, Sanfey H, Cameron JL. Prospective randomized trial of nasogastric suction in patients with acute pancreatitis. Surgery 1986; 100: 500–54.

9. Navarro S, Ros E, Aused R, et al. Comparison of fasting, nasogastric suction and cimetidine in the treatment of acute pancreatitis. Digestion 1984; 30: 224–230.

10. Fuller RK, Loveland JP, Frankel MH. An evaluation of the efficacy of nasogastric suction treatment in alcoholic pancreatitis. Am J Gastroenterol 1981; 75: 349–353.

11. Meshkinpour H, Molinari MD, Gardner L, et al. Cimetidine in the treatment of acute alcoholic pancreatitis: A randomized double-blind study. Gastroenterology 1979; 77: 687–690.

12. Maisto OE, Bremner CG. Antacids in the treatment of acute alcohol-induced pancreatitis. SA Med J 1983; 63: 351–352.

13. Choi TK, Mok F, Zhan WH, et al. Somatostatin in the treatment of acute pancreatitis: A prospective randomized controlled trial. Gut 1989; 30: 223–227.

14. Karakoyunlar O, Sivrel E, Tanir N, Denecil AG. High dose octreotide in the management of acute pancreatitis. Hepatogastroenterology 1999; 46: 1968–1972.

15. Buchler UW, Malfertheiner P, Beger HG, et al. A randomized, double-blind, multicenter trial of octreotide in moderate to severe acute pancreatitis. Gut 1999; 45: 97–104.

16. Lerch MM, Gorelick FS. Early trypsinogen activation in acute pancreatitis. Med Clin N Am 2000; 84: 549–561.

17. Yang CY, Chang-Chien CS, Liaw YF. Controlled trial of protease inhibitor gabexate mesilate in the treatment of acute pancreatitis. Pancreas 1987; 6: 698–700.

18. Harada H, Miyake H, Ochi K, Tanaka J, Kimura I. Clinical trial with a protease inhibitor gabexate mesilate in acute pancreatitis. Int J Pancreatol 1991; 9: 75–79.

19. Valderrama R, Perez-Mateo M, Navarro S, et al. Multicenter double-blind trial of gabexate mesilate in unselected patients with acute pancreatitis. Digestion 1992; 51: 65–70.

20. Messori A, Rampazzo R, Scroccaro G, et al. Effectiveness of gabexate mesilate in acute pancreatitis: A meta-analysis. Dig Dis Sci 1995; 40: 734–748.

21. Buchler M, Malfertheiner P, Uhl W, et al. Gabexate mesilate in human acute pancreatitis. German Pancreatitis Study Group. Gastroenterology 1993; 104: 1216–1219.

22. Platell C, Cooper D, Hall JC. A meta-analysis of peritoneal lavage for acute pancreatitis. J Gastroenterol Hepatol 2001; 16: 689–693.

23. Montero-Otero R, Rodriguez S, Carbo J, et al. Double blind Trial of Pirenzepine in Acute Pancreatitis. Digestion 1989; 42: 51–56.

24. Goebell H, Ammann R, Herfarth CH, et al. A double-blind trial of synthetic salmon calcitonin in the treatment of acute pancreatitis. Scand J Gastroent 1979; 14: 881–889.

25. Freeman ML, James AD, Nelson DB, et al: Risk Factors for post-ERCP pancreatitis: a prospective multicenter study. Gastrointest Endos 2001; 54: 425–434.

26. Shimizu Y, Takahashi H, Deura M, et al. Prophylactic effects of preoperative administration of gabexate mesilate on post-ERCP pancreatitis. Gendai Iryo 1979; 11: 540–544.

27. Salamon V, Kuntz HD, May B, eds. Wirkung Des Suntehetischen Proteinase-Inhibitors FOY Workshop, 1981. Wolf G and Sohn, Dusseldorf, Germany;1982: 132–135.
28. Cavallini G, Tittobello A, Frulloni L, et al. Gabexate for the prevention of pancreatic damage related to endoscopic retrograde cholangiopancreatography. Gabexate in digestive endoscopy-Italian Group. N Engl J Med 1996; 335; 961–963.
29. Andriuilli A, Leandro G. Niro A, et. al. Gastrointest Endosc 2000; 51: 1–7.
30. Andruilli A, Clemente R, Solmi L, et. al. Gastrointest Endosc, 2002; 56: 488–495.
31. De Plama GD, Catanzano C. Use of corticosteroids in the prevention of post-ERCP pancreatitis: results of a controlled prospective study. Am J Gastroenterol 1999; 94: 982–985.
32. Budzynska A, Markek T, Nowak A, et al. A prospective, randomized, placebo-controlled trial of prednisone and allopurinol in the prevention of ERCP-induced pancreatitis. Endoscopy 2001; 33: 766–772.
33. Borsch G, Bergbauer M, Nebel W, Sbin G. Effect of somatostatin on amylase level and pancreatitis rate following ERCP. Med Welt 1984; 35: 109–112.
34. Saari A, Kivilaakso E, Schroder T. The influence of somatostatin on pancreatic irritation after pancreatography: an experimental and clinical study. Surg Res Commun 1988; 2: 271–278.
35. Person B, Slezak P. Efendic S, Haggmark A. Can somatostatin prevent injection pancreatitis after ERCP? Hepatogastroenterology 1992; 39: 259–261.
36. Tung-Ping Poon R, Yeng C, Lo CM, et al. Prophylactic effect of somatostatin on post-ERCP pancreatitis: a randomized controlled trial. Gastrointest Endosc 1999; 49: 593–598.
37. Bordas JM, Toledo-Pimentel V, Llach J. Effects of bolus somatostatin in preventing pancreatitis after endoscopic pancreatography: results of a randomized study. Gastrointest Endosc 1998; 47: 230–234.
38. Bordas JM, Toledo V, Nondelo F, Rodes J. Prevention of pancreatic reactions by bolus somatostatin administration in patients undergoing endoscopic retrograde cholangio-pancreatography and endoscopic sphincterotomy. Horm Res 1988; 29: 106–108.
39. Binmoeller KF, Harris AG, Dumas R, et al. Does the somatostatin analogue octreotide protect against ERCP-induced pancreatitis? Gut 1992; 33: 1129–1133.
40. Arvanitidis D, Hatzipanayiotis J, Koutsounopoulos G, Frangou E. The effect of octreotide on the prevention of acute pancreatitis and hyperamylasemia after diagnostic and therapeutic ERCP. Hepatogastro 1998; 19: 248–252.
41. Testoni PA, Bagnolo F, Andriulli A, Bernasconi G, et al. Octreotide 24-h prophylaxis at high risk for post-ERCP pancreatitis: results of a multicenter, randomized, controlled trial. Aliment Pharmacol Ther 2001; 15: 965–972.
42. Manolakopoulos S, Avgerinos A, Vlacholgiannakos J, et al. Octreotide versus hydrocortisone versus placebo in the prevention of post-ERCP pancreatitis: a multi-center randomized controlled trial. Gastrointest Endosc 2002; 55: 470–475.
43. Staritz M, Poralla T, Dormeyer HH, Meyer zum Buschenfelde KH. Effect of glyceryl trinitrate on the sphincter of Oddi motility and baseline pressure. Gut 1985; 26: 194–197.
44. Sudhindran S, Bromwich E, Edwards PR. Prospective randomized double-blind placebo-controlled trial of glyceryl trinitrate in endoscopic retrograde cholangiopancreatography-induced pancreatitis. Br J Surg 2001; 88: 1178–1182.
45. Moreto M, Zaballa M. Prospective randomized double-blind placebo-controlled trial of glyceryl trinitrate in endoscopic retrograde cholangiopancreatography-induced pancreatitis. Br J Surg 2002; 89: 628–629.

46. Gabryelewicz A, Kosidlo S, Prokopowicz J, Peokopowicz K. Does heparin modify protease-antiprotease balance in acute experimental pancreatitis in rats? Hepatogastro 1986; 33: 79–92.

47. Dobosz M, Hac S, Minonskowska L, et al. Microcirculatory disturbances of the pancreas in caerulein-induced acute pancreatitis in rats with reference to L-arginine, heparin, and procaine treatment. Pharmacol Res 1997; 36: 123–128.

48. Rabenstein T, Sylvia R, Framke B, et al. Complications of endoscopic sphincterotomy: Can heparin prevent acute pancreatitis after ERCP? Gastrointest Endosc 2002; 55: 476–483.

49. Deviere J, Le Moine O, Van Laethem JL, et al. Interleukin 10 reduces the incidence of pancreatitis after therapeutic endoscopic retrograde cholangiopancreatography. Gastroenterology 2001; 120: 498–505.

50. Dumot JA, Conwell DL, Zuccaro G, et al. A randomized, double-blind study of interleukin 10 for the prevention of ERCP-induced pancreatitis. Am J Gastroenterol 2001; 96: 2098–2102.

51. Murray B, Carter R, Imrie C, et al. Diclofenac reduces the incidence of acute pancreatitis after endoscopic retrograde cholangiopancreatography. Gastroenterology 2003; 124: 1786–1791.

52. Smithline A, Silverman W, Rogers D, et. al. Effect of prophylactic main pancreatic duct stenting on the incidence of biliary endoscopic sphincterotomy-induced pancreatitis in high risk patients. Gastrointest Endosc 1993; 39: 652–657.

53. Sherman S, Earl D, Bucksot L, et al. Does leaving a main pancreatic duct stent in place reduce the incidence of pre cut biliary sphincterotomy pancreatitis? Am J Gastroenterol 1995; 90: 1614.

54. Tarnasky P, Yuko P, Cunningham JT, et al. Pancreatic stenting prevents pancreatitis after biliary sphincterotomy in patients with sphincter of Oddi dysfunction. Gastroenterology 1998; 115: 1518–1524.

55. Aizawa T, Ueno N. Stent placement in the pancreatic duct prevents pancreatitis after endoscopic sphincter dilation for removal of bile duct stones. Gastrointest Endosc 2001; 54: 209–213.

56. Fazel A, Quadri A, Catalano M, et al. Does a pancreatic duct stent prevent post ERCP pancreatitis? A prospective randomized study. Gastrointest Endosc 2003; 57: 291–294.

57. Singh P, Sivak M, Agarwal D, et al. Prophylactic pancreatic stenting for prevention of post ERCP pancreatitis: A meta-analysis of controlled trials. Gastrointest Endosc 2003; 57: AB89.

6   Treatment of Severe Acute Pancreatitis

Peter Draganov, MD

INTRODUCTION

Acute pancreatitis (AP) is a protean disease capable of wide clinical variation, ranging from mild discomfort to overwhelming organ failure and death. This chapter introduces definitions, discusses the diagnosis of severe AP (SAP), and examines in detail the various therapeutic options for management of patients with SAP.

DEFINITIONS

The variability in presentation and clinical course has plagued the study and management of AP since its original clinical description. It is crucial for practicing clinicians in the care of individual patients, as well as to academicians seeking to compare interinstitutional data, to have a classification system that is clinician-friendly and universally

From: *Pancreatitis and Its Complications*
Edited by: C. E. Forsmark © Humana Press Inc., Totowa, NJ

Table 1
Acute Pancreatitis Definitions According to the Atlanta Conference

Category	Definition
Severe acute pancreatitis	Severe acute pancreatitis is associated with organ failure and/or local complications, such as necrosis, abscess, or pseudocyst
Acute fluid collections	Acute fluid collections occur early in the course of acute pancreatitis, are located in or near the pancreas, and always lack a wall of granulation or fibrous tissue
Pancreatic necrosis	Pancreatic necrosis is a diffuse or focal area(s) of nonviable pancreatic paren-chyma,which is typically associated with peripancreatic fat necrosis
Acute pseudocyst	A pseudocyst is a collection of pancreatic juice enclosed by a wall of fibrous or granulation tissue, which arises as a consequence of acute pancreatitis, pancreatic trauma, or chronic pancreatitis
Pancreatic abscess	A pancreatic abscess is a circumscribed intra-abdominal collection of pus, usually in proximity to the pancreas, containing little or nopancreaticnecrosis, which arises as a consequence of acute pancreatitis or pancreatic trauma
Pancreatic phlegmon, infected pseudocyst, hemorrhagic pancreatitis, persistent acute pancreatitis	The use of these ambiguous terms is discouraged

accepted. In the fall of 1992, following 3 days of group meetings and open discussions, unanimous consensus on a series of definitions and a clinically based classification system for AP was achieved by a diverse group of 40 international authorities from six medical disciplines and 15 countries (Table 1; 1). Since the meeting occurred in Atlanta, Georgia, this classification is frequently referred to as the "Atlanta consensus."

Severe Acute Pancreatitis

According to the Atlanta consensus, SAP is associated with organ failure and/or local complications, such as necrosis, abscess, or pseudocyst, coupled with unfavorable early prognostic signs (Ranson's criteria).

Organ Failure

The most important indicator of severity in AP is the presence of organ failure. The consensus definitions of organ failure include the presence of shock (systolic blood pressure <90 mmHg), pulmonary insufficiency (PaO$_2$ <60 mmHg), renal failure (creatinine >2 mg/dL after initial rehydration), and gastrointestinal (GI) bleeding (>500 mL/24 h). Systemic complications, such as disseminated intravascular coagulation and hypocalcemia, may also be seen but are not part of the consensus definitions.

Local Complicatios

Pancreatic necrosis: Pancreatic necrosis is a diffuse or focal area of nonviable pancreatic parenchyma, which is typically associated with peripancreatic fat necrosis. Most patients with severe pancreatitis have pancreatic necrosis. The necrosis may remain sterile or become infected (infected necrosis). Infected necrosis is a mixture of devitalized tissue, fluid, pus, and bacteria.

Acute fluid collections: Acute fluid collections occur early in the course of AP, are located in or near the pancreas, and always lack a wall of granulation or fibrous tissue. Most acute fluid collections regress spontaneously, whereas others progress to become an abscess or pseudocyst *(2)*.

Pancreatic abscess: A pancreatic abscess is a circumscribed intra-abdominal collection of pus, usually in proximity to the pancreas that contains little or no pancreatic necrosis, which arises as a consequence of AP. The term "pancreatic abscess" has been used improperly in the past for all forms of pancreatic infection. The distinction between pancreatic abscess and infected necrosis is critical for two reasons: the mortality risk for infected necrosis is double that for pancreatic abscess *(3)* and the specific therapy for each condition may be markedly different *(4)*.

Acute pseudocyst: A pseudocyst is a collection of pancreatic juice enclosed by a wall of fibrous or granulation tissue. Formation of a pseudocyst requires at least 4 weeks from the onset of AP *(5)*. In this regard, an acute pseudocyst is a fluid collection that arises in association with an episode of AP, is of more than 4 week duration, and is surrounded by a defined wall. Fluid collections of less than 4 week duration that lack a defined wall are more properly termed "acute fluid collections."

These definitions are now used routinely in both clinical practice and clinical research. Several other terms, including "phlegmon" and "infected pseudocyst," have been abandoned either because no consensus on their definition could be reached (phlegmon), or because an alternative term was more appropriate (i.e., pancreatic abscess instead of infected pseudocyst).

DIAGNOSIS OF SEVERE ACUTE PANCREATITIS

The diagnosis of SAP is based on the detection of systemic and/or local complications.

Systemic Complications

Systemic complications are usually easy to detect if clinicians actively monitor for them. All patients with AP should be routinely monitored for the presence of hypotension, renal failure, pulmonary insufficiency, GI bleeding, disseminated intravascular coagulation, and hypocalcemia. In a recent retrospective series of 67 patients with SAP, the most common systemic complications were respiratory failure (44%), acute renal failure (35%), and shock (20%; 6). Although these complications are discussed separately, it is not unusual for patients to have multiple complications concurrently or sequentially.

Shock (systolic blood pressure <90 mmHg) carries a poor prognosis *(7)*. Patients suffering from AP show indirect signs of hypovolemia; the filling pressure of the right heart and pulmonary capillary wedge pressure, as a parameter for the pressure in the left atrium, are lowered *(8)*. Once shock has occurred, it can convert edematous pancreatitis to necrotizing pancreatitis *(9)*. The mechanism of this effect remains unclear. As hypoperfusion seems to be a critical factor in the progression of the disease, adequate fluid replacement and resuscitation is an important therapeutic principle. Although there are no controlled clinical studies that verify the hypothesis of a shock-induced conversion of pancreatic edema into necrosis, breaking this vicious cycle is considered by most clinicians of paramount therapeutic importance.

Respiratory failure is characterized by arterial hypoxemia (PaO_2 <60 mmHg). The spectrum of pulmonary complications ranges from isolated arterial hypoxemia without clinical symptoms or radiological abnormalities to severe life-threatening adult respiratory distress syndrome *(10,11)*. The development of radiographic abnormalities, such as pleural effusions (most are left-sided), atelectasis, elevation of the diaphragm, or focal pulmonary infiltrates, are associated with higher rates of respiratory failure than that associated with hypoxia alone. Adult respiratory distress syndrome is the most serious respiratory complication of AP and carries a mortality rate that may exceed 60% *(10)*.

Renal failure carries a mortality rate of more than 50% *(12)*. The pathogenesis of renal failure is complex and not completely understood. Although hypovolemia and shock are considered to be major etiological factors in the pathogenesis; a decreased glomerular filtration rate and renal plasma flow have been shown even after the correction of volume depletion *(12,13)*. Early correction of hypovolemia is critical in attempting to prevent renal failure.

Biochemical and metabolic abnormalities like hypocalcemia *(7,14,15)*, hyperglycemia *(7,15)*, hyperlipidemia *(16)*, and coagulation abnormalities *(17,18)* are seen in 28–52% of cases with AP. Both hypocalcemia and hyperglycemia indicate poor prognosis and are included in the Ranson criteria *(7,19)*. Hyperlipidemia is associated with AP as a possible etiological factor or consequence *(20)*. It is often impossible to decide during an AP attack whether the lipid abnormalities are primary or secondary. For that reason, if the etiology of the episode of AP is unclear, repeating the lipid profile is recommended after the attack of pancreatitis is resolved. Generally, however, levels of triglyceride above 1000 mg/dL are required to initiate AP, whereas levels of less than 300 mg/dL are seen as a consequence of AP. Coagulation disorders can vary from a hypercoagulable state presenting with thrombosis *(17)* to coagulopathy that presents with bleeding *(18)*. Some studies have attempted to use the coagulation abnormalities as a prognostic factor *(21,22)*. The development of disseminated intravascular coagulation appears to worsen prognosis, although it is not a strong independent predictor of mortality. Trials with the protease inhibitor, aprotinin, or heparin have not given positive results and specific therapy of the coagulation disorders is not currently available.

GI bleeding is relatively uncommon, occurring in 4–8% of AP episodes *(15,23)*. The usual causes are gastric or duodenal ulcerations, gastritis, and varices. Varices may be present owing to underlying cirrhosis or as a result of splenic vein thrombosis (a well-recognized complication of AP; *24,25*). This produces a "left-sided" portal hypertension with gastric varices out of proportion to esophageal varices. Bleeding from a pseudoaneurysm in the wall of a pseudocyst is usually seen in chronic pancreatitis (CP) but can also occur in AP *(26)*.

Local Complications

Local complications of AP, including acute fluid collections, pancreatic abscess, pseudocyst and pancreatic necrosis, are best detected by dynamic intravenous contrast-enhanced computed tomography (CECT; *27*). The severity of pancreatitis can be graded by computed tomography (CT; *28–30*). A CT severity index can be calculated based on these findings (*see* Chapter 2). Although not every patient with severe pancreatitis on CT will develop organ failure, the chance of organ failure increases with the severity of CT appearance. The higher the CT severity index is, the worse the prognosis *(29,31)*. In a prospective study the incidence of organ failure increased significantly with the increases of CT score *(32)*. It is of critical importance to obtain an intravenous CECT to properly evaluate a patient for local complications of AP. A noncontrast CT will be of very limited value, because it will not detect pancreatic necrosis. Although CT is very helpful in the management of patients with AP, not every patient with AP needs CT. After all, most patients with AP recover uneventfully. One obvious consideration is the issue of cost. That issue aside, there has been a concern that the use of intravenous contrast media in the initial course of AP might increase or extend pancreatic necrosis. Decreased pancreatic capillary flow rates and worsening pancreatitis have been observed in two animal studies *(33,34)*. One retrospective study found that patients who underwent CECT had longer hospitalization than those who did not *(35)*, yet this could easily have been because of selection bias. In a cohort analytic study, an increased incidence of local and systemic complications was observed in patients with mild AP who underwent CECT *(36)*. Because prospective and randomized human studies are unavailable, it is reasonable to reserve CECT scans for patients with SAP, those with smoldering AP that is slow to improve, or in those with suspected local septic complications. The dilemma clinicians face is that CT is indicated in patients with SAP and, in contrast, one of the prerequisites of SAP is the presence of local complications best detected by CT scan. There are no firm guidelines on which patient should recieve a CT scan. One could argue that CT scans are useful in every patient, which may relate that those with SAP need a CT to document severity and that a normal or near-normal CT in those with mild AP would reassure the responsible clinician and allow one to triage that patient to a less expensive venue (e.g., a general floor bed rather than in intermediate care unit or intensive care unit). However, obtaining a CT scan on every patient might use health care resources unwisely. One reasonable approach is to reserve CT for patients with unfavorable early prognostic signs and/or patients who develop systemic complications of AP. On the other hand, if the early prognostic signs are favorable and systemic complications are absent, then CT scan may not be indicated.

The most commonly used early prognostic signs are the Ranson's criteria (*see* Chapter 2) and the Acute Physiology And Chronic Health Evaluation (APACHE II) scoring system. In many clinicians' experience, the APACHE II system is complex and difficult to use in every-day patient care, but it has an important role as a research tool. The Ranson's criteria are somewhat easier to use and are reasonably accurate at predicting the severity of AP at the extremes of the scoring system. If a patient has 0 or 1 criteria, they will almost certainly recover uneventfully and likely do not require a CECT scan. A patient with more than 4 criteria score will most likely develop SAP. Most patients, unfortunately, fall in the middle category of 2–4 criteria. At this level, the mortality is still a significant at 10–15%, but the Ranson criteria cannot identify which patient with a 4 criteria score will develop organ failure and die and which patient with

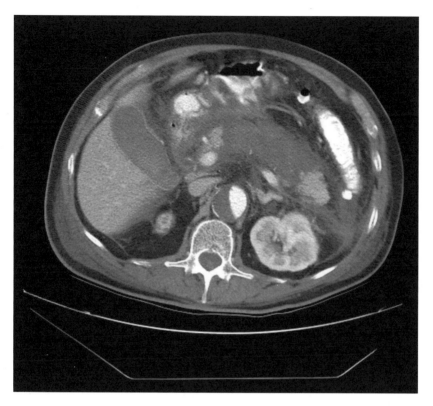

Fig. 1. A computed tomography (CT) demonstrates a large area of pancreas in the mid-body of the gland, which does not opacify with intravenous contrast. A small amount of opacified pancreas can be seen in the head and tail. This CT finding is consistent with necrosis of the majority of the body of the gland.

this criteria will recover without incident. Nonetheless, a recent meta-analysis evaluated the discriminant power of Ranson's signs in the prediction of AP severity and outcome when compared to clinical judgment *(37)*. Nineteen studies (*n* = 2728) for severity prediction and 10 (*n* = 1513) for prognosis were included. The Ranson's criteria show a poor predictive power for severity and outcome of AP and did not differ from that of clinical judgment. The Ranson (and other multiple factor scoring systems) are perhaps best useful in deciding who does not need a CECT scan, but they can also guide clinicians in triage by identifying a group of patients who are more likely to benefit from intensive care unit or intermediate care unit admission.

Pancreatic necrosis develops in approximately 10–20% of patients with AP (Fig. 1; *38*). Of those, approximately 30–35% will develop infected necrosis, which is usually documented during the second or third week of illness and occasionally beyond this timeframe. Pancreatic infection should be suspected among patients with necrotizing pancreatitis when there is ongoing systemic toxicity, including persisting leukocytosis and fever and/or unresolved organ failure. When pancreatic infection is suspected, a CT-guided percutaneous aspiration with Gram stain and culture should be performed. CT-guided percutaneous aspiration has proven to be a safe and accurate method to distinguish infected from sterile necrosis (39). In a longitudinal study of 194 patients with unequivocal AP, pancreatic necrosis developed in 20%. All patients with documented necrosis underwent fine-needle aspiration and infection was documented in 71% of the patients (38). Once suspected, documentation of infected necrosis via percutaneous fine-needle aspiration is of paramount importance for two reasons: it has poor prognostic implications, and it requires prompt specific therapy (see the next section and Chapter 7).

THERAPY OF SEVERE ACUTE PANCREATITIS

Most patients with SAP and all patients with systemic complications should be monitored in an intensive care unit under the coordinated care of a multidisciplinary team. To date, no specific therapy has been shown to be effective for SAP. The lack of specific therapy underscores why skillful supportive care becomes paramount and consequently the need for gastroenterologists to coordinate the care with intensivists, surgeons, and radiologists. Several drugs have been evaluated by prospective controlled trials and found ineffective in the treatment of AP. The list, by no means complete, includes glucagon (40–43), atropine (44), H-2 receptor antagonists (45–47), protease inhibitors, such as aprotinin and gabexate (48–51), calcitonin (52), and somatostatin and its analog octreotide (53–56). The latest disappointment is the platelet-activating factor antagonist lexipafant (57). Although still not reported in manuscript form, a recent randomized double-blind, placebo-controlled, multicenter trial involving more than 1500 patients showed that lexipafant had no effect on the incidence of organ failure, local complications, or death (58).

Therefore, at present, meticulous supportive care and treatment of local and systemic complications as they arise remains the cornerstone of therapy in patients with SAP.

The Role of Fasting in Severe Acute Pancreatitis

Most patients with AP cannot tolerate oral intake secondary to abdominal pain, nausea, and vomiting. Null per os is routinely recommended in all patients with AP and particularly in those with SAP. However, the role of fasting as a way to rest the pancreas and reduce the severity of AP has not been established. Theoretically, this would reduce cholecystokinin (CCK)-stimulated pancreatic secretion. It has been demonstrated that CCK-stimulated pancreatic secretion is nearly abolished in four different experimental models of AP. This probably explains the reason why maneuvers aimed to "rest the pancreas" have failed to demonstrate any therapeutic benefit (59). There are no firm criteria when to reintroduce oral intake in patients with SAP. The decision is based on clinical judgment. The usual criteria used are that abdominal pain has resolved or substantially decreased, organ dysfunction (if present) has improved, and the patient is hungry. Some authors recommend that the elevation of serum amylase/lipase or persistent inflammatory changes seen on CT should not discourage the clinician from feeding a hungry asymptomatic patient. Two prospective nonblinded studies showed that resolution of inflammatory changes on CT scan and elevation of amylase and lipase may not take place for several months (60,61). In a recent multicenter prospective study from France, longer duration of initial pain, high CT severity index, and serum lipase concentrations more than three times the upper limit of normal 1 day before refeeding were independently associated with and increased the risk of pain relapse (62).

The Role of Nasogastric Tube Suctioning in Severe Acute Pancreatitis

In the past, it was believed that removing acid-dependent stimulation of the pancreas would "rest" the inflamed organ and promote recovery, but there is no evidence to support such a belief. Two relatively small prospective randomized trials have examined the role of nasogastric (NG) tube suction in the management of AP (63,64). In both trials, no benefit from NG tube suction was observed. In these studies, stratification of severity was done on clinical grounds rather than CT findings and precludes us the ability to separate necrotizing from interstitial pancreatitis. Current consensus based on clinical trials suggests a limited use of NG suction in patients with significant ileus and to provide symptomatic relief in patients with vomiting (65).

The Role of Intravenous Fluid Therapy in Severe Acute Pancreatitis

Fluid resuscitation is a cornerstone in the management of SAP. It is believed that correction of intravascular volume loss may protect against hypotension, acute renal failure, and may preserve the pancreatic microcirculation. The pancreatic vessels are particularly poor at responding to ischemia, and the pancreas is prone to ischemia-related injury. In the early treatment of SAP, the replacement fluid of choice is normal saline, and 5–6 L are required each day. It is advisable to use colloid replacement (e.g., albumin) if the serum albumin falls below 2.0 g/L. Packed red blood cells should be used to maintain a hematocrit of approximately 30%. Occasionally, patients with SAP may require in excess of 10 L daily to maintain an adequate intravascular volume. The adequacy of fluid resuscitation is usually judged based on clinical parameters, including patient's intake and output, vital signs, renal function, electrolytes, and hematocrit. The role of a pulmonary artery catheter (Swan-Ganz) has not been formally evaluated in randomized trials, and the decision to use it in patients with SAP should be individualized. In general, the use of pulmonary artery catheter monitoring should be considered if there are substantial fluid requirements, the cardiovascular status is unstable, and there is deterioration of respiratory function.

The Role of Symptomatic Pain Medications in Severe Acute Pancreatitis

The majority of patients with AP suffer from severe abdominal pain that requires narcotic analgesics for symptomatic relief. Because most patients are nauseated, and many pateints have significant vomiting, intravenous administration is the preferred route. Pain medications can be given when needed or via patient-controlled anesthesia. A variety of narcotic agonist agents are available, all can increase the pressure of the sphincter of Oddi, and, in theory, might impede drainage from the pancreas that leads to worsening pancreatitis. Morphine has a more pronounced effect in increasing sphincter pressures and is avoided by some physicians as a first choice for symptomatic pain therapy in AP. There is currently no evidence that morphine actually worsens pancreatitis. A frequently used narcotic is meperidine, but it should not be used in high dosages in patients with renal impairment because one of the meperidine metabolites is excreted via the kidney. If that metabolite accumulates, as it can in patients with renal failure, it can cause seizures. Also, using meperidine and imipenem in combination should be avoided, as both drugs can cause seizures. This is particularly true in patients with renal failure. My biased choice of narcotic agonist in patients with AP is hydromorphone, because seizures are less likely and it has less pronounced effects on the sphincter of Oddi.

The Role of Nutritional Support in Severe Acute Pancreatitis

Patients with SAP may not be able to receive oral nourishment for a few weeks and need nutritional support. Two controversial issues regarding nutritional support in patients with SAP remain unresolved. The first issue is the proper timing of initiation of nutritional support. One school of thought is that as patients with severe SAP will not be able to initiate full oral intake for at least a few weeks, nutritional support early in the course should be considered. In contrast, total parenteral nutrition (TPN), which is the most commonly used system of nutrient supplementation in this country, is associated with several complications that tend to increase with increased duration of TPN use. The second controversial issue is the preferred route of providing exogenous nutrients, either TPN or enteral jejunal feeding. Some retrospective studies suggest that pancreatitis patients given early TPN are at increased risk for sepsis and pancreatic infection *(66–68)*. A prospective study has demonstrated that enteral feeding infused distal to the ligament of Treitz is associated with a decreased rate of complications, including infection when compared to TPN *(69)*. Most studies demonstrate enteral feeding is less expensive than TPN. However, a recent evidence-based review suggests that although there is a trend toward reductions in the adverse outcomes of AP after administration of enteral feeding, there are clearly insufficient data to draw firm conclusions about the effectiveness and safety of enteral feeding versus TPN *(70)*. Since that review was published, another randomized trial showed that hypocaloric enteral feeding seems to be safer and less expensive than TPN. In this study, patients with more than 3 Ranson's criteria fed enterally had a decreased duration of nutritional support. In the enteric nutrition group, the mean duration of feeding was 6.8 days, and in the TPN group, 12.8 days ($p = 0.03$). A trend toward shorter hospital stay was noted in the enteral nutrition group but the difference did not reach statistical significance (12.8 days versus 20.1 days; *71*). Presently, there is accumulating evidence that enteral feeding using a tube placed beyond the ligament of Treitz is safer and less expensive than TPN. Enteral feeding using a nasojejunal tube should be strongly considered in patients with SAP who do not have such a severe ileus to preclude such therapy.

The Role of Endoscopic Retrograde Cholangiopancreatography in Severe Biliary Acute Pancreatitis

Acute biliary (gallstone) pancreatitis is defined as AP with a finding of gallstones and in the absence of other known causes, especially alcohol. Acute biliary pancreatitis is the most common cause of AP and likely accounts for well over half of the cases. Most patients with acute biliary pancreatitis have mild-to-moderate clinical disease and recover spontaneously within a few days, presumably as stones pass. In contrast, 20–25% experience severe pancreatitis with mortality up to 10%. Bacteremia, cholangitis, and infected necrosis are more common, whereas the incidence of pseudocyst formation, splenic vein thrombosis, and pancreatic ascites is less than that in alcoholic pancreatitis. Although the association is well-established, the exact means by which gallstones cause AP is a subject of much debate. All theories revolve around the presence of stones in the common bile duct or their passage via the ampulla of Vater. Most patients with acute biliary pancreatitis have already passed the offending common bile duct stone into the duodenum at the onset of the illness. Some patients have persistent or multiple bile duct stones, and in these patients, there is both a predisposition to concomitant cholangitis as well as a tendency toward more severe pancreatitis. By extracting the stones from the common bile duct and performing biliary sphincterotomy one could hope to improve the outcome of biliary pancreatitis, prevent cholangitis, and avoid further attacks of acute biliary pancreatitis.

Four prospective randomized trials have examined the role of endoscopic retrograde cholangiopancreatography (ERCP) versus conservative management in acute biliary pancreatitis. A study from the United Kingdom found no difference in outcomes in the patients with mild disease, but in patients with severe disease, a significant reduction of complications and mortality in the ERCP group was seen when compared with the conservative therapy group (24% versus 61% complications and 4% versus 18% mortality; 72). A study from Hong Kong in AP (biliary and others like Ascaris worm-induced) found that biliary sepsis was higher in the conservatively treated group. In the group predicted to have severe pancreatitis, the benefit was most marked from ERCP (73). This study did not demonstrate a reduction in mortality in the overall groups, but it did demonstrate significantly less mortality in the subgroup that actually had gallstones (about two thirds of the entire group). A study from Poland found a significant reduction of both complications and mortality in the ERCP/sphincterotomy group as compared with the conservative management group (17% versus 36% complications and 2% versus 13% mortality). The ERCP was particularly beneficial if performed within 24 hours. The benefits of sphincterotomy were present in patients with mild as well as with severe pancreatitis, although the trend was more pronounced in patients with severe disease. (This study has never been published in manuscript form.) A final study from Germany found no benefit from ERCP. Notably, patients with jaundice and cholangitis (most likely to benefit from ERCP) were excluded from enrollment (74). These studies are discussed in more detail in Chapter 3. The results of these trials are not uniform. Clinicians can draw their own conclusions, but the following list reflects the author's conclusions and represents areas of general agreement. Patients with acute biliary pancreatitis fall in one of three groups.

1. Patient most likely to benefit from ERCP are those with severe biliary AP or with bile duct stones documented on imaging study (transabdominal ultrasound, CT, magnetic resonance cholangiopancreatography, or endoscopic ultrasound), or those who have developed coexistent cholangitis.

2. Patients that may benefit from ERCP are those with smoldering pancreatitis or strong suspicion of retained bile duct stones (judged by persistent elevation of liver chemistries, dilated bile duct, but no direct evidence of ductal stones).
3. Patients most likely to not benefit from ERCP are those with resolved acute biliary pancreatitis prior to planned elective laparoscopic cholecystectomy.

The Role of Antibiotics in Severe Acute Pancreatitis

Over the years, many trials have evaluated the role of antibiotics in patients with AP, and the results have been contradictory. A number of reasons may have contributed to conflicting results, which include the use of different antibiotics, inclusion of patients with varying severity of AP, and different definitions of severity and local complications of AP. Despite these difficulties, the following recommendations can be made:

1. Antibiotics are not indicated in patients with mild (interstitial) AP.
2. Antibiotics are indicated in patients with documented infection, including cholangitis, infected pancreatic necrosis, and infected pseudo-cyst. The choice of antibiotic preferably should be based on bacterial identification and sensitivity testing.
3. The use of antibiotics remains controversial in patients with SAP and documented necrosis, but without documented infection. If used, broad-spectrum empiric antibiotic coverage should be considered in patients with noninfected pancreatic necrosis with the following possible regimens based on trial evidence: imipenem alone (two trials), cefuroxime alone (one trial), a combination of ceftazidime, amikacin, and metronidazole (one trial), or a combination of ofloxacin and metronidazole (one trial). Antibiotics were beneficial in four recently completed studies *(75)*. Imipenem significantly reduced pancreatic and nonpancreatic sepsis ($p \leq 0.01$; *76*); cefuroxime reduced all infectious complications ($p < 0.01$) and deaths ($p = 0.0284$; *77*); a regimen of ceftazidime, amikacin, and metronidazole reduced all infectious complications ($p < 0.03$; *78*); and protocol use of imipenem significantly reduced pancreatic infection compared with nonprotocol antibiotics ($p = 0.04$) and no antibiotics ($p < 0.001$).

A recent meta-analysis on controlled trials that compared antibiotic prophylaxis with no prophylaxis in patients with acute necrotizing pancreatitis showed significant reduction in sepsis by 21% (number needed to treat [NNT] = 5) and mortality by 12.3% (NNT = 8; *79*). There was also a nonsignificant trend toward a decrease in local pancreatic infections. Several recent reports have noted the development of fungal superinfection of pancreatic necrosis in patients receiving these broad-spectrum regiments. Proponents and opponents of antibiotic prophylaxis have nearly equal ammunition to argue for or against the practice. In the author's opinion, early antibiotic prophylaxis in patients with necrotizing pancreatitis is reasonable if there is significant necrosis (more than one third of gland necrotic), and the patient is likely to remain hospitalized for a significant period of time. Although a regimen utilizing imipenem is most often used at my institution, the best drug and duration of therapy are unknown.

TREATMENT OF INFECTED PANCREATIC NECROSIS

Intravenous antibiotics should be initiated in patients with documented infected pancreatic necrosis. In these cases, the choice of antibiotic is best guided by the identification and sensitivity testing of the offending microorganism. The treatment of choice for infected necrosis is surgical debridement *(80–82)*. This approach is based on clinical experience that infected necrosis is usually fatal without debridement, delay in surgery increases mortality, and at least half of the deaths in necrotizing pancreatitis are as a result of pancreatic infection. To date, no prospective randomized trial has been conducted that compares surgery with medical therapy, and such a study will likely never be done. The anecdotal experience with radiological and endoscopic drainage is growing *(83–86)*. The role of these approaches remains under active study. There are a few reports of successful management with antibiotics alone, yet this approach is not recommended. At present, they should be considered as a therapeutic alternative in patients deemed not to be surgical candidates. Currently, radiological and endoscopic drainage attempts at therapy of infected pancreatic necrosis should be limited to major tertiary centers in the setting of ongoing clinical trials.

Therapy of SAP remains a formidable challenge. Until a specific therapeutic agent is discovered, meticulous supportive care remains the cornerstone for success. This therapy includes appropriate triage to a intensive care unit, a multidisciplinary care team, intense clinical surveillance to detect complications and organ failure, and the judicious use of CT to guide therapy.

REFERENCES

1. Bradley EL 3rd. A clinically based classification system for acute pancreatitis. Summary of the International Symposium on Acute Pancreatitis, Atlanta, GA, September 11 through 13, 1992. Arch Surg 1993; 128: 586–590.
2. Siegelman SS, Copeland BE, Saba GP, et al. CT of fluid collections associated with pancreatitis. Am J Roentgenol 1980; 134: 1121–1132.
3. Bittner R, Block S, Buchler M, et al. Pancreatic abscess and infected pancreatic necrosis. Different local septic complications in acute pancreatitis. Dig Dis Sci 1987; 32: 1082–1087.

4. VanSonnenberg E, Wittich GR, Casola G, et al. Percutaneous drainage of infected and noninfected pancreatic pseudocysts: experience in 101 cases. Radiology 1989; 170: 757–761.

5. Bradley EL, Gonzalez AC, Clements JL Jr. Acute pancreatic pseudocysts: incidence and implications. Ann Surg 1976; 184: 734–737.

6. Johnson DH, Arteaga CL. Gefitinib in recurrent non-small-cell lung cancer: an IDEAL trial? J Clin Oncol 2003; 21: 2227–9.

7. Ranson JH, Rifkind KM, Turner JW. Prognostic signs and nonoperative peritoneal lavage in acute pancreatitis. Surg Gynecol Obstet 1976; 143: 209–219.

8. Beger HG, Bittner R, Buchler M, et al. Hemodynamic data pattern in patients with acute pancreatitis. Gastroenterology 1986; 90: 74–79.

9. Kyogoku T, Manabe T, Tobe T. Role of ischemia in acute pancreatitis. Hemorrhagic shock converts edematous pancreatitis to hemorrhagic pancreatitis in rats. Dig Dis Sci 1992; 37: 1409–1417.

10. Interiano B, Stuard ID, Hyde RW. Acute respiratory distress syndrome in pancreatitis. Ann Intern Med 1972; 77: 923–926.

11. Ranson JH, Turner JW, Roses DF, et al. Respiratory complications in acute pancreatitis. Ann Surg 1974; 179: 557–566.

12. Werner MH, Hayes DF, Lucas CE, et al. Renal vasoconstriction in association with acute pancreatitis. Am J Surg 1974; 127: 185–190.

13. Goldstein DA, Llach F, Massry SG. Acute renal failure in patients with acute pancreatitis. Arch Intern Med 1976; 136: 1363–1365.

14. Allam BF, Imrie CW. Serum ionized calcium in acute pancreatitis. Br J Surg 1977; 64: 665–668.

15. Imrie CW, Whyte AS. A prospective study of acute pancreatitis. Br J Surg 1975; 62: 490–494.

16. Cameron JL, Capuzzi DM, Zuidema GD, et al. Acute pancreatitis with hyperlipemia: the incidence of lipid abnormalities in acute pancreatitis. Ann Surg 1973; 177: 483–489.

17. Vogel RM, Keohane M. Renal vascular abnormalities in acute pancreatitis. Arch Intern Med 1967; 119: 610–616.

18. Greipp PR, Brown JA, Gralnick HR. Defibrination in acute pancreatitis. Ann Intern Med 1972; 76: 73–76.

19. Ranson JH, Rifkind KM, Roses DF, et al. Prognostic signs and the role of operative management in acute pancreatitis. Surg Gynecol Obstet 1974; 139: 69–81.

20. Dominguez-Munoz JE, Malfertheiner P, Ditschuneit HH, et al. Hyperlipidemia in acute pancreatitis. Relationship with etiology, onset, and severity of the disease. Int J Pancreatol 1991; 10 :261–267.

21. Salomone T, Tosi P, Palareti G, et al. Coagulative disorders in human acute pancreatitis: role for the D-dimer. Pancreas 2003; 26: 111–116.

22. Jacobs ML, Daggett WM, Civette JM, et al. Acute pancreatitis: analysis of factors influencing survival. Ann Surg 1977; 185: 43–51.

23. Marks IN, Bank S, Louw JH, et al. Peptic ulceration and gastrointestinal bleeding in pancreatitis. Gut 1967; 8: 253–259.

24. Little AG, Moossa AR. Gastrointestinal hemorrhage from left-sided portal hypertension. An unappreciated complication of pancreatitis. Am J Surg 1981; 141: 153–158.

25. Madsen MS, Petersen TH, Sommer H. Segmental portal hypertension. Ann Surg 1986; 204: 72–77.

26. Stroud WH, Cullom JW, Anderson MC. Hemorrhagic complications of severe pancreatitis. Surgery 1981; 90: 657–665.

27. Lankisch PG, Struckmann K, Assmus C, et al. Do we need a computed tomography examination in all patients with acute pancreatitis within 72 h after admission to hospital for the detection of pancreatic necrosis? Scand J Gastroenterol 2001; 36: 432–436.

28. Balthazar EJ, Robinson DL, Megibow AJ, et al. Acute pancreatitis: value of CT in establishing prognosis. Radiology 1990; 174: 331–336.

29. Balthazar EJ, Freeny PC, vanSonnenberg E., et al. Imaging and intervention in acute pancreatitis. Radiology 1994; 193: 297–306.

30. Freeny PC. Incremental dynamic bolus computed tomography of acute pancreatitis. Int J Pancreatol 1993; 13:147–158.

31. Balthazar EJ, Robinson DL, Megibow AJ, et al. Acute pancreatitis: value of CT in establishing prognosis. Radiology 1990; 174: 331–336.

32. Lankisch PG, Pflichthofer D, Lehnick D. No strict correlation between necrosis and organ failure in acute pancreatitis. Pancreas 2000; 20: 319–322.

33. Schmidt J, Hotz HG, Foitzik T, et al. Intravenous contrast medium aggravates the impairment of pancreatic microcirculation in necrotizing pancreatitis in the rat. Ann Surg 1995; 221: 257–264.

34. Foitzik T, Lewandrowski KB, Fernandez-del Castillo C, et al. Exocrine hyperstimulation but not pancreatic duct obstruction increases the susceptibility to alcohol-related pancreatic injury. Arch Surg 1994; 129: 1081–1085.

35. McMenamin DA, Gates LK Jr. A retrospective analysis of the effect of contrast-enhanced CT on the outcome of acute pancreatitis. Am J Gastroenterol 1996; 91: 1384–1387.

36. Carmona-Sanchez R, Uscanga L, Bezaury-Rivas P, et al. Potential harmful effect of iodinated intravenous contrast medium on the clinical course of mild acute pancreatitis. Arch Surg 2000; 135: 1280–1284.

37. De Bernardinis M, Violi V, Roncoroni L, et al. Discriminant power and information content of Ranson's prognostic signs in acute pancreatitis: a meta-analytic study. Crit Care Med 1999; 27: 2272–2283.

38. Bradley EL 3rd, Allen K. A prospective longitudinal study of observation versus surgical intervention in the management of necrotizing pancreatitis. Am J Surg 1991; 161: 19–24.

39. Banks PA, Gerzof SG, Langevin RE, et al. CT-guided aspiration of suspected pancreatic infection: bacteriology and clinical outcome. Int J Pancreatol. 1995; 18: 265–270.

40. Knight MJ, Condon JR, Day JL. Possible role of glucagon in pathogenesis of acute pancreatitis. Lancet 1972; 1: 1097–1099.

41. Anonymous. Death from acute pancreatitis. M.R.C. multicentre trial of glucagon and aprotinin. Lancet 1977; 2: 632–635.

42. Waterworth MW, Barbezat GO, Bank S. Glucagon in treatment of acute pancreatitis. Lancet 1974; 1: 1231.

43. Durr HK, Maroske D, Zelder O, et al. Glucagon therapy in acute pancreatitis. Report of a double-blind trial. Gut 1978; 19: 175–179.

44. Cameron JL, Mehigan D, Zuidema GD. Evaluation of atropine in acute pancreatitis. Surg Gynecol Obstet 1979; 148: 206–208.

45. Broe PJ, Zinner MJ, Cameron JL. A clinical trial of cimetidine in acute pancreatitis. Surg Gynecol Obstet 1982; 154: 13–16.

46. Meshkinpour H, Molinari MD, Gardner L, et al. Cimetidine in the treatment of acute alcoholic pancreatitis. A randomized, double-blind study. Gastroenterology 1979; 77: 687–690.

47. Hadas N, Wapnick S, Grosberg SJ. Cimetidine in pancreatitis. N Engl J Med 1978; 299: 487.

48. Trapnell JE, Rigby CC, Talbot CH, et al. A controlled trial of Trasylol in the treatment of acute pancreatitis. Br J Surg 1974; 61: 177–182.

49. Trapnell JE, Talbot CH, Capper WM. Trasylol in acute pancreatitis. Am J Dig Dis 1967; 12: 409–412.

50. Imrie CW, Benjamin IS, Ferguson JC, et al. A single-centre double-blind trial of Trasylol therapy in primary acute pancreatitis. Br J Surg 1978; 65: 337–341.

51. Buchler M, Malfertheiner P, Uhl W, et al. Gabexate mesilate in human acute pancreatitis. German Pancreatitis Study Group. Gastroenterology 1993; 104: 1165–1170.

52. Goebell H, Ammann R, Herfarth C, et al. A double-blind trial of synthetic salmon calcitonin in the treatment of acute pancreatitis. Scand J Gastroenterol 1979; 14: 881-889.

53. Usadel KH, Leuschner U, Uberla KK. Treatment of acute pancreatitis with somatostatin: a multicenter double blind study. N Engl J Med 1980; 303: 999–1000.

54. Choi TK, Mok F, Zhan WH, et al. Somatostatin in the treatment of acute pancreatitis: a prospective randomised controlled trial. Gut 1989; 30: 223–227.

55. Bordas JM, Toledo V, Mondelo F, et al. Prevention of pancreatic reactions by bolus somatostatin administration in patients undergoing endoscopic retrograde cholangio-pancreatography and endoscopic sphincterotomy. Horm Res 1988; 29: 106–108.

56. Uhl W, Buchler MW, Malfertheiner P, et al. A randomised, double blind, multicentre trial of octreotide in moderate to severe acute pancreatitis. Gut 1999; 45: 97–104.

57. Johnson CD, Kingsnorth AN, Imrie CW, et al. Double blind, randomised, placebo controlled study of a platelet activating factor antagonist, lexipafant, in the treatment and prevention of organ failure in predicted severe acute pancreatitis. Gut 2001; 48: 62–69.

58. Larvin M and the international lexipifant study group. A double blind randomised controlled multi-centre trial of lexipifant in acute pancreatitis. Pancreas 2001; 23 (abstract): 448

59. Marshall JB. Acute pancreatitis. A review with an emphasis on new developments. Arch Intern Med 1993; 153: 1185–1198.

60. Lankisch PG, Haseloff M, Becher R. No parallel between the biochemical course of acute pancreatitis and morphologic findings. Pancreas 1994; 9: 240–243.

61. Seidensticker F, Otto J, Lankisch PG. Recovery of the pancreas after acute pancreatitis is not necessarily complete. Int J Pancreatol 1995; 17: 225–229.

62. Levy P, Heresbach D, Pariente EA, et al. Frequency and risk factors of recurrent pain during refeeding in patients with acute pancreatitis: a multivariate multicentre prospective study of 116 patients. Gut 1997; 40: 262–266.

63. Naeije R, Salingret E, Clumeck N, et al. Is nasogastric suction necessary in acute pancreatitis? Br Med J 1978; 2: 659–660.

64. Loiudice TA, Lang J, Mehta H, et al. Treatment of acute alcoholic pancreatitis: the roles of cimetidine and nasogastric suction. Am J Gastroenterol 1984; 79: 553–558.

65. Reynaert MS, Dugernier T, Kestens PJ. Current therapeutic strategies in severe acute pancreatitis. Intensive Care Med 1990; 16: 352–362.

66. Grant JP, James S, Grabowski V, et al. Total parenteral nutrition in pancreatic disease. Ann Surg 1984; 200: 627–631.

67. Runkel NS, Rodriguez LF, Moody FG. Mechanisms of sepsis in acute pancreatitis in opossums. Am J Surg 1995; 169: 227–232.

68. Medich DS, Lee TK, Melhem MF, et al. Pathogenesis of pancreatic sepsis. Am J Surg 1993; 165: 46–50.

69. Kalfarentzos F, Kehagias J, Mead N, et al. Enteral nutrition is superior to parenteral nutrition in severe acute pancreatitis: results of a randomized prospective trial. Br J Surg 1997; 84:1665–1669.

70. Al-Omran M, Groof A, Wilke D. Enteral versus parenteral nutrition for acute pancreatitis. Cochrane Database Syst Rev 2001; 2: CD002837.

71. Abou-Assi S, Craig K, O'Keefe SJ. Hypocaloric jejunal feeding is better than total parenteral nutrition in acute pancreatitis: results of a randomized comparative study. Am J Gastroenterol 2002; 97: 2255–2262.

72. Neoptolemos JP, Carr-Locke DL, London N, et al. ERCP findings and the role of endoscopic sphincterotomy in acute gallstone pancreatitis. Br J Surg 1988; 75: 954–960.

73. Fan ST, Lai EC, Mok FP, et al. Early treatment of acute biliary pancreatitis by endoscopic papillotomy. N Engl J Med 1993; 328: 228–232.

74. Folsch UR, Nitsche R, Ludtke R, et al. Early ERCP and papillotomy compared with conservative treatment for acute biliary pancreatitis. The German Study Group on Acute Biliary Pancreatitis. N Engl J Med 1997; 336: 237–242.

75. Kramer KM, Levy H. Prophylactic antibiotics for severe acute pancreatitis: the beginning of an era. Pharmacotherapy 1999; 19: 592–602.

76. Pederzoli P, Bassi C, Vesentini S, et al. A randomized multicenter clinical trial of antibiotic prophylaxis of septic complications in acute necrotizing pancreatitis with imipenem. Surg Gynecol Obstet 1993; 176: 480–483.

77. Sainio V, Kemppainen E, Puolakkainen P, et al. Early antibiotic treatment in acute necrotising pancreatitis. Lancet 1995; 346: 663–667.

78. Delcenserie R, Yzet T, Ducroix JP. Prophylactic antibiotics in treatment of severe acute alcoholic pancreatitis. Pancreas 1996; 13: 198–201.

79. Sharma VK, Howden CW. Prophylactic antibiotic administration reduces sepsis and mortality in acute necrotizing pancreatitis: a meta-analysis. Pancreas 2001; 22: 28–31.

80. Banks PA. Practice guidelines in acute pancreatitis. Am J Gastroenterol 1997; 92: 377–386.

81. Farkas G, Marton J, Mandi Y, et al. Progress in the management and treatment of infected pancreatic necrosis. Scand J Gastroenterol Suppl 1998; 228: 31–37.

82. Rau B, Uhl W, Buchler MW, et al. Surgical treatment of infected necrosis. World J Surg 1997; 21: 155–161.

83. Baron TH, Morgan DE. Endoscopic transgastric irrigation tube placement via PEG for debridement of organized pancreatic necrosis. Gastrointest Endosc 1999; 50: 574–577.

84. Monkemuller KE, Baron TH, Morgan DE. Transmural drainage of pancreatic fluid collections without electrocautery using the Seldinger technique. Gastrointest Endosc 1998; 48: 195–200.

85. Baron TH, Harewood GC, Morgan DE, et al. Outcome differences after endoscopic drainage of pancreatic necrosis, acute pancreatic pseudocysts, and chronic pancreatic pseudocysts. Gastrointest Endosc 2002; 56: 7–17.

86. Baron TH, Thaggard WG, Morgan DE, et al. Endoscopic therapy for organized pancreatic necrosis. Gastroenterology 1996; 111: 755–764.

7

Pancreatic Necrosis and Infections in Patients With Acute Pancreatitis

Michael L. Kendrick, MD and Michael G. Sarr, MD

CONTENTS

INTRODUCTION
DEFINITION
PRESENTATION/DIAGNOSIS
MANAGEMENT
OPERATIVE MANAGEMENT
LONG-TERM SEQUELA
QUALITY OF LIFE
REFERENCES

INTRODUCTION

The majority of patients with acute pancreatitis (AP) have a mild "edematous" form of the disease with a self-limited course devoid of serious local or systemic sequelae. However, in 3–5% of patients (10–20% in tertiary referral centers), a more severe form involving pancreatic and/or peripancreatic necrosis occurs. Necrotizing pancreatitis is the most severe form and is the predominant cause of serious morbidity and mortality in the spectrum of patients with AP. One of the most serious complications of necrotizing pancreatitis is infection of the necrosis, occurring in 15–30% of patients. This "superinfection" is important, because it significantly increases morbidity and mortality.

From: *Pancreatitis and Its Complications*
Edited by: C. E. Forsmark © Humana Press Inc., Totowa, NJ

99

With growing understanding of the etiopathogenesis of AP, many novel therapies are in development, and the optimal management of necrotizing pancreatitis continues to evolve. In recent decades, the clinical outcome of these patients has improved owing to advances in critical care management, as well as our knowledge of the natural history of the disease process, and careful selection and timing of patients for surgical intervention. This section describes the presentation, diagnosis, management, and outcomes of patients with acute necrotizing pancreatitis and the associated complications of superinfection.

DEFINITION

In an effort to standardize the terminology in AP and its complications, an international consensus conference of world authorities established the "Atlanta classification" *(1)*. Necrotizing pancreatitis was classified as sterile necrosis, infected necrosis, or pancreatic abscess. Sterile necrosis implies pancreatic or peripancreatic necrosis without proven infection. Infected necrosis is documented when the nonviable pancreatic or peripancreatic tissue has culture-proven bacterial or fungal superinfection. Pancreatic abscess is defined as a localized collection of purulent material in the absence of significant necrosis. Although these definitions have been adopted (albeit, not universally), ostensibly allowed a common terminology, and were well-meaning, there are some problems with the latter term of "pancreatic abscess." By the strict definition of the Atlanta classification, a pancreatic abscess would be quite unusual. Most patients with necrotizing pancreatitis do not have a single localized area of suppurative infection without necrosis, but rather, they have a combination of necrosis and suppurative changes, especially later in the course of the disease (3–6 weeks after the onset of pancreatitis). Although these patients would be considered as having "infected necrosis," they represent a different clinical scenario from the other group of patients with infected necrosis who become clinically evident usually 1–3 weeks after the onset of pancreatitis. This latter group harbor necrosis that is infected but has not yet progressed to suppurative changes. Indeed, a pancreatic abscess as defined by the Atlanta classification would be best represented by the formerly used term of an infected pseudocyst.

PRESENTATION/DIAGNOSIS

The diagnosis of necrotizing pancreatitis is based on the suspicion and exclusion of other abdominal catastrophes. The onset of disease is usually quite abrupt and progresses rapidly over the initial 48 hours. Patients complain of severe abdominal pain and manifest tachycardia, fluid sequestration, and fever. An increased serum amylase or lipase activity is supportive of the diagnosis within the first 2–4 days in the absence of an intra-abdominal upper gut perforation. Thus, in large part, the diagnosis is based on clinical suspicion and is a diagnosis of exclusion.

Severe necrotizing pancreatitis progresses through two main phases. The initial phase is characterized by a noninfective systemic inflammatory response syndrome (SIRS) that predominates in the first 2 weeks of the illness that may lead to multisystem organ failure. The second phase is associated with either slow resolution and eventual reabsorption of the necrosis (3–6 months) or with a more aggressive course with superinfection of the pancreatic and/or peripancreatic necrosis, leading to the sepsis syndrome and progressive organ failure *(2)*. Patients in this latter phase account for the vast majority of the mortality in AP. The pathophysiology of each phase is different, and the optimal management differs accordingly. The incidence of organ failure correlates with both the extent of necrosis and the presence of superinfection of the associated necrosis. In those patients with evidence of pancreatic necrosis greater than 50% on contrast-enhanced computed tomography (CECT) *(see* below), local complications and systemic organ failure involving lungs, kidneys, liver, gut, and cardiovascular organs may develop early in the course of disease *(3)*.

In an attempt to maximize care, several staging systems have been proposed to predict the severity and prognosis of patients with AP initially in the course of the disease. The two well-known staging systems of Ranson *(4)* and Imrie *(5)* are based on multiple clinical, biochemical, and hematologic indices obtained in the first 48 hours of disease onset and can predict severity and outcome of patients with AP with reasonable accuracy (80–85%). Limitations of these systems are the necessity of 48-hour assessment prior to categorization and the inability to monitor clinical progression or response to treatment throughout the course of disease. As a result, these early staging or prognostic systems have been replaced in some centers by the Acute Physiology And Chronic Health Evaluation (APACHE-II) grading system that can accurately predict severity and outcome of patients with AP. This scoring system is a dynamic and allows immediate stratification of patients upon admission and repeated assessments throughout the course of illness *(6)*. An APACHE-II score of 6 is considered predictive of severe pancreatitis. A modification of this system, which includes body mass index, has been suggested as well (APACHE-O), because some studies suggest a higher incidence of severe necrotizing pancreatitis in the obese patient *(7,8)*. These systems are discussed in Chapter 2.

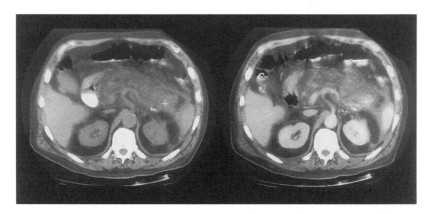

Fig. 1. Computed tomography of a patient with necrotizing pancreatitis at the same anatomic level before **(A)** and after **(B)** intravenous administration of the contrast agent. Note in **B** the lack of enhancement (signifying absence of blood flow) in much of the body and tail of the pancreas.

A number of single-factor indicators have also been evaluated in the hope of being able to predict severity of AP within the first 6–12 hours of onset of the disease. The rationale for believing such an approach to be feasible originates from the observation based on computed tomography (CT) that the necrosis (or at least the initial signs of parenchymal nonperfusion, i.e., irreversible ischemia) is an early process that is already established at the time of clinical presentation. Various nonspecific early response factors, such as interleukins (IL), IL-6 and IL-8, and polymorphonuclear elastase, have been shown to peak in the first 24 hours and can discriminate between mild and severe pancreatitis *(9,10)*. C-reactive protein is likely the best discriminator of disease severity, but it also requires a 48-hour assessment after the onset of symptoms and has been shown to be as accurate as the more clinically based, multifactor scoring systems *(9,11)*. Attempts to identify a pancreas-specific factor (e.g., amylase, lipase, and so on) with the ability to predict severity have been discouraging. One recent pancreas-specific candidate is trypsin activation peptide, which can be assessed in the urine and may be helpful *(12)*.

The diagnosis of pancreatic necrosis and the complication of superinfection begins with clinical assessment. Patients with a severe course based on hemodynamic and laboratory profiles, progressive fluid requirements, and intensive supportive care should be suspected of having necrotizing pancreatitis. Dynamic CECT is the mainstay in the objective diagnosis of pancreatic and peripancreatic necrosis and is able to accurately estimate the extent of necrosis *(13)* (Fig. 1). The presence of extravisceral air within the pancreatic or peripancreatic necrosis as

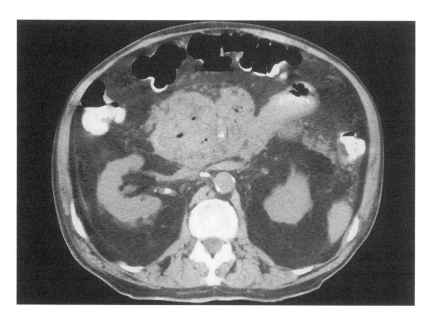

Fig. 2. Computed tomography of a patient with infected pancreatic necrosis. Note the presence of extraluminal peripancreatic gas pathognomonic of infection. (Reprinted with permission from ref. *13a*.)

demonstrated by CT is virtually pathognomonic of infected necrosis, but it is an uncommon finding (Fig. 2; *13a*). Suspicion of pancreatic infection based on signs of sepsis warrants evaluation by CT or percutaneous, ultrasound-guided, fine-needle aspiration *(14,15)*. Debate continues regarding the optimal timing and frequency of aspiration, as there exists a theoretic risk of introducing organisms into the otherwise sterile necrosis. Although this risk remains to be substantiated, routine early pancreatic aspiration in patients who have clinically stable pancreatic necrosis is not indicated as it will likely not change immediate management.

Ultimately, approximately 30% of patients with necrotizing pancreatitis will develop infection. Superinfection of the necrotic process has been shown to be a time-dependent complication. Bacterial contamination rates have been estimated to be as high as 24% at 1 week, 36% at 2 weeks, and 71% at 3 weeks postonset of necrotizing pancreatitis in those patients eventually undergoing operative treatment *(16)*. Because septic complications resulting from bacterial infection of pancreatic necrosis account for more than 80% of deaths in AP *(17)*, early recognition and treatment of the infected necrosis assume paramount importance. Multiple routes of bacterial infection have been implicated, but evidence suggests that the predominant route of infection is via a colonic source; whether "superinfection" in humans occurs via bacterial translocation, intermittent bacteremia, lymphatic drainage, or direct transperitoneal spread remains undefined.

Necrosis of extrapancreatic tissue alone with viable pancreatic tissue occurs in up to 19% of patients with necrotizing pancreatitis *(18)*. Although this may portend a more favorable prognosis, treatment follows the same principles as for pancreatic necrosis.

MANAGEMENT

The initial management approach for patients with pancreatic necrosis is primarily nonoperative with aggressive cardiorespiratory resuscitation and attempts at prevention of secondary complications related to hemodynamic instability. Prompt restoration and maintenance of circulating volume and arterial oxygen tension during the initial 48–72 hours are the main objectives, but full intensive care of other failing organ systems is required. Severe pancreatitis is often accompanied by SIRS, resulting from a cascade of proinflammatory mediators that leads to multiorgan system failure. When this response is not abated by natural defenses or therapeutic intervention, progression to sepsis often ensues, particularly when infection complicates necrosis (usually during the second and third week).

Intravenous administration of a broad-spectrum antibiotic should probably begin early (within 24–48 hours) in patients with necrotizing pancreatitis in an attempt to prevent subsequent pancreatic superinfection. Two principles guide the initial antibiotic selection: appropriate spectrum and ability to penetrate pancreatic parenchyma. The carbapenems, such as imipenem, have been shown to decrease the incidence of superinfection, and in several studies, mortality as well *(19–21)*. We administer imipenem to all patients with severe acute pancreatitis (SAP) (APACHE-II score of 6 or higher). The optimal duration of antibiotic treatment is unknown, but most pancreatologists consider 2–3 weeks to be appropriate. The prophylactic use of broad-spectrum antibiotics has increased the presence of *Candida* species, complicating necrosis in 5–24% of patients who develop infection; fungal infection is also associated with an increased mortality *(22,23)*. Whether antifungal prophylaxis is beneficial remains unclear; however, treatment of documented fungal infection is imperative. The role of antibiotics in severe pancreatitis is also discussed in Chapter 6.

Despite intriguing preliminary preclinical trials, no inflammatory modifiers (platelet activating factor antagonists, IL receptor antagonists, and so on) have had a significant clinical effect on mortality in patients with SAP. Although much of the pathogenesis of the development and progression of SIRS and the sepsis syndrome is understood, the inflammatory cascade has already been initiated and amplified by the time the diagnosis is made. Thus, monotherapy directed at one of the early mediators, such as tumor necrosis factor or platelet-activating factor, or the use of monoclonal antibodies directed at a specific inflammatory cytokine or IL is likely doomed to fail because the cascade of multiple factors has become broad and multifactorial by the time treatment is initiated. A more rational approach might be to not target the inflammatory cascade in the pancreas (the damage has already occurred by the time the diagnosis is made), but rather, institute a more global approach using inhibitors of systemic, particularly hepatic and pulmonary monocyte function, in an attempt to blunt the extrapancreatic amplification of the release of pancreatic-derived cytokines in the liver, lungs, and gut.

The nutritional needs of the patient also require consideration early in the course of necrotizing pancreatitis. Total parenteral nutrition should be started initially with conversion to enteral nutrition as soon as possible and delivered intrajejunally as opposed to intraduodenally. Several experimental studies demonstrate that severe pancreatitis promotes bacterial overgrowth in the gut lumen, alters the gut mucosal barrier, and increases permeability. This process leads to bacterial translocation from the gut in rodents with consequent superinfection of pancreatic necrosis and mortality *(24,25)*. In patients with severe pancreatitis, several randomized studies have suggested a reduction of complications and possibly mortality from early enteral feeding delivered beyond the ligament of Treitz *(26)*. The intuitive advantages of enteral over parenteral nutrition include reduced cost, maintenance of gut integrity, and avoidance of catheter-related sepsis (especially fungal infections).

During the second week of severe pancreatitis, the continued requirement of intensive care management with marginal or no clinical improvement should prompt evaluation for extensive necrosis and/or superinfection. The use of CECT is paramount at this point and defines the extent of necrosis, suggesting signs of pancreatic superinfection and guiding percutaneous fine-needle aspiration for the culture of necrotic tissue. The use of CECT early in the course of pancreatitis (first 7 days) when superinfection is unlikely, will not change the management, and is unnecessary unless the diagnosis remains doubtful.

Without evidence of superinfection, management continues to be supportive. Severe clinical deterioration within the first 7–10 days often initiates surgical necrosectomy in desperation as a "last ditch" resort. Currently, however, there is no evidence that this approach decreases mortality. Ongoing failure to clinically improve in patients with sterile necrosis is a controversial topic with some surgeons advocating necrosectomy after 3 weeks *(27)*. Yet, others maintain that operative intervention is rarely, if ever, indicated in the absence of infection *(28)*. Once diagnosis of infected necrosis has been established, however, the current standard of care is surgical necrosectomy and debridement. The pendulum has swung from early operative debridement to delayed operative intervention whenever possible. This delay in operative intervention in the stable patient provides time for the necrotic process to fully demarcate, allowing a safer and more complete debridement while allowing the preservation of viable pancreas. This delayed operative approach is supported by a prospective randomized study showing decreased morbidity and mortality when the necrosectomy is delayed as long as possible *(29)*. The optimal timing for operative necrosectomy may be 1 month to 6 weeks with the best patient outcome *(28,30)*. Thus, after documented infection, the preferred approach seems to be continued aggressive, nonoperative management as long as there is hemodynamic stability; percutaneous aspiration for culture and sensitivity may allow targeted antibiotic therapy to suppress bacteremia and sepsis, as well as allow delayed operative intervention. Necrosectomy may then be planned later in the course of disease (20–40 days) when the necrotic process has ceased, viable and nonviable tissues are well-defined, and the infected necrotic tissues are organized.

Unlike the early phase of infected necrosis that often lacks suppuration, the later phases of infected necrosis using the Atlanta classification occurs more commonly as a late complication of necrotizing pancreatitis (>4 weeks) and may have suppurative changes in the background of associated necrosis (although the bacteriology is similar). In our experience, pancreatic abscess by the Atlanta classification occurs in much less than 5% of patients with acute necrotizing pancreatitis. The clinical severity and mortality of patients with pancreatic abscess is much less than that for infected necrosis, because by the Atlanta classification, this entity represents a localized abscess without significant necrosis (Fig. 3; *30a*). Pancreatic abscess can be treated with appropriate percutaneous interventional management *(31,32)*. Laparoscopic minimal access debridement of more confined areas of organized necrosis has been proposed recently *(33)* and may be appropriate in selected patients (*see* next section).

OPERATIVE MANAGEMENT

Although the techniques of operative necrosectomy are similar, multiple techniques have been reported to manage the operative bed afterward. Means for allowing either ongoing debridement, evacuation of the exudative response, and controlled egress of "leaking" pancreatic exocrine secretions from areas of injured pancreatic parenchyma are

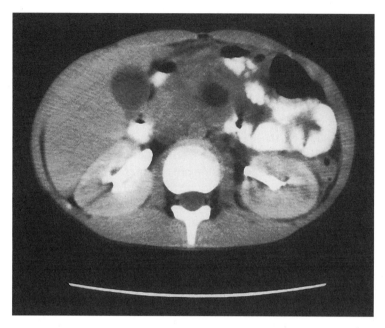

Fig. 3. Computed tomography of a patient with a pancreatic abscess. (Reprinted with permission from ref. *30a.*)

very important in allowing the necrotizing process to abate and the peripancreatic area to eventually heal. Methods of controlled open drainage (laparostomy or marsupialization of the lesser sac), wide-closed peripancreatic drainage, continuous postoperative-closed peripancreatic lavage, and planned repeated necrosectomy with delayed primary closure over drains have all been described *(2,30,34–36)*. Overall results are similar, where the differences exist predominantly with the incidence and type of various complications. We prefer an approach of planned repeated necrosectomy, which appears to have a lesser incidence of recurrent intra-abdominal abscesses, albeit requiring an additional one to three reoperations for operative debridement *(2)*. The controversy regarding management of the pancreatic and peripancreatic bed after necrosectomy is becoming less of an issue given the trend of delayed operation, which increases the likelihood of a complete initial necrosectomy with primary closure; reoperations (planned or unplanned) are less likely.

CECT serves as an invaluable intraoperative guide to necrosectomy by defining the site and extent of the necrosis and directing a complete operative necrosectomy, especially in areas remote from the pancreas (perinephric space, paracolic gutters, suprapancreatic retroperitoneum, and small bowel mesentery). Emphasis must be placed on identifying, unroofing, debriding, and draining all areas of pancreatic and peripancreatic necrosis.

The necrosectomy begins with the appropriate incision, preferably a midline incision, because it allows the best exposure to all potential remote areas of necrosis. Initial exploration of the abdominal cavity involves a systematic and comprehensive evaluation of all known and potential pancreatic and peripancreatic spaces, as well as directed exploration as guided by the CECT. The entire pancreas, paracolic gutters, infracolic root of the small bowel mesentery, transverse mesocolon, and the suprapancreatic retroperitoneum are all carefully assessed. Adequate exposure entails entering the lesser sac through the gastrocolic omentum and, if necessary, mobilizing the ascending and descending colon to approach extensive retroperitoneal necrosis extending down to the paracolic gutters. Mobilization of the spleen is rarely ever necessary and may be hazardous. With the necrosis identified, blunt manual dissection of all necrotic material is performed; careful attention must be paid to the major vessels. Aggressive necrosectomy of tissue adherent to inflamed, viable, hypervascular tissue is dangerous and must be carefully contemplated to avoid bleeding. These areas are often best left *in situ* and debrided at a subsequent re-exploration 2 days later, when better demarcation with autoseparation has occurred.

After completing the necrosectomy, we prefer to use blunt liquid debridement using a type of gentle jet irrigation (Water-Pik irrigator, Surgilav, model 201, Stryker, Kalamazoo, MI) to remove devitalized tissue and residual bacteria. If the surgeon is satisfied that the necrosectomy is complete and/or optimal, the abdomen is closed primarily over drains. Soft closed-suction Silastic® drains are placed in each anatomic area of débrided necrosis. Drains are exteriorized through separate stab incisions in the lateral abdominal wall. Generally, we also place a gastrostomy tube and feeding jejunostomy tube (usually a needle catheter gastrojejunostomy; *2,37*).

If it is apparent that the necrotic process is still in evolution, or the necrosectomy was incomplete owing to adherent friable tissue, the debrided areas are packed with moistened gauze, and any exposed vessels are protected from direct contact with the gauze packs by a sheet of Silastic®. Soft closed suction drains are then placed on top of the gauze packing to evacuate any serous drainage until the next planned re-exploration 2 days later. The abdominal wall closure is then completed with a zipper sewn to the fascial edges for ease of re-exploration, thereby minimizing repeated trauma to the fascial edges. Open laparostomy "closures," while preventing the possibility of an abdominal compartment syndrome, allow the fascial edges to separate, often preventing a delayed primary closure. Use of a zipper not only maintains the abdominal domain but keeps the fascial edges close together between operative debridements, thereby facilitating a delayed primary closure after the necrosectomy is fully completed. Reoperation is then planned 48 hours later, and exploration/debridement is repeated in the same systematic and comprehensive manner as previously performed. With cessation of ongoing necrosis and confirmation of a complete necrosectomy, the abdomen is definitively closed over drains.

LONG-TERM SEQUELA

In-hospital morbidity and mortality have been the main focus of outcome in patients with necrotizing pancreatitis. As mortality has improved from the 40–70% rate of the 1960s and 1970s to the current mortality of 10–20%, more interest has emerged in defining the long-term clinical outcome and quality of life.

Some extent of endocrine pancreatic insufficiency has been reported in approximately 50% of patients (38–40). Although overt diabetes mellitus develops in up to 25% of patients, abnormal glucose tolerance is found in an additional 10–25%. Endocrine insufficiency is more frequent in patients with alcohol versus gallstone-induced necrotizing pancreatitis (64% vs 22%), likely because of chronic and repeated pancreatic parenchymal damage secondary to alcohol abuse.

As with endocrine insufficiency, exocrine insufficiency is more common in patients with alcohol-induced necrotizing pancreatitis. Even though a certain degree of exocrine insufficiency can be documented via formal tests of pancreatic function in 70–100% of cases, clinically significant steatorrhea is present in only 16–20% (40–42).

The natural history of endocrine and exocrine pancreatic insufficiency is not well-defined. We evaluated our experience in 44 patients successfully treated with necrotizing pancreatitis who were followed for a mean of 5 years (40). Endocrine insufficiency was present in 50%, and clinically significant exocrine insufficiency (steatorrhea) was found in 25%. Most patients manifested signs of pancreatic endocrine insufficiency prior to hospital discharge and in the remaining patients, within 2 years. Endocrine function tended to either deteriorate with time or remain stable but did not improve in any patients. In contrast, exocrine function tended to improve with time in 45% of patients. Patients with either endocrine (52%) or exocrine pancreatic insufficiency (66%) were more likely to have had extensive pancreatic parenchymal necrosis than those with maintenance of normal pancreatic function (27%).

Recurrent episodes of AP may occur in 5–30% of patients who survive necrotizing pancreatitis and is seen predominantly in association with alcoholic pancreatitis in patients continuing alcohol consumption and those with hereditary pancreatitis *(43)*. For patients with gallstone pancreatitis, recurrent pancreatitis is quite unusual *(40)*.

The incidence of abdominal wall hernias after surgical treatment of necrotizing pancreatitis ranges from 4 to 39%, with the incidence varying depending on the technique of operative management. The loss of abdominal wall fascia because of repeated abdominal explorations, fistulas, and extensive intraperitoneal inflammation poses a challenging repair. Initial management of these hernias should be conservative to allow sufficient resolution of the inflammatory process and assure that further intervention for debridement or management of intra-abdominal sepsis is not indicated. We generally wait 6–12 months prior to consideration of repair. Most of these hernias require a mesh-based repair to allow closure.

QUALITY OF LIFE

Despite the sequela of necrotizing pancreatitis, most patients are able to return to work and report an excellent or good outcome. In our experience, decreased performance status (9%) and inability to return to work (23%) was associated with a higher APACHE-II score on admission *(40)*. Thus, regardless of the time and resource-consuming care required for patients with necrotizing pancreatitis, the expected quality of life and productivity of most patients with necrotizing pancreatitis justifies the aggressive management.

REFERENCES

1. Bradley EL III. A clinically based classification system for acute pancreatitis. Arch Surg 1993; 128: 586–590.
2. Tsiotos GG, Luque-de Leon E, Söreide JA, et al. Management of necrotizing pancreatitis by repeated operative necrosectomy using a zipper technique. Am J Surg 1998; 175: 91–98.
3. Isenmann R, Rau B, Schoenberg MH, et al. Determinants of organ failure (OF) in patients with necrotizing pancreatitis (NP). Gastroenterology 1998; 114 (Abstract): A470.
4. Ranson JHC, Rifkind KM, Roses DF, et al. Prognostic signs and the role of operative management in acute pancreatitis. Surg Gynecol Obstet 1974; 139: 69–81.
5. Imrie CW, Benjamin IS, Ferguson JC, et al. A single centre double blind trial of Trasylol therapy in primary acute pancreatitis. Br J Surg 1978; 65: 337–341.
6. Wilson C, Heath DI, Imrie CW. Prediction of outcome in acute pancreatitis: a comparative study of APACHE-II clinical assessment and multiple factor scoring systems. Br J Surg 1990; 77: 1260–1264.
7. Johnson CD, Toh SKC, Campbell MJ. Combination of APACHE-II score and an obesity score (APACHE-O) for the prediction of severe acute pancreatitis. Pancreatology 2004; 4: 1–6.
8. Lankisch PG, Schirren CA. Increased body weight as a prognostic parameter for complications in the course of acute pancreatitis. Pancreas 1990; 5: 626–629.

9. Pezzilli R, Billi P, Minero R, et al. Serum interleukin 6, interleukin 8 and α2 microglobulin in early assessment of severity of acute pancreatitis. Comparison with C reactive protein. Dig Dis Sci 1995; 40: 2341–2348.

10. Dominguez-Munoz JE, Carballo F, Garcia MJ. Clinical usefulness of polymorphonuclear elastase in predicting the severity of acute pancreatitis: results of a multicentre study. Br J Surg 1991; 78: 1230–1234.

11. Wilson C, Heads A, Shenkin A, Imrie CW. C-reactive protein, antiproteases and compliment factors as objective markers of severity in acute pancreatitis. Br J Surg 1989; 76: 177–181.

12. Gudgeon AM, Heath DI, Hurley P, et al. Trypsinogen activation peptide assay in the early severity prediction of acute pancreatitis. Lancet 1990; 335: 4–8.

13. Johnson CD, Stephens DH, Sarr MG. Necrotic pancreatitis: re-emphasis of the importance of contrast-enhanced CT. Am J Radiol 1991; 156: 93–95.

13a. Tsiotos GG, Sarr MG. Management of fluid collections and necrosis in acute pancreatitis. Curr Gastroenterol Rep 1999; 1: 139–144.

14. Banks PA, Gerzof SG, Langevin RE, et al. CT-guided aspiration of suspected pancreatic infection: bacteriology and clinical outcome. Int J Pancreatol 1995; 18: 265–270.

15. Rau B, Pralle U, Mayer JM, Beger HG. The role of fine-needle aspiration in the diagnosis of infected pancreatic necrosis: an 8-year experience. Br J Surg 1998; 85: 179–184.

16. Beger HG, Bittner R, Block S, Buchler M. Bacterial contamination of pancreatic necrosis: A prospective clinical study. Gastroenterology 1986; 91: 433–438.

17. Isenmann R, Buchler MW. Infection and acute pancreatitis. Br J Surg 1994; 81: 1707–1708.

18. Sakorafas GH, Tsiotos GG, Sarr MG. Extrapancreatic necrotizing pancreatitis with viable pancreas: a previously under-appreciated entity. J Am Coll Surg 1999; 188: 643–648.

19. Buchler M, Malfertheiner P, Friess H, et al. Human pancreatic tissue concentration of bacterial antibiotics. Gastroenterology 1992; 103: 1902–1908.

20. Pederzoli P, Bassi C, Vesentini S, Campedelli A. A randomized multicenter clinical trial of antibiotic prophylaxis of septic complications in acute necrotizing pancreatitis with imipenem. Surg Gynecol Obstet 1993; 176: 480–483.

21. Bassi C, Falconi M, Talamini G, et al. Controlled clinical trial of perfloxacin versus imipenem in severe acute pancreatitis. Gastroenterology 1998; 115: 1513–1517.

22. Grewe M, Tsiotos GG, Luque-de Leon E, Sarr MG. Fungal infection in acute necrotizing pancreatitis. J Am Coll Surg 1999; 188: 408–414.

23. Isenmann R, Schwarz M, Rau B, et al. Characteristics of infection with Candida species in patients with necrotizing pancreatitis. W J Surg 2002; 26: 372–376.

24. Runkel NS, Moody FG, Smith GS, et al. The role of the gut in the development of sepsis in acute pancreatitis. J Surg Res 1991; 51: 18–23.

25. Gianotti L, Munda R, Alexander JW, et al. Bacterial translocation: a potential source for infection in acute pancreatitis. Pancreas 1993; 8: 551–558.

26. Kalfarentzos F, Kehagias J, Mead N, et al. Enteral feeding is superior to parenteral nutrition in severe acute pancreatitis: results of a randomized prospective trial. Br J Surg 1997; 84: 1665–1669.

27. Rattner DW, Legermate DA, Lee MJ, et al. Early surgical debridement of symptomatic pancreatic necrosis is beneficial irrespective of infection. Am J Surg 1992; 163: 105–110.

28. Buchler MW, Gloor B, Muller CA, et al. Acute necrotizing pancreatitis: treatment strategy according to the status of infection. Ann Surg 2000; 232: 6196–6226.

29. Mier J, Leon EL, Castillo A, et al. Early versus late necrosectomy in severe necrotizing pancreatitis. Am J Surg 1997; 173: 71–75.
30. Fernandez-del Castillo C, Rattner DW, Makary MA, et al. Debridement and closed packing for the treatment of necrotizing pancreatitis. Ann Surg 1998; 228: 676–684.
30a. Vitas GJ, Sarr MG. Selected management of pancreatic pseudocysts: operative versus expectant management. Surgery 1992; 111: 123–130.
31. Bittner R, Block S, Buchler M, Beger HG. Pancreatic abscess and infected necrosis: Different local septic complications in acute pancreatitis. Dig Dis Sci 1987; 32: 1082–1087.
32. Mithofer K, Mueller PR, Warshaw AL. Interventional and surgical treatment of pancreatic abscess. W J Surg 1997; 21: 162–168.
33. Carter CR, McKay CJ, Imrie CW. Percutaneous necrosectomy and sinus tract endoscopy in the management of infected pancreatic necrosis: an initial experience. Ann Surg 2000; 232: 175–180.
34. Davidson ED, Bradley EL III. Marsupialization in the treatment of pancreatic abscess. Surgery 198: 252–256.
35. Sarr MG, Nagorney DM, Mucha P, et al. Acute necrotizing pancreatitis: management by planned, staged pancreatic necrosectomy debridement and delayed primary wound closure over drains. Br J Surg 1991; 78: 576–581.
36. Beger HG, Buchler M, Bittner R, et al. Necrosectomy and postoperative local lavage in necrotizing pancreatitis. Br J Surg 1988; 75: 207–212.
37. Sarr MG, Mayo S. Needle catheter jejunostomy: an unappreciated and misunderstood advance in the care of patients after major abdominal operations. Mayo Clin Proc 1988; 63: 565–572.
38. Doepel M, Eriksson J, Halme L, et al. Good long-term results in patients surviving acute pancreatitis. Br J Surg 1993; 80: 1583–1586.
39. Norback IH, Auvinen OA. Long-term results after pancreas resection for acute necrotizing pancreatitis. Br J Surg 1985; 72: 687–689.
40. Tsiotos GG, Luque-de Leon E, Sarr MG. Long-term outcome of necrotizing pancreatitis treated by necrosectomy. Br J Surg 1998; 85: 1650–1653.
41. Mitchell CJ, Playforth MJ, Kelleher J, McMahon MJ. Functional recovery of the exocrine pancreas after acute pancreatitis. Scand J Gastroenterol 1983; 18: 15–18.
42. Bozkurt T Maroske D, Adler G. Exocrine pancreatic function after recovery from necrotizing pancreatitis. Hepato-Gastroenterol 1995; 42: 55–58.
43. Seidensticker F, Otto J, Lankisch PG. Recovery of the pancreas after acute pancreatitis is not necessarily complete. Int J Pancreatol 1995; 17: 225–229.

8 Pancreatic Fluid Collections and Pseudocysts in Patients With Acute Pancreatitis

Michael F. Byrne, MA, MB, ChB, MRCP and John Baillie, MB, ChB, FRCP

CONTENTS

INTRODUCTION

Acute pancreatitis (AP) has a wide range of pathological features, radiological appearances, and treatment options *(1)*. In most cases, it is a mild and self-limiting disease. However, severe disease develops in approximately 20% of patients associated with local and systemic complications *(2–5)*. Fluid collections commonly complicate AP and occur in up to half of cases of patients with moderate-to-severe cases *(6,7)*. These fluid collections are associated with increased morbidity and mortality *(8)* and represent an exudative or serous reaction to injury of

From: *Pancreatitis and Its Complications*
Edited by: C. E. Forsmark © Humana Press Inc., Totowa, NJ

the pancreas. Around 50% of these acute fluid collections resolve spontaneously within 6 weeks *(7,9,10)*. Between 10 and 15% may progress to pseudocyst formation after developing a capsule, and pseudocysts present further potential clinical and management problems.

This chapter reviews the pathophysiology, clinical presentation, investigation and management of acute fluid collections, and pancreatic pseudocysts. Additionally, other cystic lesions of the pancreas are briefly discussed.

FLUID COLLECTIONS IN ACUTE PANCREATITIS

Acute Fluid Collections

Understanding the pancreatic ductal anatomy when a pancreatic fluid collection is present enables appropriate management. Disruption of the pancreatic duct or acinar integrity is necessary to allow formation of a pancreatic fluid collection *(11,12)*. These collections may consist of enzyme-rich pancreatic juice with or without necrotic debris *(9)*. By definition, they lack a definite wall, may be single or multiple, and usually develop early in the course of AP *(7)*. They can be intra- or extrapancreatic *(12,13)*: intrapancreatic collections can occur anywhere in the pancreatic head, body, or tail *(14)*; extrapancreatic locations include the lesser sac, around the spleen and liver, pararenal spaces, peritoneal cavity, and the mediastinum *(14–16)*. The presentation of extrapancreatic collections is variable, depending on the location of the fluid. For example, patients may develop gastric outlet obstruction or have findings that mimic hepatomegaly or splenomegaly. Pancreatic ascites can occur owing to leakage of pancreatic exocrine secretions into the peritoneal cavity, which typically follows major pancreatic ductal disruption *(14)*.

As a rule, nearly 50% of these collections settle spontaneously *(7)*, but those that persist may develop into pseudocysts, abscesses, or sterile necrotic collections *(9)*.

Pseudocysts

Pseudocysts are the most common cystic lesions in the pancreas and result from episodes of AP or as part of chronic pancreatitis. Only acute pseudocysts are considered here. Pancreatic cysts other than pseudocysts are described later in this chapter.

A pancreatic pseudocyst is a collection of pancreatic juice encased by granulation tissue and collagen occurring in or around the pancreas as a result of autodigestive fat necrosis in AP or ductal leakage *(17–19)*. Development of an acute pseudocyst requires at least 4 weeks *(9)* and is usually preceded by, and should be differentiated from, an AP fluid collection *(20)*. Pseudocysts lack a true epithelial lining. By definition,

Table 1
Complications of Pseudocysts

Infection
Pancreatic fistulas
Gastrointestinal or urinary obstruction
Jaundice
Pseudoaneurysm formation
Pancreatic ascites
Rupture (peritonitis)
Splenic or portal vein thrombosis

pseudocysts contain fluid, but they also often contain debris. There is some overlap between pseudocysts and organized pancreatic necrosis, in which there is solid material frequently surrounded by fluid (20).

Pseudocysts present in a variety of ways: failure of an episode of pancreatitis to resolve; persistently high-serum amylase levels; persistent pain, pressure or fullness, vomiting or jaundice from pressure on adjacent organs, such as stomach, duodenum, and bile duct (9,18,20). Occasionally, a smooth epigastric mass may be palpable.

COMPLICATIONS OF PSEUDOCYSTS

The potential complications of untreated pseudocysts are listed in Table 1 (7,14,20,21). Infection, usually with gut flora, occurs in up to 10% of pseudocysts. If left untreated, this may progress to peritonitis and/or systemic sepsis. Pseudocysts may also rupture into a neighboring viscus (stomach, duodenum, or colon) or directly into the peritoneal cavity, presenting as an acute abdominal emergency or as pancreatic ascites or pleural effusion. Pancreatic ascites is rich in amylase and protein. A rare but rightly feared complication of pancreatic pseudocysts is erosion into a major artery (typically, the splenic artery), resulting in the development of a pseudoaneurysm and subsequent bleeding. When there is communication between the pseudoaneurysm and pancreatic duct, massive gastrointestinal bleeding (hemosuccus pancreaticus) can result (22,23). Not infrequently, portal or splenic vein thrombosis may complicate pancreatitis and pseudocysts (24). Thrombosis of the splenic vein may produce a segmental or left-sided portal hypertension with isolated gastric varices.

IMAGING OF PANCREATIC FLUID COLLECTIONS/ PSEUDOCYSTS

Pseudocysts are usually diagnosed using transabdominal ultrasound (US) or computed tomography (CT; Fig. 1) and, more recently, magnetic

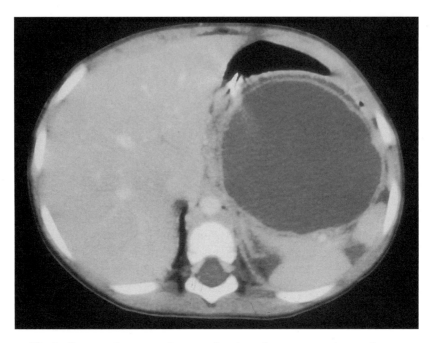

Fig. 1. Computed tomography scan showing a large pancreatic pseudocyst.

resonance imaging (MRI) and endoscopic ultrasound (EUS) *(20,25–27)*. However, it should be noted that true pancreatic cysts (benign or malignant) can be mistaken for pseudocysts. Fine-needle aspiration (FNA) under EUS or CT guidance has increased the diagnostic accuracy of these imaging modalities *(28,29)*. EUS-guided FNA has been shown to be useful in distinguishing the various cystic lesions of the pancreas; in one study, it had an 89% sensitivity for detecting malignant cysts *(29)*. Pseudocyst fluid usually has high-amylase levels and low levels of tumor markers, such as carcinoembryonic antigen (CEA) and CA19-9.

CT and EUS are also able to provide valuable information about the likely severity of pancreatic damage, such as echogenicity and degree of peripancreatic fluid in the setting of AP. One study showed that a score based on the EUS appearance of the pancreas in AP correlated well with the number of days in the hospital and in intensive care *(30)*. EUS may also allow the distinction of necrotizing from edematous AP and more accurate prognostic predictions *(31)*, but further studies are needed before EUS can be recommended as a tool to reliably prove this important distinction. Another study using a CT scoring system devised by Balthazar *(32)* showed that the presence and extent of extrapancreatic fluid collections as detected by CT are indicators of severe AP *(13)*. This CT-based study also confirmed previous suggestions that involvement of the anterior and posterior pararenal spaces by extrapancreatic fluid collections indicated the most severe prognosis *(13,33)*.

TREATMENT

Acute Fluid Collections

Acute fluid collections are very common early in the course of AP; the majority regress spontaneously within weeks *(7,9,10)*. Drainage of these immature collections with no clear wall of granulation tissue is not recommended *(9)* unless they are large and symptomatic, causing pain or obstructive complications, such as hydronephrosis or gastric outlet obstruction, or there is a concern about infection, in which case a diagnostic tap is indicated. If the collections mature and persist beyond 4–6 weeks, they become pseudocysts and are treated as discussed in the following section.

Pancreatic Pseudocysts

MEDICAL MANAGEMENT

No clear consensus exists regarding the optimal management of asymptomatic pseudocysts. Because up to 40–50% of acute pseudocysts resolve spontaneously within 6 weeks, an expectant policy with asymptomatic pseudocysts may be warranted *(7,9)*. Vitas et al. reviewed a series of 68 pancreatic pseudocysts that were managed expectantly *(34)*. There were serious complications in 9% of patients, all within the first 8 weeks. In this series, 80% of cysts less than 6-cm diameter resolved without intervention. One suggested policy is that small pseudocysts (<6 cm), asymptomatic pseudocysts, and uncomplicated pseudocysts can be managed expectantly *(35)*. However, this belief is not universally held. Some series show a complication rate as high as 60% in medically managed pseudocysts that fail to resolve by 12 weeks *(7,21)*. It seems reasonable to withhold intervention unless symptoms arise or the pseudocyst is clearly enlarging on serial measurement *(36)*. It has been recommended that if interventional therapy is considered, 4–6 weeks should be allowed for the pseudocyst to mature *(9)*. Yet, early intervention may be dictated by changes in the patient's condition. The interventional options available are now described.

INTERVENTIONAL MANAGEMENT

Case Selection for Intervention. The indications for drainage of acute pseudocysts include ongoing symptoms, complications, progressive

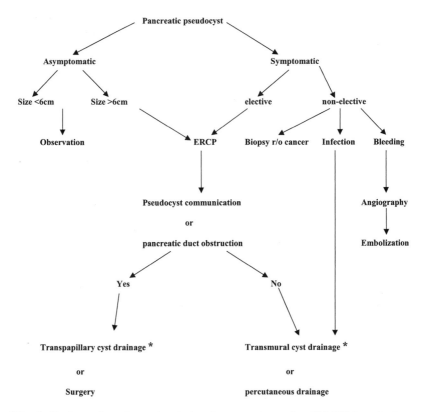

Fig. 2. Endoscopic retrograde cholangiopancreatography (ERCP)-based algorithm for the management of pancreatic pseudocysts. Modified from Ahearne et al. *(37)*. *Refer to Table 2.

enlargement, or suspicion of malignancy *(20)*. Before intervening, it is important to consider the likelihood that the apparent pseudocyst may actually be a cystic tumor, taking into account the radiological and FNA features described previously.

Pseudocysts can be drained endoscopically, radiologically, or surgically. Essential information required in choosing the appropriate intervention pertains to the pancreatic ductal anatomy. It is important to know if there is a pancreatic duct obstruction or stricture, and if there is communication between a pseudocyst and the pancreatic duct *(14)*. In the presence of either of these features, percutaneous drainage is more likely to fail or result in recurrence, as continued pancreatic secretion will keep the cyst from resolving if ductal integrity is not restored. An endoscopic retrograde cholangiopanecreatography (ERCP)-based algorithm was proposed by Ahearne et al. from our institution in 1992 *(37)*, which suggested that all patients with pseudocysts

Table 2
Do's and Don'ts of Endoscopic Pseudocyst Drainage

Do's
1. Confirm that lesion actually is a pseudocyst.
2. Collaborate with surgical and radiological colleagues.
3. Fully inform patient of risks.
4. Use EUS if available.
5. Make small puncture and enlarge with a balloon. Maintain access with wire. Use large double pigtail stents.
6. Keep patient overnight for observation.
7. Repeat endoscopy to remove stents once pseudocyst decompression is confirmed.

Don'ts
1. Don't do the procedure unless skilled in advanced ERCP. Don't evacuate necrotic material.
2. Don't perform endoscopic drainage for multiple pseudocysts as there is high risk of introducing infection.
3. Don't perform endoscopic drainage procedure on asymptomatic, frail, elderly population. Watch and wait.
4. Don't make a large hole in the stomach or duodenum with a needle knife. Make a small puncture and dilate with balloon to minimize the bleeding risk.
5. Don't hesitate to discontinue procedure if problems are encountered. Don't attempt blind puncture.
6. Don't lose patients to follow-up.
7. Don't forget that the apparent pseudocyst may actually be a cystic neoplasm. Be sure of the diagnosis before attempting drainage.

EUS, endoscopic ultrasound; ERCP, endoscopic retrograde cholangiopancreato-graphy.

treated electively should first have ERCP to appropriately allocate treatment. In this algorithm, if there was main pancreatic duct obstruction or pseudocyst communication, surgical treatment was indicated, whereas those pseudocysts that did not communicate and were unassociated with duct obstruction could be safely treated with percutaneous drainage. In the emergency situation where immediate drainage is indicated, it was suggested that the patient should be stabilized with the least invasive procedure, and definitive treatment should be performed later if necessary.

This algorithm was suggested before endoscopic drainage of pseudocysts became more widely accepted. A modified ERCP-based algorithm that takes the major therapeutic options into account is shown in Fig. 2. The same principles relating to ductal anatomy apply, but endoscopic drainage can justifiably be attempted in the majority of cases (assuming

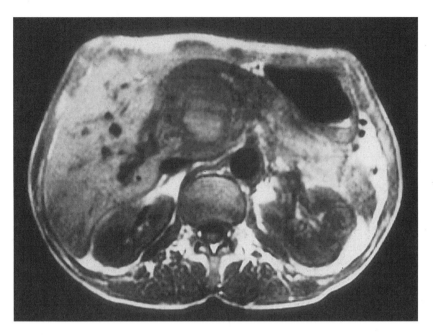

Fig. 3. Magnetic resonance imaging image of a pancreatic pseudocyst with an associated pseudoaneurysm.

applicability of a transmural or transpapillary approach as detailed below; *see* Table 2). It should be noted that if preoperative ERCP is performed, any instrumented fluid collections should be drained as soon as logistically possible and preferably within 72 hours, as these collections may become colonized *(14)*.

It is also critical to know about the presence of underlying pancreatic necrosis. If there is solid material or debris in the pseudocyst, this should be considered a contraindication to endoscopic or radiological drainage, because this material may not be readily removed, and the risk of infection is high *(38)*. Endoscopic drainage of so-called "organized pancreatic necrosis" has been described by Baron et al. but the complication rate was high *(39)*. At present, endoscopic necrosectomy remains experimental and should not be attempted in routine clinical practice. Partially liquefied necrotic collections may be confused for pseudocysts. Some believe that if a fluid collection contains any solid material (as seen on CT or MRI), this is not a true pseudocyst and should be regarded as suspicious for necrosis *(38)*. Further management of these so-called "necromas" should employ the same principles as those applied to management of obvious pancreatic necrosis, which is discussed in Chapter 7.

Finally, in the selection of patients for intervention, it is crucial to exclude the possibility of a pseudoaneurysm prior to treatment (Fig. 3). Fatal hemorrhage has complicated endoscopic "drainage" of unsuspected pancreatic pseudoaneurysms. It is reported that pseudoaneurysms can occur in up to 10% of pseudocysts (40,41), although experienced pancreatologists would find this a surprisingly high number. Pseudoaneurysms can usually be detected by dynamic CT scanning, although if there is any concern about missing a pseudoaneurysm, selective mesenteric angiography is the definitive test. Pseudoaneurysms should be embolized before surgery is attempted owing to the high risk of catastrophic bleeding.

ENDOSCOPIC THERAPY

Endoscopic therapy of pancreatic pseudocysts has been reported in many studies since the first description by Rodgers in 1975 (42). Two main endoscopic approaches—transmural and transpapillary—are used, depending on ductal anatomy (19,43–47).

If the pseudocyst communicates with the main pancreatic duct, drainage can be achieved by placing a small stent into the pancreatic duct (transpapillary cyst drainage; 48–50). Although experience with this approach is less than with transmural cyst drainage, some feel it is the most appropriate way to deal with communicating pseudocysts, particularly if they are relatively small. Pseudocysts communicate with the pancreatic duct in 55–69% of cases (51,52). The transpapillary approach is less invasive and potentially safer than transmural drainage. In some but not all series, a pancreatic sphincterotomy is first performed (19,53,54). Then, a soft-tipped guidewire is placed across the ductal disruption; a 5-Fr or 7-Fr gauge straight stent is advanced over the guidewire (53,54). It is not clear whether these stents work by occluding the ductal leak or simply by equalizing the pressure between the pancreatic duct and the duodenum. Thus, it is not clear whether transpapillary stents actually need to bridge the fistula or not. In some series, if a pseudocyst was large, a nasopancreatic drain was placed for approximately 5 days to achieve direct cyst drainage (48,53). Intravenous antibiotics should be given prior to these procedures. Repeat CT or transabdominal US should be performed 4–6 weeks later (19) and, if follow-up ERCP confirms pseudocyst resolution and unimpeded pancreatic duct drainage, the stent is removed. It is important to deal with any downstream pancreatic duct stones or stricture at initial or follow-up ERCP, because failure to do so will likely result in pseudocyst recurrence (14,19). In Kozarek's series, stents were left in situ for an average of 6 weeks with a range of 1–18 months (53). However, pancreatic stents left in place for more than 4–6 weeks have the potential to cause side branch injury and focal pancreatitis, and if they become blocked, patients may develop septicemia. Recent studies that evaluated the transpapillary technique for pseudocyst drainage have reported success rates similar to those for transgastric drainage *(45,47,55)*, and the transpapillary approach has a lower incidence of bleeding and perforation.

The other endoscopic approach to pseudocyst drainage is transmural. If the pseudocyst is not communicating with the pancreatic duct, and there is an endoscopically visible bulge, or CT predicts the site of compression of the pseudocyst on the stomach or duodenum, a transgastric or transduodenal approach is indicated *(19,44–47,54)*. If no endoscopically visible bulge is noted, a safe and suitable access must be identifiable by EUS. Indeed, where EUS is available, it should be used to target the access site. A fistula must be created to drain pseudocysts directly into the stomach or duodenum. The pseudocyst should be punctured with a standard needle catheter (22-gauge needle, 7-Fr catheter), fluid aspirated (and sent for cytology and culture), and contrast-instilled to confirm entry into the cyst *(56;* Fig. 4). The distance from the gut lumen to the pseudocyst lumen should be no greater than 10 mm when contemplating endoscopic cyst-gastrostomy or cyst-duodenostomy *(57,58)*. Thereafter, a small incision is made using a needle knife papillotome and a wire advanced into the cyst. This opening is dilated to 5–10 mm with a balloon and two double pigtail stents are placed. Bleeding and perforation can complicate entry through the gastric or duodenal wall *(44,56,59)*. More recently, a Seldinger technique without electrocautery has been compared to standard needle-knife electrocautery *(60)*.The results suggest that this technique is equally effective but also safer when compared to the standard needle-knife technique. Once the pigtail stents are in place, management is similar to that for transpapillary drainage. Cyst size is monitored radiologically, and the stents are removed endoscopically once complete drainage has been confirmed.

An early study by Cremer et al. in 1989 showed success and recurrence rates for transgastric and transduodenal pseudocyst drainage of 100 and 18%, and 96 and 9%, respectively *(57)*. Complications were low for transduodenal drainage but reported as 18% for transgastric procedures. Since this study, the reported success rates for endoscopic pseudocyst drainage have varied widely between 70 and 94% with overall complication rates between 11 and 24%. Recurrence rates range from 4 to 23% *(20,45,54,55)*.

EUS has augmented the endoscopic management of pancreatic pseudocysts *(61–63)*. Unaided endoscopic cystogastrostomy is done in a relatively "blind" fashion. If no significant intragastric bulge is

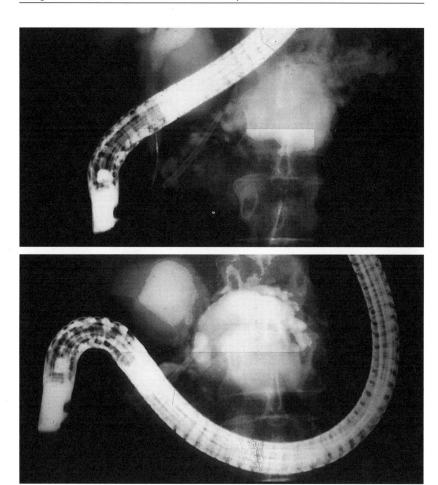

Fig. 4. Endoscopic retrograde cholagiopancreatography image of a large dumb-bell-shaped pancreatic pseudocyst filled with contrast.

observed, there is an increased risk of perforation or bleeding *(52)*. EUS is useful for locating a puncture site devoid of vessels and other structures, and the site is marked by biopsy *(64)* or tattooing. In the series of 32 patients described by Fockens et al. *(62)*, preinterventional EUS provided essential information that resulted in a major change in therapeutic management in one third of patients. Some argue that endoscopic drainage should not be done without prior endosonographic examination. It has been shown with newer interventional echoendo-scopes that pseudocyst drainage is possible using EUS techniques alone (Fig. 5; *65*).

Endoscopic pseudocyst drainage is a very useful procedure in selected cases if certain "do's" and "don'ts" are observed (*see* Table 2).

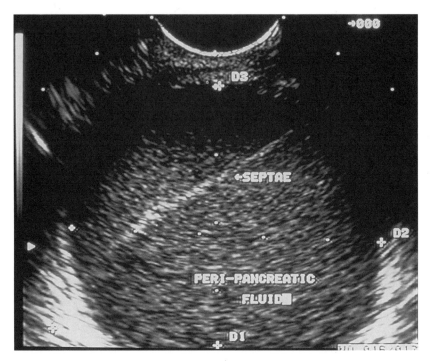

Fig. 5. Aspiration of a pseudocyst under endoscopic ultrasound guidance.

PERCUTANEOUS THERAPY

Before the advent of endoscopic decompression, the only alternative to surgical drainage of pseudocysts was percutaneous drainage. Using US guidance, external drainage with an internal–external catheter or internal cystogastric drainage with a double-pigtail catheter can be performed percutaneously *(66–68)*. Percutaneous aspiration is relatively easy to perform. However, simple aspiration without drain placement had a high recurrence rate (63%) and overall failure rate (54%) in a collation of nine studies *(69)*. Percutaneous drainage with catheter placement, again performed under US guidance, is usually successful in resolving the pseudocysts (70–90%; *66,70,67*), with a recurrence rate of 8–25% *(71–74)*. This approach is thought to be particularly indicated for infected pseudocysts *(75)*. But, there can be difficulties in maintaining catheter drainage, and the introduction of new infection may be a problem *(71,76)*. The other major problem with percutaneously placed external catheters is that up to one fourth of such placements will result in the formation of a pancreatic-cutaneous fistula, especially if there is communication between the pseudocyst and pancreatic duct *(74,77)*. The overall complication rate from percutaneous drainage is estimated in some series as high as 16% *(67,71,76,78)* of cases. Use of octreotide and/or placement of progressively smaller catheters may encourage closure of these fistulas *(77,79)*. Careful patient selection, including preintervention ERCP to outline the ductal anatomy, will minimize these problems. External drainage catheters are usually removed after 2–6 weeks, but they are sometimes left in place for up to 6 months to achieve complete drainage. The presence of distal pancreatic ductal disruption or obstruction is considered by some to be a relative contraindication to percutaneous drainage, as these patients tend to develop persistent pancreatic-cutaneous fistulas *(37)*.

An US-guided percutaneous approach can be used to place pigtail stents for prolonged internal cystogastric drainage (until the pseudocyst collapses and seals off [*80–82*]). This approach employs the same principle as endoscopic cystogastrostomy, which is done as an outpatient procedure under local anesthesia. The pseudocyst should preferably be greater than 5-cm diameter and adherent to the posterior wall of the stomach *(68)*. Monthly screening US examinations allow the physician to decide when to remove the stent endoscopically.

SURGICAL THERAPY

Historically, if pseudocyst drainage became necessary because of increasing size, symptoms, or complications, surgical intervention was the only option *(14,69,71,83)*. Currently, surgery for pseudocyst treatment is indicated only in patients in whom endoscopic or percutaneous drainage is not feasible and in those patients suspected of having a cystic tumor. As a rule, surgical pseudocyst drainage uses a technique of internal drainage with a reported morbidity of 15–30% and a mortality of less than 3% *(84,85,86)*. Surgery allows pseudocyst drainage, debridement of any surrounding necrotic material, and correction of ductal problems *(36)*. The pseudocyst recurrence rate after surgical treatment ranges between 10 and 20% *(84–86)*. It is difficult to make direct comparisons between nonsurgical and surgical drainage of pseudocysts, as in many surgical series, the sicker patients were excluded and drained percutaneously. In cases of duct obstruction or persistent disruption, some have advocated surgical treatment over endoscopic or percutaneous approaches *(83)*. If there is disruption or disconnection of the pancreas in the head, a proximal pancreatic resection is necessary. If, in contrast, pancreatic duct disruption occurs in the neck or body of the gland, a distal resection is performed.

There are still hospitals with little or no expertise in the latest endoscopic or percutaneous techniques for pseudocyst drainage. Although there are indications for one technique over another depending on the particular situation, local expertise still plays a significant role in deciding which drainage procedure will be employed.

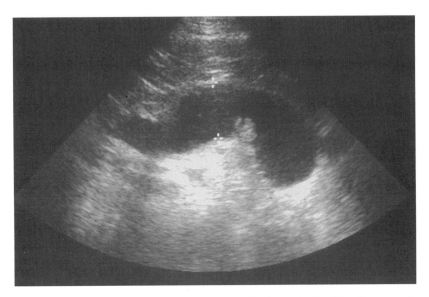

Fig. 6. Transabdominal ultrasound image showing a markedly dilated pancreatic duct in a patient with a pancreatic mucinous cystadenocarcinoma.

CYSTIC LESIONS OF THE PANCREAS

Classification

Unlike pseudocysts, true pancreatic cysts have an epithelial lining; they can be broadly divided into non-neoplastic cysts and primary neoplastic cysts *(87–90)*. Overall, true cysts account for approximately 10–15% of all pancreatic cystic lesions *(91)*. The non-neoplastic cysts include simple cysts and duplication cysts. Cysts that are malignant include mucinous cystadenocarcinoma (Fig. 6) and adenocarcinoma with cystic degeneration. Those regarded as premalignant lesions include mucinous cystadenoma and intraductal papillary mucinous tumor (formerly mucinous ductal ectasia). Cystic neoplasms regarded as benign include serous cystadenomas (microcystic adenoma) (Fig. 7) and dermoid lymphangiomas. Approximately 10% of pancreatic cysts are neoplastic *(87)*. Cystic tumors of the pancreas account for only about 1% of all pancreatic cancers *(91,92)*. Cystic neoplasms of the pancreas can present in a number of ways: abdominal pain, weight loss, anorexia, jaundice, and a palpable mass. They may also be asymptomatic and detected incidentally. The most common and clinically important of the cystic tumors are serous and mucinous cystadenomas and mucinous cystadenocarcinomas. Serous cystadenomas may be multiple in cases of the von Hippel-Lindau disease *(93)*, an autosomally dominant inherited condition in which there are associated central nervous system

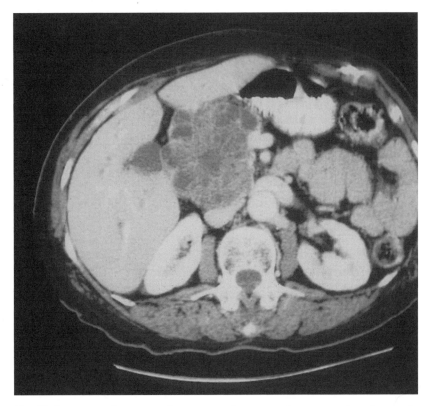

Fig. 7. A computed tomography tomography scan of a pancreatic microcystic adenoma (serous cystadenoma).

hemangioblastomas and retinal angiomas. This disorder is associated with other tumors, such as pheochromocytoma and renal cell cancer *(94)*.

Diagnosis

Although rare, cystic tumors of the pancreas are now more frequently diagnosed because of modern imaging techniques (*87*). The largest clinical problem associated with these cystic neoplasms is in being mistaken for pseudocysts and treated inappropriately. Accurate diagnosis is consequently critical. The classic history is that of an incidentally discovered or minimally symptomatic cystic lesion in a middle-aged or elderly patient with no previous history of pancreatitis and no risk factors for pancreatitis. A definite histological diagnosis cannot be made until a cystic lesion has been totally resected. However, certain radiological features aid appropriate diagnosis. ERCP findings may contribute to the diagnosis. For example, ductal obstruction or stenosis in the presence of cysts suggest malignancy, as does a lack or communication between the cyst and the pancreatic duct *(87,89)*. Traditionally, imaging of these cystic lesions of the pancreas has been with CT, MRI, or more recently, EUS. CT will reliably detect cystic structures but has variable success for distinguishing benign from malignant disease *(95,96)*. For EUS imaging, it has been suggested that well-defined, simple, uniloculated cysts are likely benign and that complex cystic lesions with thick walls and septations or with solid matter protruding into the cyst lumen are often malignant *(97)*. Some reports have suggested that the nature of a pancreatic cyst can be predicted with greater than 90% accuracy using EUS findings alone *(97,98)*. However, as highlighted in a recent study, EUS alone cannot be considered the gold standard *(99)*. Although some limitations of this study were highlighted in an accompanying editorial *(100)*, nonetheless, it shows that further advances are required in the diagnosis and management of pancreatic cysts. One advance has been the use of fine-needle aspiration under CT or EUS guidance. A recent multicenter study showed that the combination of fluid cytology, CEA levels, and EUS features increased the sensitivity of EUS for diagnosing malignant cysts to 89% *(29)*. It must be remembered that a negative FNA does not exclude malignancy. There has also been some concern that FNA of cystic lesions may lead to a higher rate of infection than FNA of solid lesions *(101)*. Further study is needed to elucidate this, but we currently recommend the use of prophylactic antibiotics for FNA procedures *(102)*.

Clinical differentiation between benign and malignant cystic pancreatic tumors remains difficult, as does the differentiation between true cysts and pseudocysts. Despite clear advances in the imaging of these lesions, the poor specificity of radiological imaging has led some to suggest, in view of the risk of malignancy within these cystic lesions and favorable outcome with resection, that all suspected cystic tumors of the pancreas should be resected *(103,104)*.

Treatment

As a rule, most cystic neoplasms of the pancreas are relatively slow growing *(87)*. Curative surgery may be possible if lesions are detected at an early stage. Certainly, if there is any doubt in the diagnosis, surgery should be strongly considered. Serous cystadenomas are essentially benign; there has been only one report of malignancy developing in such a lesion *(87)*. The most appropriate treatment may be simple observation in high-operative risk patients, specifically the elderly. If these lesions cause symptoms or there is uncertainty about the diagnosis, surgical resection is indicated.

Mucinous cystic neoplasms (subclassified as cystadenomas and cystadenocarcinomas) can contain both benign and malignant epithelium

(105,106). As such, they should all be considered as potentially malignant, and surgical resection is the treatment of choice. The 2-year survival rate for patients with invasive mucinous cystadenocarcinoma in one series was 67% *(107)*, which is significantly better than for pancreatic ductal adenocarcinoma. For less invasive and less differentiated mucinous cystic neoplasms, 5- to 12-year survival rates after resection range from 40 to 75% *(89,90,108)*. Left untreated, the prognosis likely approaches that of unresected pancreatic adenocarcinoma *(109)*. Thus, it is very important to consider surgery if there is any doubt to the nature of a cystic tumor to avoid missing a potentially treatable neoplasm.

SUMMARY

Intrapancreatic and extrapancreatic fluid collections are common in the early course of AP and often resolve spontaneously. If collections persist, they may become infected and progress to necrotic collections or abscesses, or they can become surrounded by granulation tissue and evolve into pseudocysts. Pseudocysts can be managed expectantly if they are uncomplicated, asymptomatic, and do not increase in size. If intervention is indicated, current management favors endoscopic drainage techniques that compare favorably to percutaneous and surgical drainage. An appreciation of ductal anatomy is critical in guiding appropriate intervention, and in the elective management of pseudocysts, an ERCP should first be performed. Adhering to certain guidelines lessens the complications of endoscopic intervention. The increasing use of EUS will certainly play a key role in improving the safety of endoscopic drainage. It is likely that newer echoendoscopes will allow direct pseudocyst drainage without the need for a separate endoscopic procedure. With that said, in any one center, the most appropriate form of drainage (endoscopic, percutaneous, or surgical) will be determined by the local expertise available.

True pancreatic cysts represent approximately 15% of all pancreatic cystic neoplasms, and these cysts can be benign or malignant. Use of fine-needle aspiration under CT and EUS has increased the diagnostic accuracy of malignant lesions. Unlike pancreatic cancer, this is critical, as many early pancreatic cystic neoplasms have a good prognosis if resected. Thus, it is crucial to determine the nature of a pancreatic cystic lesion. If there is any doubt at all, surgical resection is indicated unless the patient is not a surgical candidate.

REFERENCES

1. Beckingham IJ, Bornman PC. ABC of diseases of liver, pancreas, and biliary system. Acute pancreatitis. Br Med J 2001; 322: 595–598.

2. Beger HG, Isenmann R. Surgical management of necrotizing pancreatitis. Surg Clin North Am 1999; 79: 783–800.
3. Steinberg W, Tenner S. Acute pancreatitis. N Engl J Med 1994; 330: 1198–1210.
4. Baron, TH, Morgan DE, Acute necrotizing pancreatitis. N Engl J Med 1999. 340:1412–1417.
5. Tsiotos GG, Luque-de Leon, Soreide JA, et al. Management of necrotizing pancreatitis by repeated operative necrosectomy using a zipper technique. Am J Surg 1998; 175: 91–98.
6. Kourtesis G, Wilson SE, Williams RA. The clinical significance of fluid collections in acute pancreatitis. Am Surg 1990; 56: 796–9.
7. Johnson CD. Timing of intervention in acute pancreatitis. Postgrad Med J 1993; 69: 509–15.
8. Anderson MC, Adams DB. Pancreatic pseudocysts. When to drain, when to wait. Postgrad Med 1991; 89: 199–206.
9. Baron TH, Morgan DE. The diagnosis and management of fluid collections associated with pancreatitis. Am J Med 1997; 102: 555–563.
10. Barthet M, Bugallo M, Moreira LS, et al. Management of cysts and pseudocysts complicating chronic pancreatitis. A retrospective study of 143 patients. Gastroenterol Clin Biol 1993; 17: 270–276.
11. Becker V, Pathological anatomy and pathogenesis of acute pancreatitis. World J Surg 1981; 5: 303–313.
12. Segal I, Epstein B, Lawson HH, et al. The syndromes of pancreatic pseudocysts and fluid collections. Gastrointest Radiol 1984; 9: 115–122.
13. Lankisch PG, Struckmann K, Lehnick D. Presence and extent of extrapancreatic fluid collections are indicators of severe acute pancreatitis. Int J Pancreatol 1999; 26: 131–136.
14. Traverso LW, Kozarek RA. Interventional management of peripancreatic fluid collections. Surg Clin North Am 1999; 79: 745–757.
15. Siegelman SS, Copeland BE, Saba GP, et al. CT of fluid collections associated with pancreatitis. AJR Am J Roentgenol 1980; 134: 1121–1132.
16. Cameron JL. Chronic pancreatic ascites and pancreatic pleural effusions. Gastroenterology 1978; 74: 134–140.
17. Kloppel G, Maillet B. The morphological basis for the evolution of acute pancreatitis into chronic pancreatitis. Virchows Arch A Pathol Anat Histopathol 1992; 420: 1–4.
18. Kloppel G, Pseudocysts and other non-neoplastic cysts of the pancreas. Semin Diagn Pathol 2000; 17: 7–15.
19. Howell DA, Elton E, Parsons WG. Endoscopic management of pseudocysts of the pancreas. Gastrointest Endosc Clin N Am 1998; 8: 143–162.
20. Lehman GA. Pseudocysts. Gastrointest Endosc 1999; 49: S81–584.
21. Bradley EL, Clements JL Jr, Gonzalez AC. The natural history of pancreatic pseudocysts: a unified concept of management. Am J Surg 1979; 137: 135–141.
22. Risti B, Marincek B, Jost R, et al. Hemosuccus pancreaticus as a source of obscure upper gastrointestinal bleeding: three cases and literature review. Am J Gastroenterol 1995; 90: 1878–1880.
23. Suter M, Doenz F, Chapuis G, et al. Haemorrhage into the pancreatic duct (Hemosuccus pancreaticus): recognition and management. Eur J Surg 1995; 161: 887–892.
24. Lankisch PG. The spleen in inflammatory pancreatic disease. Gastroenterology 1990; 98: 509–516.
25. Snady H. Endoscopic ultrasonography in benign pancreatic disease. Surg Clin North Am 2001; 81: 329–344.

26. Shams, J, Stein A, and Cooperman AM. Computed tomography for pancreatic diseases. Surg Clin North Am, 2001. 81(2): p. 283–306.
27. Fulcher AS, Turner MA. MR pancreatography: a useful tool for evaluating pancreatic disorders. Radiographics 1999; 19: 5–24; discussion 41–44; quiz 148–149.
28. Luning M, Kursawe R, Schopke W, et al. CT guided percutaneous fine-needle biopsy of the pancreas. Eur J Radiol 1985; 5: 104–108.
29. Brugge WR, Saltzman JR., Scheiman JM, et al. Diagnosis of cystic neoplasms of the pancreas by EUS: The report of the cooperative pancreatic cyst study. Gastrointest Endosc 2001; 53(Abstract): AB71.
30. Chak A, Hawes RH, Cooper GS, et al. Prospective assessment of the utility of EUS in the evaluation of gallstone pancreatitis. Gastrointest Endosc 1999; 49: 599–604.
31. Sugiyama M, Atomi Y. Acute biliary pancreatitis: the roles of endoscopic ultrasonography and endoscopic retrograde cholangiopancreatography. Surgery 1998; 124: 14–21.
32. Balthazar EJ, Robinson DL, Megibow AJ, et al. Acute pancreatitis: value of CT in establishing prognosis. Radiology 1990; 174: 331–336.
33. Rotman N, Chevret S, Pezet D, et al. Prognostic value of early computed tomographic scans in severe acute pancreatitis. French Association for Surgical Research. J Am Coll Surg 1994; 179: 538–44.
34. Vitas GJ, Sarr MG. Selected management of pancreatic pseudocysts: operative versus expectant management. Surgery 1992; 111: 123–130.
35. Haber GB. Endoscopic drainage of pancreatic pseudocysts. Proc ASGE Postgrad Course, 1994. 1(Abstract).
36. Yeo CJ, Bastidas JA, Lynch-Nyhan A, et al. The natural history of pancreatic pseudocysts documented by computed tomography. Surg Gynecol Obstet 1990; 170: 411–417.
37. Ahearne PM, Baillie JM, Cotton PB, et al. An endoscopic retrograde cholangiopancreatography (ERCP)-based algorithm for the management of pancreatic pseudocysts. Am J Surg 1992; 163: 111–116.
38. Hariri M, Slivka A, Carr-Locke DL, et al. Pseudocyst drainage predisposes to infection when pancreatic necrosis is unrecognized. Am J Gastroenterol 1994; 89: 1781–1784.
39. Baron TH, Thaggard WG, Morgan DE, et al. Endoscopic therapy for organized pancreatic necrosis. Gastroenterology 1996; 111: 755–764.
40. el Hamel A, Parc R, Adda G, et al. Bleeding pseudocysts and pseudoaneurysms in chronic pancreatitis. Br J Surg 1991; 78: 1059–1063.
41. Pitkaranta P, Haapiainen R, Kivisaari L, et al. Diagnostic evaluation and aggressive surgical approach in bleeding pseudoaneurysms associated with pancreatic pseudocysts. Scand J Gastroenterol 1991; 26: 58–64.
42. Rogers BH, Cicurel NJ, Seed RW. Transgastric needle aspiration of pancreatic pseudocyst through an endoscope. Gastrointest Endosc 1975; 21: 133–134.
43. Kozarek RA. Endoscopic therapy of complete and partial pancreatic duct disruptions. Gastrointest Endosc Clin N Am 1998; 8: 39–53.
44. Smits ME, Rauws EA, Tytgat GN, et al. The efficacy of endoscopic treatment of pancreatic pseudocysts. Gastrointest Endosc 1995; 42: 202–207.
45. Libera ED, Siqueira ES, Morais M, et al. Pancreatic pseudocysts transpapillary and transmural drainage. HPB Surg 2000; 11: 333–338.
46. Vidyarthi G, Steinberg SE. Endoscopic management of pancreatic pseudocysts. Surg Clin North Am 2001; 81: 405–410.
47. Vitale GC, Lawhon JC, Larson GM, et al. Endoscopic drainage of the pancreatic pseudocyst. Surgery 1999; 126: 616–623.

48. Barthet M, Sahel J, Bodiou-Bertei C, et al. Endoscopic transpapillary drainage of pancreatic pseudocysts. Gastrointest Endosc 1995; 42: 208–213.
49. Catalano MF, Geenen JE, Schmalz MJ, et al. Treatment of pancreatic pseudocysts with ductal communication by transpapillary pancreatic duct endoprosthesis. Gastrointest Endosc 1995; 42: 214–218.
50. Mallavarapu R, Habib TH, Elton E, et al. Resolution of mediastinal pancreatic pseudocysts with transpapillary stent placement. Gastrointest Endosc 2001; 53: 367–370.
51. Kolars JC, Allen MO, Ansel H, et al. Pancreatic pseudocysts: clinical and endoscopic experience. Am J Gastroenterol 1989; 84: 259–264.
52. Sahel J, Bastid C, Pellat B, et al. Endoscopic cystoduodenostomy of cysts of chronic calcifying pancreatitis: a report of 20 cases. Pancreas 1987; 2: 447–453.
53. Kozarek RA, Ball TJ, Patterson DJ, et al. Endoscopic transpapillary therapy for disrupted pancreatic duct and peripancreatic fluid collections. Gastroenterology 1991; 100: 1362–1370.
54. Binmoeller KF, Seifert H, Walter A, et al. Transpapillary and transmural drainage of pancreatic pseudocysts. Gastrointest Endosc 1995. 42: 219–224.
55. De Palma GD, Galloro G, Puzziello A, et al. [Personal experience in the endoscopic treatment of pancreatic pseudocysts. Long-term results and analysis of prognostic factors]. Minerva Chir 2001 56: 475–481.
56. Howell DA, Holbrook RF, Bosco JJ, et al. Endoscopic needle localization of pancreatic pseudocysts before transmural drainage. Gastrointest Endosc 1993; 39: 693–698.
57. Cremer M, Deviere J, Engelholm L. Endoscopic management of cysts and pseudocysts in chronic pancreatitis: long-term follow-up after 7 years of experience. Gastrointest Endosc 1989; 35: 1–9.
58. Ryan ME. Endoscopic management of a pancreatic pseudocyst during pregnancy. Gastrointest Endosc 1992; 38: 605–608.
59. Donnelly PK, Lavelle J, Carr-Locke D. Massive haemorrhage following endoscopic transgastric drainage of pancreatic pseudocyst. Br J Surg 1990; 77: 758–759.
60. Monkemuller KE, Baron TH, Morgan DE. Transmural drainage of pancreatic fluid collections without electrocautery using the Seldinger technique. Gastrointest Endosc 1998; 48: 195–200.
61. Kozarek RA, Brayko CM, Harlan J, et al. Endoscopic drainage of pancreatic pseudocysts. Gastrointest Endosc 1985; 31: 322–327.
62. Fockens P, Johnson TG, van Dullemen HM, et al. Endosonographic imaging of pancreatic pseudocysts before endoscopic transmural drainage. Gastrointest Endosc 1997; 46: 412–416.
63. Norton ID, Clain JE, Wiersema MJ, et al. Utility of endoscopic ultrasonography in endoscopic drainage of pancreatic pseudocysts in selected patients. Mayo Clin Proc 2001; 76: 794–798.
64. Gerolami R, Giovannini M, Laugier R. Endoscopic drainage of pancreatic pseudocysts guided by endosonography. Endoscopy 1997; 29: 106–108.
65. Seifert, H, Dietrich C, Schmitt T, et al. Endoscopic ultrasound-guided one-step transmural drainage of cystic abdominal lesions with a large-channel echo endoscope. Endoscopy 2000; 32: 255–259.
66. D'Agostino HB, vanSonnenberg E, Sanchez RB, et al. Treatment of pancreatic pseudocysts with percutaneous drainage and octreotide. Work in progress. Radiology 1993; 187: 685–8.
67. Neff R. Pancreatic pseudocysts and fluid collections: percutaneous approaches. Surg Clin North Am 2001; 81: 399–403.

68. Sever M, Vidmar D, Surlan M, et al. Percutaneous drainage of pancreatic pseudo-cyst into the stomach. Surg Endosc 1998; 12: 1249–1253.
69. Gumaste UV, Dave PB. Pancreatic pseudocyst drainage—the needle or the scalpel? J Clin Gastroenterol 1991; 13: 500–505.
70. Barkin JS, Hyder SA. Changing concepts in the management of pancreatic pseu-docysts. Gastrointest Endosc 1989; 35: 62–64.
71. Grace PA, Williamson RC. Modern management of pancreatic pseudocysts. Br J Surg 1993; 80: 573–581.
72. Andersson R, Janzon M, Sundberg I, et al. Management of pancreatic pseudo-cysts. Br J Surg 1989; 76: 550–2.
73. Freeny PC, Lewis GP, Traverso LW, et al. Infected pancreatic fluid collections: percutaneous catheter drainage. Radiology 1988; 167: 435–441.
74. Adams DB , Anderson MC. Percutaneous catheter drainage compared with inter-nal drainage in the management of pancreatic pseudocyst. Ann Surg 1992; 215: 571–578.
75. Baril NB, Ralls PW, Wren SM, et al. Does an infected peripancreatic fluid collec-tion or abscess mandate operation? Ann Surg 2000; 231: 361–367.
76. Agha FP. Spontaneous resolution of acute pancreatic pseudocysts. Surg Gynecol Obstet 1984; 158: 22–26.
77. Fotoohi M, D'Agostino HB, Wollman B, et al. Persistent pancreatocutaneous fis-tula after percutaneous drainage of pancreatic fluid collections: role of cause and severity of pancreatitis. Radiology 1999; 213: 573–578.
78. Malecka-Panas E, Juszynski A, Chrzastek J, et al. Pancreatic fluid collections: diagnostic and therapeutic implications of percutaneous drainage guided by ultra-sound. Hepatogastroenterology 1998; 45: 873–878.
79. Pederzoli P, Bassi C, Falconi M, et al. Conservative treatment of external pancre-atic fistulas with parenteral nutrition alone or in combination with continuous intravenous infusion of somatostatin, glucagon or calcitonin. Surg Gynecol Obstet 1986; 163: 428–432.
80. Hancke S, Henriksen FW. Percutaneous pancreatic cystogastrostomy guided by ultrasound scanning and gastroscopy. Br J Surg 1985; 72: 916–917.
81. Davies RP, Cox MR, Wilson TG, et al. Percutaneous cystogastrostomy with a new catheter for drainage of pancreatic pseudocysts and fluid collections. Cardiovasc Intervent Radiol 1996. 19: 128–131.
82. Bilbao JI, Alejandre PL, Longo JM, et al. Percutaneous transgastric cystoduo-denostomy in the treatment of a pancreatic pseudocyst: a new approach. Cardiovasc Intervent Radiol 1995; 18: 422–425.
83. Weltz C, Pappas TN. Pancreatography and the surgical management of pseudo-cysts. Gastrointest Endosc Clin N Am 1995; 5: 269–279.
84. Grimm H, Binmoeller KF, Soehendra N. Endosonography-guided drainage of a pancreatic pseudocyst. Gastrointest Endosc 1992; 38: 170–171.
85. Lohr-Happe A, Peiper M, Lankisch PG. Natural course of operated pseudocysts in chronic pancreatitis. Gut 1994; 35: 1479–1482.
86. Kohler H, Schafmayer A, Ludtke FE, et al, Surgical treatment of pancreatic pseu-docysts. Br J Surg 1987; 74: 813–815.
87. Meyer W, Kohler J, Gebhardt C. Cystic neoplasms of the pancreas—cystadenomas and cystadenocarcinomas. Langenbecks Arch Surg 1999; 384: 44–49.
88. Talamini MA, Pitt HA, Hruban RH, et al. Spectrum of cystic tumors of the pan-creas. Am J Surg 1992; 163: 117–23 124.
89. Warshaw AL, Compton CC, Lewandrowski K, et al. Cystic tumors of the pan-creas. New clinical, radiologic, and pathologic observations in 67 patients. Ann Surg 1990; 212: 432–445.

90. ReMine SG, Frey D, Rossi RL, et al. Cystic neoplasms of the pancreas. Arch Surg 1987; 122: 443–446.
91. Fernandez-del Castillo C, Warshaw AL. Current management of cystic neoplasms of the pancreas. Adv Surg 2000; 34: 237–248.
92. Cubilla AL, Fitzgerald PJ. Cancer of the exocrine pancreas: the pathologic aspects. CA Cancer J Clin 1985; 35: 2–18.
93. Hammel PR, Vilgrain V, Terris B, et al. Pancreatic involvement in von Hippel-Lindau disease. The Groupe Francophone d'Etude de la Maladie de von Hippel-Lindau. Gastroenterology 2000; 119: 1087–1095.
94. Sims KB. Von Hippel-Lindau disease: gene to bedside. Curr Opin Neurol 2001; 14: 695–703.
95. Friedman AC; Lichtenstein JE, Dachman AH. Cystic neoplasms of the pancreas. Radiological-pathological correlation. Radiology 1983; 149: 45–50.
96. Itoh S, Ishiguchi T, Ishigaki T, et al. Mucin-producing pancreatic tumor: CT findings and histopathologic correlation. Radiology 1992; 183: 81–86.
97. Koito K, Namieno T, Nagakawa T, et al. Solitary cystic tumor of the pancreas: EUS-pathologic correlation. Gastrointest Endosc 1997; 45: 268–276.
98. Maguchi H, Osanai M, Yanagawa N, et al. Endoscopic ultrasonography diagnosis of pancreatic cystic disease. Endoscopy 1998; 30 (Suppl 1): A108–A110.
99. Ahmad NA, Kochman ML, Lewis JD, et al. Can EUS alone differentiate between malignant and benign cystic lesions of the pancreas? Am J Gastroenterol 2001. 96: 3295–3300.
100. Hernandez LC, Bhutani MS. Endoscopic ultrasound and pancreatic cysts: a sticky situation! Am J Gastroenterol 2001; 96: 3229–3230.
101. Wiersema MJ, Vilmann P, Giovannini M, et al. Endosonography-guided fine-needle aspiration biopsy: diagnostic accuracy and complication assessment. Gastroenterology 1997; 112: 1087–1095.
102. Bhutani MS. Endoscopic ultrasound in pancreatic diseases. Indications, limitations, and the future. Gastroenterol Clin North Am 1999; 28: 747–770.
103. Ooi LL, Ho GH, Chew SP, et al. Cystic tumours of the pancreas: a iagnostic dilemma. Aust N Z J Surg 1998; 68: 844–6.
104. Martin I, Hammond P, Scott J, et al. Cystic tumours of the pancreas. Br J Surg 1998. 85: 1484–1486.
105. Delcore R, Thomas JH, Forster J, et al. Characteristics of cystic neoplasms of the pancreas and results of aggressive surgical treatment. Am J Surg 1992; 164: 437–442.
106. Katoh H, Rossi RL, Braasch JW, et al. Cystadenoma and cystadenocarcinoma of the pancreas. Hepatogastroenterology 1989; 36: 424–430.
107. Wilentz RE, Albores-Saavedra J, Zahurak M, et al. Pathologic examination accurately predicts prognosis in mucinous cystic neoplasms of the pancreas. Am J Surg Pathol 1999; 23: 1320–1327.
108. Le Borgne J, de Calan L, Partensky C. Cystadenomas and cystadenocarcinomas of the pancreas: a multiinstitutional retrospective study of 398 cases. French Surgical Association. Ann Surg 1999; 230: 152–161.
109. Fernandez-del Castillo C, Warshaw AL. Cystic tumors of the pancreas. Surg Clin North Am 1995; 75: 1001–1016.

II   CHRONIC PANCREATITIS

9 Epidemiology of Chronic Pancreatitis

Albert B. Lowenfels, MD
and Patrick Maisonneuve, ING

CONTENTS

INTRODUCTION

Despite decades of research, the epidemiology of chronic pancreatitis (CP) remains mysterious. As in other parts of the digestive tract, it is reasonable to assume that CP develops after numerous antecedent bouts of acute pancreatitis (AP). Although generally accepted, it is difficult to document this logical sequence of events.

The etiology of CP is not completely known. In approximately 70–80% of patients, alcohol (or alcohol and smoking) is the probable cause, but it is not clear why so few heavy drinkers develop CP, or what factors predict the development of CP instead of chronic alcoholic cirrhosis.

This section reviews the data relating to the epidemiology of CP.

From: *Pancreatitis and Its Complications*
Edited by: C. E. Forsmark © Humana Press Inc., Totowa, NJ

Table 1
Number of First-Listed Hospital Discharges for Acute and Chronic
Pancreatitis (in Thousands) in the United States: 1999

				Age group (years)		
	Total	Male	Female	15–44	45–64	≥65
Acute pancreatitis	191	92	99	70	67	52
Chronic pancreatitis	27	8	12	8	7	–
Ratio acute/chronic	7.1	11.5	8.2	8.8	9.6	–

Data from ref. 1.

DESCRIPTIVE EPIDEMIOLOGY

The frequency and descriptive epidemiology of CP is poorly documented likely because: (1) The diagnosis of CP is observer-dependent; (2) the criteria for a definitive diagnosis varies from center to center and depends on the type and extent of diagnostic investigations carried out; (3) disagreement concerning the test that should be considered as the "gold standard" for the diagnosis of CP.

From hospital discharge data, information can be accumulated about the frequency of this disorder. Table 1 presents data from the United States that compares the number of patients with a hospital discharge diagnosis of CP to the number of patients with a discharge diagnosis of AP (1). In all groups, AP is more common than CP.

The same data source can be used to estimate discharge rates for patients with CP and examine time trends. Discharge rates range from about 6 to 10 per 100,000 persons per year with some fluctuation, and there are no clear time trends during the period from 1990 to 1999. The frequency of CP as recorded in different countries varies widely, but, as noted previously, it is difficult to determine how much of this variation is related to regional differences in diagnostic criteria or to the use of different denominators. Some studies have reported prevalence rates of about 3–5 per 1000 in hospitalized patients (2). Within European populations, the incidence of recently diagnosed cases per 100,000 population varies widely (3). Because alcohol consumption in combination with smoking are the major causes of CP (see below), one would predict that the frequency of CP would be closely related to variation in these two lifestyle variables.

From data reported from more than 2000 patients with CP diagnosed and treated at major referral centers in the United States and Europe, some of the main characteristics of the disease can be determined. (4; Table 2). The mean age at diagnosis of CP was 44.6 years and, as in

Table 2
Characteristics of 2015 Patients With Chronic Pancreatitis

Variable	Percent of patients with characteristic
Age at diagnosis	
<40	35%
40–59	50%
≥60	15%
Gender	
Male	79%
Female	21%
Pancreatitis type	
Alcoholic	78%
Nonalcoholic	22%
Diabetes	
Present	52%
Absent	48%
Calcification	
Present	37%
Absent	63%
Cirrhosis	
Present	10%
Absent	90%
Alcohol consumption	
Nonconsumer	12%
<5 drinks/day	26%
≥5 drinks/day	62%
Smoking status	
Ever	86%
Never	14%
Surgery[*]	
Yes	48%
No	52%
Cancer diagnosed during follow-up[*]	
No	89%
Yes	11%
Pancreas cancer	3%
Other cancer	8%

Data from ref. *4*.
[*]During mean follow-up of 7.4 years.

other series, males accounted for nearly 80% of the total group. Alcoholic pancreatitis, the most common type, was diagnosed in 1515 (75%) of patients, and most patients were heavy drinkers, consuming five or more drinks per day. Eighty-six percent of all patients were or had been smokers—much higher than the prevalence of smoking in the background population. During a mean follow-up period of 7.4 years, 11% of patients developed cancer, of which 3% were primary pancreatic tumors and 8% developed in other organs.

Regarding racial factors, we have studied the frequency of alcoholic cirrhosis and alcoholic pancreatitis in white and black populations (5). The findings suggest that there are differences in the occurrence of these two diseases in different racial groups: blacks who drink heavily are more likely to develop pancreatitis, whereas whites who consume large amounts of alcohol are more likely to develop alcoholic cirrhosis. The cause for these racial differences are unknown, but the reason may be related to racial differences in ability to detoxify carcinogens contained in tobacco smoke (6) or possibly from a result of different exposure patterns for alcohol and tobacco in varying racial groups.

ETIOLOGIC ASPECTS

Excess alcohol consumption has been linked to the onset of both AP and CP, as well as to many other digestive and nondigestive disorders. Twenty-five years ago, Durbec and Sarles noted that the logarithm of the risk of pancreatitis was linearly related to alcohol consumption (7). Recent data confirms this linear relationship as shown in the figure prepared from case-control data (8; Fig. 1). Small amounts of alcohol do not appear to cause chronic alcoholic pancreatitis, but it is not known whether or not there is a "threshold" level that must be exceeded before CP develops. Furthermore, little is known about individual variation in susceptibility to alcohol-induced CP.

Smoking and Chronic Pancreatitis

Smoking doubles the risk of pancreatic cancer (9–12) thus, it is not surprising that several studies conducted in different populations suggest that smoking is also an independent risk factor for CP (8,13–19). The results, even after corrected for alcohol consumption, show that the risk of pancreatitis in those who smoke one or more packs of cigarettes per day is about ten times higher than in light smokers or nonsmokers. The relationship may be stronger in males than in females. Both the duration and quantity of cigarettes consumed contribute to the excess risk.

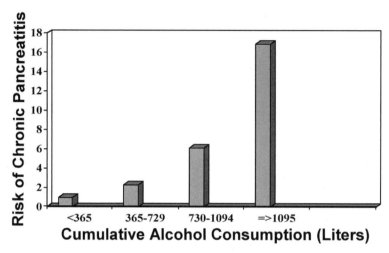

Fig. 1. Relation between alcohol consumption and risk of chronic pancreatitis. Cumulative amount of alcohol = average amount of ethanol intake per day × 365 × years of alcohol exposure. The baseline comparison group consists of nonconsumers of alcohol or consumers whose cumulative intake is less than 365 L of alcohol. Based on data from Lin and coworkers (8).

The exact mechanism to explain why smoking is related to CP has not been well-documented, but smoking appears to reduce the age at which CP is first diagnosed, and it also increases the likelihood of pancreatic calcification (Fig. 2; 15,20).

Smoking has been overlooked as an important cofactor that leads to chronic relapsing pancreatitis. Clinicians should recognize the importance of smoking as a risk factor for this disease and should urge patients who suffer from any form of pancreatitis to reduce their exposure to both tobacco and alcohol.

CHRONIC PANCREATITIS AND CANCER

Pancreatic Cancer

In many parts of the digestive tract, such as the stomach, large bowel, and liver, there is a well-developed pattern where, after many years, longstanding pre-existing benign disease progresses to cancer within the target organ. Many studies have been published to determine if this same pattern attributes to the pancreas. Gastroenterologists often remember a patient with well-documented CP who, after many years, succumbed to pancreatic cancer. Anecdotal evidence from case reports provided the stimulus for larger and stronger studies.

Several case-control studies have shown that a history of CP is more common in patients with pancreatic cancer than in control subjects. The

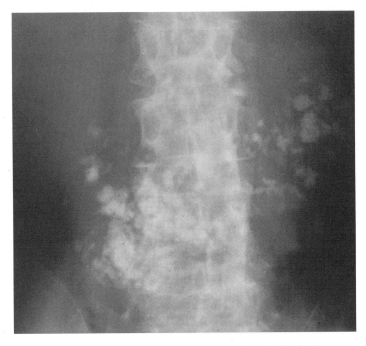

Fig. 2. In addition to alcohol, smoking also increases the risk of calcific pancreatitis.

evidence from these studies is somewhat limited because in some cancer cases, symptoms of pancreatitis can be an early manifestation of pancreatic cancer. Also, pancreatitis is an uncommon digestive event; therefore, only a few patients with pancreatic cancer will have suffered from CP. However, in general, case-control studies provide evidence that supports an association between prior attacks of CP and pancreatic cancer (21–27).

Cohort studies of patients with CP provide additional evidence for the importance of CP as an etiologic stimulus that leads to the development of pancreatic cancer. In 1993, we reported a follow-up study of more than 2000 patients with CP who were diagnosed, treated, and followed at major centers in Europe and the United States. Even after eliminating cancers arising in the first 2 years of the follow-up period, there was still an increased risk of pancreatic cancer. After a follow-up period of 7.4 years, pancreas cancer was about 16 times more common in patients with CP than in the general population (4). However, even in this high-risk population, only approximately 2% of the entire group developed pancreatic cancer. The findings in a similar, more recent, study based on a longer follow-up period were nearly identical (28). Other study types, such as record linkage studies, have also found that pancreatitis results in an increased risk of pancreatic cancer, although the estimated risk was somewhat lower than in cohort studies (29–31).

Table 3
Chronic Pancreatitis and Genetic Mutations

	Cationic trypsinogen (PRSS1)	Serine protease inhibitor (SPINK1)	CFTR
Affected chromosome	7	5	7
Inheritance pattern	Autosomal dominant	Complex: might only act as disease modifier	Autosomal recessive
Frequency in population	Extremely rare	1–3%	5%
Frequency in CP patients	About 1%	About 12%	≥20% in patients with ICP
Presence in patients with ACP	Rarely found	6%	No
Cumulative risk of pancreas cancer	40%	Likely around 5%	Likely around 5%

CP, chronic pancreatitis; CFTR, cystic fibrosis transmembrane conductance regulator; ICP, idiopathic chronic pancreatitis; ACP, alcoholic pancreatitis.

Hereditary pancreatitis (HP) is a rare autosomal dominant inherited disorder, causing symptoms and signs that closely resemble more common types of pancreatitis. HP is characterized by frequent attacks of AP, which begin during childhood or early adult life and eventually lead to CP. The cumulative lifetime risk of pancreatic cancer in these patients has been estimated to be near 40% (32). The explanation for this dramatic increase in risk is unknown.

Other Cancers

Although there appears to be a high risk of pancreatic cancer in patients with CP, the burden of other tumors is much higher. For example, in our CP cohort of 2015 subjects, 159 patients developed nonpancreatic cancer during the mean follow-up observation period when compared to 56 patients with pancreatic cancer. Most of the nonpancreatic tumors were related to smoking—an additional important risk factor for alcoholic pancreatitis (33).

GENETIC EPIDEMIOLOGY OF CHRONIC PANCREATITIS

Although chronic alcoholism is the most frequent cause of CP, mutations in several genes can also cause CP (Table 3). In 1952, Comfort and Steinberg first described a kindred with relapsing pancreatitis, which affected multiple family members and appeared to follow an autosomal dominant inheritance pattern *(34)*. In 1996, Whitcomb and coworkers discovered the cause to be a mutation in the cationic trypsinogen gene located on chromosome 7 *(35)*. The signs and symptoms of this rare hereditary type of pancreatitis are similar to more common types of pancreatitis, but the age of onset is usually before age 20, a strong family history exists, and the risk of pancreatic cancer is high.

Mutations in a pancreatic secretory trypsin inhibitor gene, *PSTI* or *SPINK1*, have also been linked to pancreatitis. The frequency of this mutation is increased in both idiopathic chronic pancreatitis (ICP) and in alcoholic chronic pancreatitis (ACP), but it is unclear whether *SPINK1* causes pancreatitis directly or by acting as a disease modifier— perhaps by increasing susceptibility to other genetic or environmental factors *(36–41)*.

Cystic fibrosis transmembrane conductance regulator *(CFTR)* mutations are now believed to cause ICP but not ACP. Genetic mutations were detected in nearly half of a sample of patients with ICP when compared to a background frequency of approximately 5% *(42)*. After detailed testing, most patients were found to carry at least one mutated gene, and some were compound heterozygotes with one mild *CFTR* mutation.

The issue of genetic testing for patients with ICP has not been resolved. Because of issues like insurance discrimination, implications for nontested family members, reproductive issues, and high-risk cancer in HP, genetic testing should be preceded and followed by genetic counseling *(43)*. Commercial testing for *CFTR* mutations usually screens only for the most common mutations and will miss many of the pancreatitis-causing mutations. The genetics of CP are discussed in more detail in Chapter 10.

SUMMARY

Even though the cumulative risk of CP is low in heavy drinkers, alcohol is the most common cause of CP, accounting for 70–80% of all cases. Recent studies suggest that smoking is also an important risk factor for CP. Additionally, mutations in genes often associated with cystic fibrosis appear to increase the probability of developing ICP.

Reliable population-based estimates of the frequency of CP are not widely available, but the evidence suggests that the incidence is approximately 5–10 per 100,000 per year—considerably lower than the incidence of AP.

Evidence from several case-control, cohort, and record linkage studies confirms that patients with CP are at increased risk of pancreatic cancer, although only about 5% of patients with common forms of pancreatitis will develop pancreatic cancer. Patients with early onset of pancreatitis, as in HP, have a high risk of developing pancreatic cancer.

ACKNOWLEDGMENTS

This research was supported in part by grants from the C.D. Smithers Foundation and Solvay Pharmaceuticals.

REFERENCES

1. Popovic JR. 1999 National Hospital Discharge Survey: Annual Summary with detailed diagnosis and procedure data. U.S. Government Printing Office, Washington, DC 2001.
2. Lankisch PG, Banks PA. Chronic Pancreatitis: Epidemiology. Pancreatitis. Springer, Berlin 1998: 219–221.
3. Dite P, Stary K, Novotny I, et al. Incidence of chronic pancreatitis in the Czech Republic. Eur J Gastroenterol Hepatol 2001; 13: 749–750.
4. Lowenfels AB, Maisonneuve P, Cavallini G, et al. Pancreatitis and the risk of pancreatic cancer. International Pancreatitis Study Group. N Engl J Med 1993; 328: 1433–1437.
5. Lowenfels AB, Maisonneuve P, Grover H, et al. Racial factors and the risk of chronic pancreatitis. Am J Gastroenterol 1999; 94: 790–794.
6. Richie JP, Carmella SG, Muscat JE, et al. Differences in the urinary metabolites of the tobacco-specific lung carcinogen 4-(methynitrosamino)-1-(3-pyridyl)-1-butanone in black and white smokers. Cancer Epidemiol Biomarkers Prev 1997; 6: 783–790.
7. Durbec JP, Sarles H. Multicenter survey of the etiology of pancreatic diseases. Relationship between the relative risk of developing chronic pancreaitis and alcohol, protein and lipid consumption. Digestion 1978; 18: 337–350.
8. Lin Y, Tamakoshi A, Hayakawa T, et al. Associations of alcohol drinking and nutrient intake with chronic pancreatitis: findings from a case-control study in Japan. Am J Gastroenterol 2001; 96: 2622–2627.
9. Boyle P, Maisonneuve P, Bueno DM, et al. Cigarette smoking and pancreas cancer: a case control study of the search programme of the IARC. Int J Cancer 1996; 67: 63–71.
10. Engeland A, Andersen A, Haldorsen T, Tretli S. Smoking habits and risk of cancers other than lung cancer: 28 years' follow-up of 26,000 Norwegian men and women. Cancer Causes Control 1996; 7: 497–506.
11. Harnack LJ, Anderson KE, Zheng W, Folsom AR, Sellers TA, Kushi LH. Smoking, alcohol, coffee, and tea intake and incidence of cancer of the exocrine pancreas: the Iowa Women's Health Study. Cancer Epidemiol Biomarkers Prev 1997; 6: 1081–1086.
12. Silverman DT, Schiffman M, Everhart J, Goldstein A, Lillemoe KD, Swanson GM et al. Diabetes mellitus, other medical conditions and familial history of cancer as risk factors for pancreatic cancer. Br J Cancer 1999; 80: 1830–1837.

13. Bourliere M, Barthet M, Berthezene P, et al. Is tobacco a risk factor for chronic pancreatitis and alcoholic cirrhosis? Gut 1991; 32: 1392–1395.
14. Hartwig W, Werner J, Ryschich E, et al. Cigarette smoke enhances ethanol-induced pancreatic injury. Pancreas 2000; 21: 272–278.
15. Imoto M, DiMagno EP. Cigarette smoking increases the risk of pancreatic calcification in late-onset but not early-onset idiopathic chronic pancreatitis. Pancreas 2000; 21: 115–119.
16. Lowenfels AB. Chronic pancreatitis, pancreatic cancer, alcohol, and smoking. Gastroenterology 1984; 87: 744–745.
17. Lowenfels AB, Zwemer FL, Jhangiani S, Pitchumoni CS. Pancreatitis in a Native American Indian population. Pancreas 1987; 2: 694–697.
18. Talamini G, Bassi C, Falconi M, et al. Cigarette smoking: an independent risk factor in alcoholic pancreatitis. Pancreas 1996; 12: 131–137.
19. Yen S, Hsieh C, MacMahon B. Consumption of alcohol and tobacco and other risk factors for pancreatitis. Am J Epidemiol 1982; 116: 407–414.
20. Cavallini G, Talamini G, Vaona B, et al. Effect of alcohol and smoking on pancreatic lithogenesis in the course of chronic pancreatitis. Pancreas 1994; 9: 42–46.
21. Boyle P, Hsieh CC, Maisonneuve P, et al. Epidemiology of pancreas cancer (1988). Int J Pancreatol 1989; 5: 327–346.
22. Bueno de Mesquita HB, Maisonneuve P, Moerman CJ, Walker AM. Aspects of medical history and exocrine carcinoma of the pancreas: a population-based case-control study in The Netherlands. Int J Cancer 1992; 52: 17–23.
23. Fernandez E, La Vecchia CL, Pora M, et al. Pancreatitis and the risk of pancreatic cancer. Pancreas 1995; 11: 185–189.
24. Ghadirian P, Simard A, Baillargeon J. Cancer of the pancreas in two brothers and one sister. Int J Pancreatol 1987; 2 (Abstract): 383–391.
25. Kalapothaki V, Tzonou A, Hsieh CC, et al. Tobacco, ethanol, coffee, pancreatitis, diabetes mellitus, and cholelithiasis as risk factors for pancreatic carcinoma. Cancer Causes Control 1993; 4: 375–382.
26. La Vecchia C, Negri E, D'Avanzo B, et al. Medical history, diet and pancreatic cancer. Oncology 1990; 47: 463–466.
27. Mack TM, Yu MC, Hanisch R, Henderson BE. Pancreas cancer and smoking, beve- rage consumption, and past medical history. JNCI 1986; 76 (Abstract): 49–60.
28. Cavallini G, Frulloni L, Pederzoli P, et al. Long-term follow-up of patients with chronic pancreatitis in Italy. Scand J Gastroenterol 1998; 33: 880–889.
29. Bansal P, Sonnenberg A. Pancreatitis is a risk factor for pancreatic cancer. Gastronenterology 1995; 109: 247–251.
30. Ekbom A, McLaughlin JK, Karlsson BM, et al. Pancreatitis and pancreatic cancer: a population-based study. J Natl Cancer Inst 1994; 86: 625–627.
31. Karlsson BM, Ekbom A, Josefsson S, et al. The risk of pancreatic cancer following pancreatitis: an association due to confounding? Gastroenterology 1997; 113: 587–592.
32. Lowenfels AB, Maisonneuve P, DiMagno EP, et al. Hereditary pancreatitis and the risk of pancreatic cancer. International Hereditary Pancreatitis Study Group. J Natl Cancer Inst 1997; 89: 442–446.
33. Lowenfels AB, Maisonneuve P, Cavallini G, et al. Prognosis of chronic pancreatitis: an international multicenter study. International Pancreatitis Study Group. Am J Gastroenterol 1994; 89: 1467–1471.
34. Comfort MW, Steinberg AG. Pedigree of a family with hereditary chronic relapsing pancreatitis. Gastroenterology 1952; 21: 54–63.

35. Whitcomb DC, Gorry MC, Preston RA, et al. Hereditary pancreatitis is caused by a mutation in the cationic trypsinogen gene. Nat Genet 1996; 14: 141–145.
36. Drenth JP, te MR, Jansen JB. Mutations in serine protease inhibitor Kazal type 1 are strongly associated with chronic pancreatitis. Gut 2002; 50: 687–692.
37. Threadgold J, Greenhalf W, Ellis I, et al. The N34S mutation of SPINK1 (PSTI) is associated with a familial pattern of idiopathic chronic pancreatitis but does not cause the disease. Gut 2002; 50: 675–681.
38. Witt H, Luck W, Becker M, et al. Mutation in the SPINK1 trypsin inhibitor gene, alcohol use, and chronic pancreatitis. JAMA 2001; 285: 2716–2717.
39. Witt H, Luck W, Hennies HC, et al. Mutations in the gene encoding the serine protease inhibitor, Kazal type 1 are associated with chronic pancreatitis. Nat Genet 2000; 25: 213–216.
40. Audrezet MP, Chen JM, Le Marechal C, et al. Determination of the relative contribution of three genes-the cystic fibrosis transmembrane conductance regulator gene, the cationic trypsinogen gene, and the pancreatic secretory trypsin inhibitor gene-to the etiology of idiopathic chronic pancreatitis. Eur J Hum Genet 2002; 10: 100–106.
41. Pfutzer RH, Barmada MM, Brunskill AP, et al. SPINK1/PSTI polymorphisms act as disease modifiers in familial and idiopathic chronic pancreatitis. Gastroenterology 2000; 119: 615–623.
42. Noone PG, Zhou Z, Silverman LM, et al. Cystic fibrosis gene mutations and pancreatitis risk: relation to epithelial ion transport and trypsin inhibitor gene mutations. Gastroenterology 2001; 121: 1310–1319.
43. Etemad B, Whitcomb DC. Chronic pancreatitis: diagnosis, classification, and new genetic developments. Gastroenterology 2001; 120: 682–707.

10 Risk, Etiology, and Pathophysiology of Chronic Pancreatitis

David C. Whitcomb, MD, PhD

INTRODUCTION

Chronic pancreatitis (CP) has been defined as a continuing inflammatory disease of the pancreas characterized by irreversible morphologic changes that typically cause pain and/or permanent loss of function *(1–3)*. Rather than a single disease, CP is a syndrome of destructive inflammatory conditions that encompasses the many sequelae of long-standing pancreatic injury *(4)*. Until recently, most research and treatment energy focused on managing end-stage CP and its complications after most of the functional pancreas was destroyed, and the patient was left with endocrine and exocrine insufficiency and chronic pain. New research is focusing on identifying environmental, genetic, and other risk factors, as well as on the inflammatory and cellular mechanisms driving the process. Furthermore, efforts are underway to improve the

From: *Pancreatitis and Its Complications*
Edited by: C. E. Forsmark © Humana Press Inc., Totowa, NJ

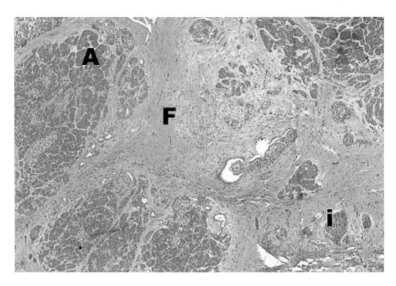

Fig. 1. Histology of chronic pancreatitis (CP). During the progression of CP the normal acini (A) are lost and replaced by progressive fibrosis (F). Note the lymphocytic infiltration associated with fibrosis. The islets (i) are relatively spared until late in the disease process.

diagnosis of CP at the earliest stages when the organ might be saved and returned toward normal.

In developed countries, CP is usually attributed to excess alcohol consumption *(4)*. However, a single factor seldom causes pancreatitis, and even prolonged excessive alcohol consumption in animal models and in most humans does not cause CP *(4)*. Instead, alcohol appears to be one of several specific environmental, metabolic, and genetic factors that play synergistic roles in increasing susceptibility to acute pancreatitis (AP) and in driving the pancreatic inflammation, fibrosis, and parenchymal destruction that eventually results in clinically recognized CP. In addition, CP may require a triggering event to initiate the inflammatory process that is a key factor in this disease *(5)*. Organizing, classifying, and understanding the major issues involved in the etiology and progression of CP will form the basis for updated methods of early detection, diagnosis, treatment, and prevention.

DIAGNOSIS

The gold standard for diagnosing CP is histology *(4)* with representative specimens demonstrating the presence of chronic inflammatory cells, acinar cell drop-out, and fibrosis (Fig. 1). Other pathological features, including duct proliferation, nerve trunk inflammation and enlargement, and distortion or loss of islets are later findings that confirm

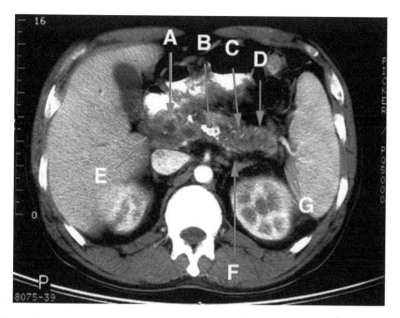

Fig. 2. Computed tomography demonstrating chronic pancreatitis (CP). Multiple complications of CP are identified through abdominal imaging techniques. This section illustrates (A) pseudocysts, (B) calcifications, (C) dilated main pancreatic duct, (D) pancreatic parenchymal atrophy, (E) dilated common bile duct, (F) splenic vein thrombosis, and (G) gastric varices. (With permission from www.pancreas.org.)

the diagnosis. Unfortunately, histology is not usually available. Instead, high-resolution imaging studies, such as computed tomography, is often used to diagnose clinically suspected CP (Fig. 2). Although major findings on imaging studies correlate with histology in moderate-to-severe CP, early diagnosis of CP remains challenging. Endoscopic ultrasound is promising, but clear and consistent criteria are yet to be developed and confirmed. Pancreatic exocrine insufficiency determined by a tubed secretin test appears to be one of the most sensitive and earliest signs of CP. However, a function test cannot always confirm the diagnosis because pancreatic insufficiency can occur without inflammation (e.g., Shwachman-Diamond syndrome and Celiac Sprue with hypoproteinemia). Thus, there remains room for improvement in the methods for diagnosing CP.

ETIOLOGY OF CHRONIC PANCREATITIS

Link Between Acute Pancreatitis and Chronic Pancreatitis

AP and CP represent opposite ends of an interrelated process. Evidence for a link between recurrent AP and CP continues to grow, bringing important insights into the mechanisms that lead to CP. The strongest evidence for this link is hereditary pancreatitis (HP; *6,7*). HP is a condition characterized by recurrent attacks of AP in approximately 80% of patients with the disease gene *(8,9)*. About half of the patients with recurrent AP progress to CP, demonstrating the connection between AP and CP. HP is caused by mutations in the cationic trypsinogen gene (protease, serine 1; *PRSS1*), causing trypsinogen to be prematurely activated to trypsin and/or preventing trypsin from being destroyed through autolysis (*see* below). Excess active trypsin inside the pancreas is pathologic because it activates other pancreatic digestive enzymes, which, in turn, cause pancreatic autodigestion and pancreatitis. Because hereditary CP appears like CP from other etiologies, and the etiology clearly involves inappropriately active trypsin and recurrent attacks of AP, the link between recurrent AP and subsequent CP is now confirmed. A similar relationship between recurrent AP and CP appears with hypertriglyceridemia, chronic hypercalcemia, and alcoholic pancreatitis. Indeed, at least one attack of AP may even be required to initiate the process that leads to CP in some cases (*see* below).

ETIOLOGY OF PANCREATITIS

Historically, CP was usually attributed to a single etiology like alcohol (~70%), idiopathic (~20%), or other rare identifiable causes (~10%). However, growing evidence suggests that alcoholic chronic pancreatitis (ACP) and idiopathic chronic pancreatitis (ICP) are complex diseases developing within the context of multiple risk factors. The evidence that ACP is a complex disease stems from the consideration of epidemiological data, animal model findings, and genetic factors. First, fewer than 10% of chronic heavy alcohol users ever develop pancreatitis *(10,11)*, whereas others develop alcoholic liver disease, neuropathy, other alcohol-associated problems, or few major consequences at all *(12)*. Second, laboratory animals fed large amounts of alcohol for prolonged periods of time fail to develop typical CP *(13,14)*, suggesting that other factors are also important. Third, the observations that heavy alcohol users from a black African background are more likely to develop pancreatic diseases than Caucasians, whereas the opposite is true for the development of liver disease *(15)*, which suggests underlying genetic susceptibility. Together, this evidence implies that ACP is a complex disease requiring cofactors, such as deleterious genetic polymorphisms, toxins, environmental stresses (particularly tobacco), or the interaction between these factors. The relative contribution of each factor may differ, and the ease of reversing or compensating for each may also differ. However, the early identification, organization, and elimination of these factors in individuals susceptible to, or developing, pancreatitis may prove to be the most inexpensive and effective therapeutic approach.

Risk Factors

Humans are highly resistant to the development of CP because numerous protective mechanisms work simultaneously and sequentially to prevent each of the pathological steps toward CP. Development of CP therefore requires either a very severe injury or the simultaneous incapacitation of several complementary protective mechanisms. Major factors that can disrupt protective mechanisms include environmental toxins, metabolic conditions, genetic variations, immune-mediated factors, and traumatic or significant duct obstruction (Table 1). Recent evidence suggests that several of these influences may occur together before CP develops *(16,17)*. In contrast, infectious diseases seldom lead to CP. The relatively obscure location of the pancreas, where it remains isolated from the external environment, and the fact that it is not associated with clearance or elimination of toxins, also protects it from a variety of direct environmental and toxic exposures experienced by the skin, respiratory system, gastrointestinal tract, liver, and kidneys. Thus, toxic–metabolic, genetic, and immune factors or duct obstruction dominate the pathophysiological landscape.

Each environmental, metabolic, or genetic factor associated with CP should be considered a *risk* factor for the development of CP. Some risk factors directly disrupt a specific protective mechanism, whereas others may disrupt several (e.g., tobacco smoking or alcohol consumption). Furthermore, the disruption or inhibition of a protective mechanism may be partial or complete, and the pancreas compensates for some insults more effectively than others. As ongoing genetic and environmental studies confirm, quantify, and identify, suspected and previously unrecognized risk factors, high-risk patients can be identified earlier, and therapeutic or preventative approaches can be initiated.

Triggering the Chronic Pancreatitis Pathological Process

There is a difference between patients with risk of a disease and those that develop a disease. In the case of CP, the difference may reflect the presence of one or two steps in a two-step process. The first step appears to be a "sentinel event" that triggers an inflammatory process within the pancreas. The second step is a prolonged or repeated injury or stress that activates the immune system and drives a progressive, destructive, and fibrotic process that ends in CP. In many cases, it has been argued that the sentinel event is an episode of AP

Table 1
Etiologic Risk Factors Associated With Chronic Pancreatitis

Toxic–Metabolic

Alcohol
Tobacco smoking
Hypercalcemia
Hyperparathyroidism
Hyperlipidemia
Chronic renal failure
Medications
    Phenacetin abuse (possibly from chronic renal insufficiency)
Toxins
    Organotin compounds (e.g., di-*n*-butyltin dichloride [DBTC])

Idiopathic

Early onset
Late onset
Tropical
    Tropical calcific pancreatitis
    Fibrocalculous pancreatic diabetes
Other

Genetic

Autosomal-dominant
    Cationic trypsinogen (*PRSS1*, e.g., codon 29 and 122 mutations)
Autosomal recessive/modifier genes
    CFTR mutations
    SPINK1 mutations

Autoimmune

Isolated autoimmune chronic pancreatitis
Syndromic autoimmune chronic pancreatitis
    Sjögrens syndrome-associated chronic pancreatitis
    Inflammatory bowel disease-associated chronic pancreatitis
    Primary biliary cirrhosis-associated chronic pancreatitis

Recurrent and Severe Acute Pancreatitis-Associated Chronic Pancreatitis

Postnecrotic (severe acute pancreatitis)
Recurrent acute pancreatitis
Vascular diseases/ischemic
Postirradiation

(continued)

Table 1 *(Continued)*

Obstructive

    Pancreatic divisum
    Sphincter of Oddi disorders (controversial)
    Duct obstruction (e.g., tumor)
    Preampullary duodenal wall cysts
    Posttraumatic pancreatic duct scars

TIGAR-O Classification system (version 1.0).
Data from ref. *4.*

(sentinel acute pancreatitis event [SAPE] hypothesis), and that fibrosis is driven by anti-inflammatory mechanisms *(5,8)*. This model will be used as a framework to discuss the various factors contributing to CP.

The Sentinel Acute Pancreatitis Event Hypothesis

The SAPE hypothesis model is illustrated in Fig. 3. On the left side of the figure, the process is described as a pathway, and on the right side, this process is illustrated. At the top of the figure is a normal pancreas, illustrated on the right as a normal acinus with acinar cells, duct cells, and quiescent (inactive) stellate cells. If a risk factor like alcohol is added, the acinar cells are injured and prone to metabolic/oxidative stress through a variety of mechanisms. However, histologically, the acinar cells and the rest of the pancreas appear remarkably normal. Fibrosis, inflammation, and destruction of acinar cells, which are the characteristics of CP, do not occur. This is likely the condition of most heavy alcohol users.

The middle section of Fig. 3 illustrates the sentinel event—an episode of AP. The sentinel event can be divided into two phases: an early proinflammatory cytotoxic phase (left side of middle acinus) and a later anti-inflammatory healing phase (right side of middle acinus). The early phase is dominated by acinar cell injury, invasion of cytotoxic lymphocytes, and monocytes/macrophages. Importantly, stellate cells are also present and become activated probably by tumor necrosis factor (TNF)-α *(18)*. In the late phase of AP, the immune system switches from proinflammatory to anti-inflammatory cytokines (e.g., interleukin-10, transforming growth factor [TGF]-β), as well as cells that serve to limit further pancreatic damage and allow the healing process to begin. As part of the healing process, active stellate cells lay down matrix proteins *(18)*, which, if this process were to continue, becomes fibrosis *(19,20)*.

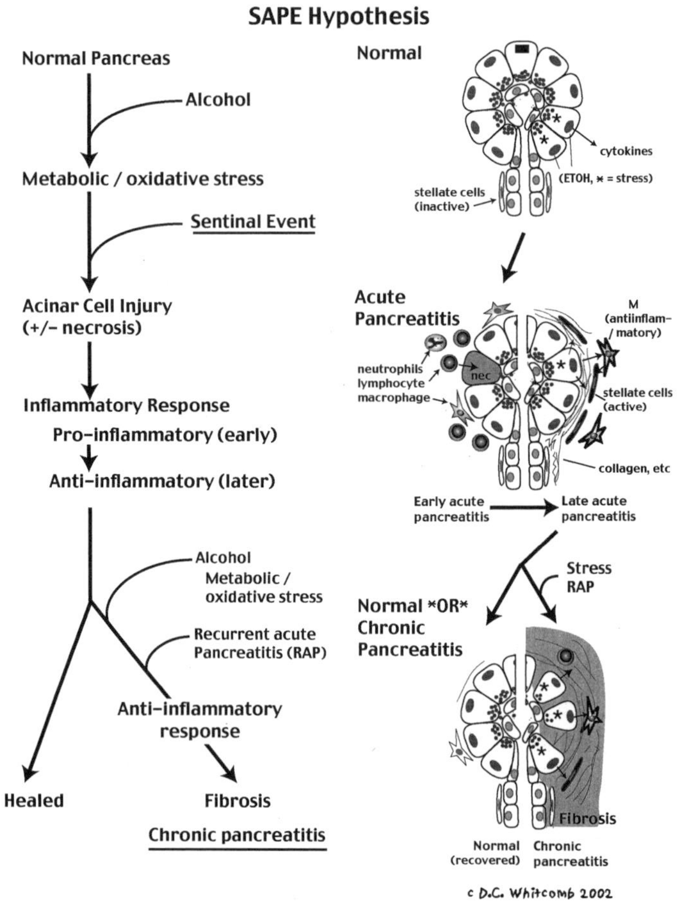

SAPE Hypothesis

Fig. 3. Sentinel acute pancreatitis event (SAPE) model. SAPE hypothesis of the etiology of chronic pancreatitis (CP). The sequential process is given on the right with corresponding cellular level illustrations of critical phases shown in three successive sections on the right. The top section represents a typical acinus under normal conditions (normal). In the presence of alcohol consumption, the acinar cells may be under metabolic stress (*), and cytokines are released (arrow), but no pathology is observed. The second section illustrates the SAPE, including early proinflammatory processes (left half of the figure) and late anti-inflammatory events (right half of the figure). Note the active lympocytes and macrophages in the early phase, and the activated stellate cells and anti-inflammatory macrophages (Mf) that dominate in the late (healing) phase. Also note the small amount of collagen that is deposited around the acinus and the continued release of cytokines by acinar cells under stress (arrow). The bottom section illustrates the recovered acinus. In the cases of biliary pancreatitis or other causes of single-episode acute pancreatitis (AP) the acinus appears normal (left side of the drawing) with residual, quiacent anti-inflammatory cells present, but slowly diminishing in number. However, with continued oxidative stress (e.g, alcohol, ischemia), recurrent pancreatitis (RAP), or similar stimuli, the tissue macrophages, and stellate cells remain active and continuously deposit collagen, matrix proteins, and other molecules that cause wide-spread fibrosis (right side of the drawing). This leads to typical CP (Adapted from ref. 5).

The lower section of Fig. 3 illustrates divergent pathways. To the left reflects healing with gradual diminution of the inflammatory cells and a return to normal. The pathway to the right illustrates progression to fibrosis and CP. The difference in pathways is determined by the presence or absence of ongoing metabolic/oxidative stress (e.g., by continued alcohol use), and/or recurrent AP (e.g., HP), or the influence of other major risk factors that result in ongoing pancreatic injury and stimulation of the inflammatory system. The difference between the acinus at the top of the figure and the bottom (postinflammatory state) is the presence of resident tissue macrophages and activated stellate cells. The presence of these cells is critical to the development of CP because the resident macrophages and other cells suppress acute inflammation by the release of anti-inflammatory cytokines, e.g., TGF-β, which drives fibrosis *(21)*. The stellate cells respond to TGF-β and other anti-inflammatory cytokines as part of the postinflammatory healing process, but if continually stimulated, they become part of a pathological process by laying down abundant extracellular matrix proteins that characterize the fibrosis of CP *(19,20)*. Thus, an appropriately severe acute pancreatitis episode plays a triggering role by initiating the critical process of recruiting the inflammatory cells into the pancreas and activating the stellate cells. From the clinician's perspective, this may be recognized as a sentinel event because it foresees the beginning of the CP pathway, and may be a signal to consider intervention.

MAJOR RISK FACTORS FOR CHRONIC PANCREATITIS

Alcohol

Alcohol consumption has been identified in many clinical case series as the most common contributing factor to CP in adults *(22–26)*. However, epidemiological data, animal data, and genetic inferences suggest that factors in addition to alcohol must be present before CP develops. On the other hand, alcohol consumption is clearly a risk factor for the development of CP *(12,25,27)*, and discontinuing alcohol use appears to slow the progression in patients with newly diagnosed alcoholic pancreatitis *(28)*.

The factors linking alcohol consumption to pancreatitis should be divided into two categories: those that increase susceptibility to AP, and those that accelerate inflammation and fibrosis. For AP, both animal models *(29)* and human studies *(30)* suggest that alcohol lowers the threshold for triggering AP and exaggerates AP once it has developed. There are multiple factors contributing to this observation and are reviewed elsewhere *(5)*. However, the risk of developing moderate AP or severe AP is clearly increased by alcohol consumption.

Alcohol also accelerates the inflammatory and fibrosis processes toward end-stage CP. Alcohol and alcoholic metabolites directly stimulate the stellate cells to secrete the complex matrix proteins (e.g., collagen and fibronectin) that are the substrate of fibrosis *(5)*. Alcohol also stimulates the immune system through the release of cytokines by stressed acinar cells. The acinar cells appear to be under constant oxidative and metabolic stress during alcohol consumption through mitochondrial injury *(31)*, production of acetaldehyde, fatty acid ethyl esters *(32,33)*, and other mechanisms. This combination of pro- and anti-inflammatory stimuli result in chronic inflammation, acinar cell loss, and fibrosis, which is eventually recognized as CP. The fact that alcohol affects both the initiation and progression of CP, and that it does so through multiple mechanisms, designates alcohol as one of the most important risk factors for developing CP. Therefore, patients with early signs of CP or with a family history of CP (*see* below) should be encouraged to stop consuming alcohol.

Tobacco Smoking

The relationship between tobacco smoking and CP has been the subject of debate for more than a decade. With few exceptions *(34)*, most evidence points to a clear association between tobacco smoking and CP *(35,36)*. These studies suggest that smoking not only increases the risk of CP, but decreases the age of onset *(37)*. The connection between tobacco smoking and alcohol consumption raised the question of whether or not these factors are independent risk factors. Recent studies suggest that tobacco smoking is an independent risk factor *(36,38)*. Therefore, patients with early signs of CP should be persuaded to stop smoking for this and other health reasons.

Chronic Renal Failure

Chronic renal failure is an important and often overlooked risk factor for CP *(4)*. Animal experiments suggest that toxins normally cleared by the kidney may be responsible for direct injury to pancreatic acinar cells *(39)*. Along with increasing the risk of CP, patients with chronic renal failure appear to have a more severe course of AP with significantly increased morbidity and mortality *(40)*. Although the relationship between chronic renal failure and CP has not been fully explained, the appearance of signs of AP and CP in a patient with chronic renal failure should prompt close attention to the management of the kidney disease.

Genetic Factors

Genetic influences are clearly major risk factors for CP. The three major genetic mutations leading to CP include mutations in the cystic fibrosis transmembrane conductant regulator gene (*CFTR*), cationic trypsinogen gene (*PRSS1*), and the pancreatic secretory trypsin inhibitor (serine protease inhibitor, Kazal-type, 1; *SPINK1*; *41*).

CYSTIC FIBROSIS TRANSMEMBRANE CONDUCTANT REGULATOR GENE MUTATIONS

The *CFTR* gene was discovered during the search for the cause of cystic fibrosis *(42–44)*. Severe mutations in *CFTR* genes, such as *CFTR* delF508, causes typical cystic fibrosis characterized by pancreatic insufficiency, maldigestion, and intestinal problems early in infancy, along with pulmonary pathology in childhood related to chronic inflammation. The *CFTR* molecule functions as a cyclic AMP-regulated anion channel with the highest permeability to chloride but also to bicarbonate that is critical to the proper function of epithelial cells lining the pancreatic duct, intestine, airway, and other sites. To date, more than 1200 mutations have been identified in the *CFTR* gene in patients with typical and atypical cystic fibrosis. The functional consequence of these mutations varies widely, resulting in the need to classify the mutations according to consequence of the mutation on the protein and its function *(45)*. Class I, II, and III mutations are severe, resulting in complete loss of function *(45,46)*. Class IV, V, and VI and progressively milder mutations *(46)*. Retention of some *CFTR* function through inheritance of one severe mutation and one mild mutation results in a clinical syndrome that differs from classic cystic fibrosis (e.g., atypical cystic fibrosis; *47,48*). In this case, the underlying genetic disorder may be completely silent until the epithelial cell-lined organs are stressed through additional genetic factors (e.g., modifier genes) or environmental insults. Indeed, many cases of ICP have been found to be associated with mild mutations in the *CFTR* gene *(16,49–51)*.

Although resent research demonstrated an association between *CFTR* mutations and some cases of ICP (or unrecognized atypical cystic fibrosis), most experts do not believe enough is known about the interpretation of results in *CFTR* genetic testing to order these tests in routine clinical settings *(49)*. Surveys of the parents of children with cystic fibrosis failed to identify an increased incidence of idiopathic pancreatitis, suggesting that having one severe *CFTR* mutation (i.e., an ~50% predicted decrease in function) is insufficient to cause AP or CP *(52)*. However, even a single severe *CFTR* mutation may increase the risk of pancreatitis when present with another mutation (*16*; e.g., *CFTR* mutation and *SPINK1* mutations, *see* below) or other pancreatic stresses, such as functional duct obstruction in pancreatic divisum. Furthermore, clinical *CFTR* tests are directed toward the most common and severe mutations; thus, important mutations associated with CP may be missed *(49)*. Finally, accurate medical and genetic counseling to patients with a single *CFTR* gene mutation on screening panels is almost uninterpretable at the present time. The addition of functional testing with nasal bioelectrical responses or other tests can be helpful in diagnosing mild cystic fibrosis, but these techniques are generally unavailable *(48,53,54)*. Therefore, *CFTR* mutations are clearly associated with idiopathic pancreatitis, but more research is needed to assist in interpreting the many possible findings and determining the proper course of action based on these results. In some cases, referral to a major center with expertise in cystic fibrosis and availability of nasal bioelectrical response measurements may also be appropriate.

CATIONIC TRYPOSINOGEN GENE MUTATIONS

Mutations in the *PRSS1* gene are responsible for approximately 60% of all cases of HP, and are also sometimes associated with ICP *(55)*. Trypsinogen is the proenzyme that becomes trypsin, a pancreatic digestive enzyme that has a key role in pancreatic physiology. Trypsin hydrolyzes peptide chains at arginine or lysine residues. The trypsin enzyme itself consists of two globular domains linked by a single peptide chain with a central arginine residue at position 122. Cutting the side chain (autolysis loop) at arginine 122 with another trypsin enzyme is the first step in the autolysis of trypsin.

Trypsin is the major enzyme that activates pancreatic digestive enzymes within the intestine. It is also the first proenzyme to be activated in the intestine because it is the only enzyme with a special four-aspartamine residue motif in the activation site, which is the target of the brush border enzyme, enterokinase. After trypsinogen is activated, it then activates most of the other pancreatic digestive enzymes, which, in turn, digest the complex molecules of a meal for absorption. Premature activation of trypsin in the pancreas with subsequent activation of other digestive enzymes is thought to be the initial step in triggering AP *(56,57)*. Therefore, the body uses a number of protective mechanisms to prevent trypsin from becoming activated, remaining activated, or prevent the spread of the activation process. Disruption of these protective mechanisms increases the risk of pancreatitis.

Mutations in the trypsinogen gene predispose to AP and CP *(7,58)*. The first mutation to be identified was in codon 122, leading to the substitution of a histidine for the key arginine (R122H) in the connecting side chain *(6)*. In this case, prematurely activated mutant trypsin cannot be destroyed through the normal self-destruction mechanism and remains active, activating itself and other digestive proenzymes in the pancreas. Interestingly, trypsin contains a calcium-binding site near R122. In a high-calcium environment, this site is occupied by the calcium ion, an interaction develops with the autolysis loop, and autolysis of trypsin is prevented. This feature is beneficial in the intestine because trypsin activity is necessary in the duodenum and jejunum, where calcium levels are high. But as calcium is absorbed in the jejunum, the large proteins are digested, and trypsin is no longer needed. The calcium-associated protection of trypsin autolysis is lost and trypsin degrades itself. However, high-calcium levels within the pancreas also protect trypsin from autodigestion and result in a condition similar to the R122H or R122C mutation.

Several other mutations have also been identified in the trypsinogen gene that lead to pancreatitis (59), and they tend to be grouped around the activation peptide region or the autolysis loop. These observations suggest that enhanced activation or reduced inhibition of trypsin is a key factor in increasing the risk for pancreatitis in affected individuals. Most of these mutations are rare with the exception of R122H and N29I (6,7).

Currently, there are no specific treatments for patients with trypsinogen mutations and pancreatitis. The diagnosis can be made by genetic testing, and guidelines have been recently published (60). The primary indications for cationic trypsinogen mutation testing include recurrent idiopathic acute pancreatitis, ICP, verification of a clinical suspicion in a family member of a kindred with known mutations, as well as to help a patient understand or validate their condition and assist individuals in making lifestyle decisions based on the known risk of pancreatitis and pancreatic cancer. Genetic testing is also used in children with unexplained pancreatitis or episodes of pancreatitis-like pain when there is significant concern about potential HP (4,60). Indeed, identification of an established pancreatitis-associated gene mutation can be valuable in expediting an often expensive and prolonged evaluation of recurrent pancreatitis in children and precludes further evaluation of elusive pancreatitis causes in adults. Currently, general recommendations include avoiding alcohol and tobacco abuse and large fatty meals. Antioxidants, vitamins, and enzyme supplements have been used with antidotal success, but formal scientific proof of their effectiveness is pending.

PANCREATIC SECRETORY TRYPSIN INHIBITOR GENE MUTATIONS

PSTI, also known as *SPINK1*, plays a major protective role in the pancreas by inhibiting prematurely activated trypsinogen (61,62). *SPINK1* is synthesized in pancreatic acinar cells and other sites (62).

SPINK1 normally inhibits trypsin by directly blocking the active catalytic site. *SPINK1* is a specific inhibitor for trypsin because it contains a key lysine that serves as "bait" for active trypsin. *SPINK1* forms a stable complex with trypsin, blocking the reactive site of trypsin. The binding is reversible, and *SPINK1* is also slowly digested by trypsin *(62)*. *SPINK1* is thought to serve as the first line of defense against trypsin, which is prematurely activated within the pancreas with trypsin autolysis at R122 acting as a fail-safe second line of protection *(6)*. The protective capacity of *SPINK1* is limited, however, because the inhibitory mechanism with trypsin requires a one-to-one relationship, and trypsin is synthesized in great excess of *SPINK1* *(62)*. However, *SPINK1* is an acute-phase reactive protein, and expression is markedly upregulated during inflammation *(63)*. This feature may limit the extent of AP attacks by providing more inhibitory capacity when it is needed the most.

A number of mutations have been identified in the *SPINK1* gene *(59)*, but the N34S mutation is the most important *(64,65)*. Interestingly, the N34S mutation is found worldwide with a incidence in most populations between 1 and 4% *(41)*. *SPINK1* mutations alone does not appear to cause pancreatitis, because the incidence of AP and CP is much lower than the incidence of *SPINK1* mutations *(41,65)*. As *SPINK1* forms the first line of defense against active trypsin, and a second fail-safe mechanism exists, widespread trypsin activation and the effects of triggering the enzyme activation cascade seldom occurs. However, if active trypsin frequently circumvents the first line of defense, the risk of pancreatitis is increased, especially if calcium levels are elevated and the second line of defense is blocked (*see* above). Thus, *SPINK1* mutations increase the risk of pancreatitis but are not directly disease-causing *(65)*.

The association between *SPINK1* mutations and various types of pancreatitis is quite variable. *SPINK1* mutations are most often seen in childhood onset CP, tropical calcific pancreatitis, and a subtype of tropical pancreatitis fibrocalculous pancreatic diabetes, where diabetes mellitus is the first major clinical sign leading to diagnosis *(66)*. Approximate frequencies include 36% of patients with fibrocalculous pancreatic diabetes, and 33% of tropical calcific pancreatitis have *SPINK1* mutations. *SPINK1* mutations are also seen in some kindreds with familial pancreatitis (6%), ACP (6%), ICP (17%, particularly at young age of onset), and young onset noninsulin dependent diabetes mellitus in Bangladesh and Southern Asia (11%). The observation that *SPINK1* mutations are associated with a variety of different types of pancreatitis, but occur in a minority of cases, suggest that common

SPINK1 mutations increase susceptibility, but also that other genetic and/or environmental risk factors are essential.

Because the risk of pancreatitis from *SPINK1* mutations in unaffected individuals is very low (<1%), genetic testing is not recommended *(4,60)*. However, testing is sometimes offered to individuals with established pancreatic disease to help determine the risk factors contributing to a case of pancreatitis. Treatments options are similar to those for cationic trypsinogen mutations (*see* above).

Autoimmune Chronic Pancreatitis

Autoimmune CP differs from other forms of chronic pancratitis in histological, morphological, and clinical features *(4)*. Autoimmune pancreatitis may be isolated or occasionally seen in association with Sjögren's syndrome *(67,68)*, primary biliary cirrhosis *(67)*, primary sclerosing cholangitis *(68–71)*, Crohn's disease and ulcerative colitis *(68,72)*, or other immune-mediated disorders.

Histologically, the ductal lesions in the pancreas resemble those seen in the salivary glands involved in autoimmune sialadenitis with destruction of the duct, fibrosis, and atrophy of the acinar tissue without calcifications *(73)*. There may be lymphocytic infiltration, plasma cells, and fibrosis *(74)*. Computed tomography or ultrasound of the pancreas usually demonstrate a diffusely enlarged gland with poor- or delayed-contrast enhancement *(74–76)*. Endoscopic retrograde cholangiopancreatography (ERCP) may show diffuse narrowing of the main pancreatic duct with an irregular duct margin *(74,76)*.

Autoantibody profiling in autoimmune pancreatitis may be helpful *(77)*, including elevated IgG4, antinuclear and antilactoferrin antibodies (~75%), anticarbonic anhydrase II antibodies (~60%), rheumatoid factor (~30%), and antismooth muscle antibodies (~18%), but not antimitochondrial antibodies. CD8- and CD4-positive cells were also elevated in the peripheral blood, suggesting a Th1 type immune response *(77)*.

Autoimmune CP therefore represents a distinct form of CP. This diagnosis is important to make because these patients appear to respond promptly to oral steroid therapy *(74,76,77)*.

Recurrent and Severe Acute Pancreatitis

Recurrent AP and SAP can lead to CP. This association has been established by careful clinicopathologic studies *(78)*, pathological arguments *(73,79)*, some animal work *(80)*, and HP *(6,7)* as noted previously. Indeed, completed recovery from SAP does not always occur *(81)*, and long-standing changes consistent with CP may be seen in these cases.

OBSTRUCTIVE CHRONIC PANCREATITIS

Obstructive CP is a distinct morphological form of CP associated with pancreatic duct dilation proximal to obstruction, atrophy of acinar cells, and a uniform diffuse fibrosis replacing the pancreatic parenchyma *(82)*. It is a pathologically distinct form of pancreatitis *(73)*. Many entities have been associated with obstructive CP, including sequelae of AP, trauma, tumor, sphincter of Oddi dysfunction, and pancreas divisum *(83–86)*. The histological and functional changes associated with this form of CP may be partially or fully reversible if the obstructive process is treated early enough *(82)*.

Chronic Pancreatitis and the Risk of Pancreatic Cancer

Long-standing CP increases the risk of pancreatic cancer *(87)*, just as long-standing ulcerative colitis increases the risk of colon cancer, chronic liver cirrhosis increases the risk of hepatocellular cancer, chronic gastritis increases the risk of gastric cancer, and so on. The risk of pancreatic cancer is increased in HP *(88)*, cystic fibrosis *(89)*, tropical pancreatitis *(90,91)* and CP in general *(87,92)*.

It appears that pancreatic cancer in these cases is similar in genetic alterations to sporadic pancreatic cancer, but that the rate of mutation accumulation in the premalignant cells is accelerated *(87)*. This process can be accelerated even faster with the addition of other risk factors. In HP, for example, the age- and sex-adjusted odds ratio of developing pancreatic cancer is doubled by tobacco smoking, and the median age of diagnosis of pancreatic cancer is 20 years earlier in smokers *(93,94)*!

To date, no effective screening method has been developed to detect and treat early pancreatic cancers in patients with CP. A consensus statement on pancreatic cancer in patients with HP was recently published *(95)* but offers little hope. Further work in this area is needed.

SUMMARY AND CONCLUSIONS

CP can be a severe and disabling disease. Treatment options for advanced cases remain limited to exogenous replacement of lost endocrine and exocrine function and attempts to control pain through medications, endoscopic therapy, surgery, and some experimental approaches. Preferably, individuals progressing toward CP could be identified early, the underlying risk factors and etiologies identified, and effective preventative strategies adopted. In general, therapies are aimed at limiting oxidative stress on the pancreas, reducing excessive pancreatic stimulation through smaller meals and pancreatic enzyme supplements, and eliminating known risk factors, such as alcohol consumption and tobacco smoking. Evidence-based guidelines are slow in coming, partly because the disease progression is often slow, patients are dissimilar, and the number of patients at any one center is limited. However, recently renewed research interest and conceptual break-throughs will likely lead to better approaches in the future.

REFERENCES

1. Sarles H. Pancreatitis: Symposium of Marseille, 1963. Karger, Basel, 1965.
2. Sarner M. Pancreatitis definitions and classification. In: Vay Liang W, Go EPD, Gardner JD, et al., eds. editor. The Pancreas: Pathobiology and Disease, second edition. Raven Press, New York, 1993: 575–580.
3. Clain JE, Pearson RK. Diagnosis of chronic pancreatitis: Is a gold standard necessary? Surg Clin North Am 1999; 79: 829–845.
4. Etemad B, Whitcomb DC. Chronic pancreatitis: Diagnosis, classification, and new genetic developments. Gastroenterology 2001; 120: 682–707.
5. Schneider A, Whitcomb DC. Hereditary pancreatitis: a model for inflammatory diseases of the pancreas. Best Pract Res Clin Gastroenterol 2002; 16: 347–363.
6. Whitcomb DC, Gorry MC, Preston RA, et al. Hereditary pancreatitis is caused by a mutation in the cationic trypsinogen gene. Nat Genet 1996; 14: 141–145.
7. Gorry MC, Gabbaizedeh D, Furey W, et al. Mutations in the cationic trypsinogen gene are associated with recurrent acute and chronic pancreatitis. Gastroenterology 1997; 113: 1063–1068.
8. Whitcomb DC. Hereditary panceatitis: New insights into acute and chronic pancreatitis. Gut 1999; 45: 317–322.
9. Whitcomb DC. Genetic predispositions to acute and chronic pancreatitis. Med Clin North Am 2000; 84: 531–547.
10. Bisceglie AM, Segal I. Cirrhosis and chronic pancreatitis in alcoholics. J Clin Gastroenterol 1984; 6: 199–200.
11. Gumaste VV. Alcoholic pancreatitis: unraveling the mystery. Gastroenterology 1995; 108: 297–299.
12. Corrao G, Bagnardi V, Zambon A, Arico S. Exploring the dose-response relationship between alcohol consumption and the risk of several alcohol-related conditions: a meta-analysis. Addiction 1999; 94: 1551–1573.
13. Perkins PS, Rutherford RE, Pandol SJ. Effect of chronic ethanol feeding on digestive enzyme synthesis and mRNA content in rat pancreas. Pancreas 1995; 10: 14–21.
14. Niebergall-Roth E, Harder H, Singer MV. A Review: Acute and chronic effects of ethanol and alcoholic beverages on the pancreatic exocrine secretion in vivo and in vitro. Alcohol Clin Exp Res 1998; 22: 1570–1583.
15. Lowenfels AB, Maisonneuve P, Grover H, et al. Racial factors and the risk of chronic pancreatitis. Am J Gastroenterol 1999; 94: 790–794.
16. Noone PG, Zhou Z, Silverman LM, et al. Cystic fibrosis gene mutations and pancreatitis risk: relation to epithelial ion transport and trypsin inhibitor gene mutations. Gastroenterology 2001; 121: 1310–1319.
17. Etemad B. Gastrointestinal complications of renal failure. Gastroenterol Clin North Am 1998; 27: 875–892.
18. Mews P, Phillips P, Fahmy R, et al. Pancreatic stellate cells respond to inflammatory cytokines: potential role in chronic pancreatitis. Gut 2002; 50: 535–541.
19. Bachem MG, Schneider E, Gross H, et al. Identification, culture, and characterization of pancreatic stellate cells in rats and humans. Gastroenterology 1998; 115: 421–432.

20. Apte MV, Haber PS, Applegate TL, et al. Periacinar stellate shaped cells in rat pancreas: identification, isolation, and culture. Gut 1998; 43: 128–133.
21. Van Laethem J, Robberecht P, Resibois A, Deviere J. Transforming growth factor beta promotes development of fibrosis after repeated courses of acute pancreatitis in mice. Gastroenterology 1996; 110: 576–582.
22. Owyang C, Levitt M. Chronic Pancreatitis. In: Yamada T, ed. Textbook of Gastroenterology. J.B. Lippencott Co, Philadelphia PA; 1991: 1874–1893.
23. Lin Y, Tamakoshi A, Matsuno S, et al. Nationwide epidemiological survey of chronic pancreatitis in Japan. J Gastroenterol 2000; 35: 136–141.
24. Mergener K, Baillie J. Chronic pancreatitis. Lancet 1997; 340: 1379–1385.
25. Dani R, Penna FJ, Nogueira CE. Etiology of chronic calcifying pancreatitis in Brazil: a report of 329 consecutive cases. Int J Pancreatol 1986; 1: 399–406.
26. Whitcomb DC, Pfützer RH, Slivka A. Alcoholic chronic pancreatitis. Curr Treatment Opin Gastroenterol 1999; 2: 273–282.
27. Durbec J, Sarles H. Multicenter survey of the etiology of pancreatic diseases. Relationship between the relative risk of developing chronic pancreatitis and alcohol, protein and lipid consumption. Digestion 1978; 18: 337–350.
28. Gullo L, Barbara L, Labo G. Effect of cessation of alcohol use on the course of pancreatic dysfunction in alcoholic pancreatitis. Gastroenterology 1988; 95: 1063–1068.
29. Pandol SJ, Periskic S, Gukovsky I, et al. Ethanol diet increases the sensitivity of rats to pancreatitis induced by cholecystokinin octapeptide. Gastroenterology 1999; 117: 706–716.
30. Jaakkola M, Sillanaukee P, Lof K, et al. Amount of alcohol is an important determinant of the severity of acute alcoholic pancreatitis. Surgery 1994; 115: 31–38.
31. Li HS, Zhang JY, Thompson BS, et al. Rat mitochondrial ATP synthase ATP5G3: cloning and upregulation in pancreas after chronic ethanol feeding. Physiol Genomics 2001; 6: 91–98.
32. Werner J, Laposata M, Fernandez, del CC, Saghir M, Iozzo RV, et al. Pancreatic injury in rats induced by fatty acid ethyl ester, a nonoxidative metabolite of alcohol. Gastroenterology 1997; 113: 286–294.
33. Pfützer RH, Tadic SD, Li HS, et al. Pancreatic cholesterol esterase, ES-10 and fatty acid ethyl ester synthase gene expression are increased in pancreas and liver, but not in brain or heart with long-term ethanol feeding in rats. Pancreas 2002; 25: 101–106.
34. Haber PS, Wilson JS, Pirola RC. Smoking and alcoholic pancreatitis. Pancreas 1993; 8: 568–572.
35. Lin Y, Tamakoshi A, Hayakawa T, et al. Cigarette smoking as a risk factor for chronic pancreatitis: a case-control study in Japan. Research Committee on Intractable Pancreatic Diseases. Pancreas 2000; 21: 109–114.
36. Talamini G, Bassi C, Falconi M, et al. Cigarette smoking: an independent risk factor in alcoholic pancreatitis. Pancreas 1996; 12: 131–137.
37. Bourliere M, Barthet M, Berthezene P, et al. Is tobacco a risk factor for chronic pancreatitis and alcoholic cirrhosis? Gut 1991; 32: 1392–1395.
38. Talamini G, Bassi C, Falconi M, et al. Alcohol and smoking as risk factors in chronic pancreatitis and pancreatic cancer. Dig Dis Sci 1999; 44: 1301–1311.
39. Lerch MM, Hoppe-Seyler P, Gerok W. Origin and development of exocrine pancreatic insufficiency in experimental renal failure. Gut 1994; 35: 401–407.
40. Pitchumoni CS, Arguello P, Agarwal N, Yoo J. Acute pancreatitis in chronic renal failure. Am J Gastroenterol 1996; 91: 2477–2482.
41. Whitcomb DC. How to think about SPINK and pancreatitis. Am J Gastroenterol 2002; 97: 1085–1088.

42. Riordan JR, Rommens JM, Kerem B, et al. Identification of the cystic fibrosis gene: cloning and characterization of complementary DNA. Science 1989; 245: 1066–1073.
43. Kerem B, Rommens JM, Buchanan JA, et al. Identification of the cystic fibrosis gene: genetic analysis. Science 1989; 245: 1073–1080.
44. Levitan IB. The basic defect in cystic fibrosis. Science 1989; 244: 1423.
45. Zielenski J, Tsui LC. Cystic fibrosis: genotypic and phenotypic variations. An Rev Genet 1995; 29: 777–807.
46. Mickle JE, Cutting GR. Genotype-phenotype relationships in cystic fibrosis. Med Clin North Am 2000; 84: 597–607.
47. Kristidis P, Bozon D, Corey M, et al. Genetic determination of exocrine pancreatic function in cystic fibrosis. Am J Hum Genet 1992; 50: 1178–1182.
48. Stern RC. The diagnosis of cystic fibrosis. N Engl J Med 1997; 336: 487–491.
49. Cohn JA, Bornstein JD, Jowell PS. Cystic fibrosis mutations and genetic predisposition to idiopathic chronic pancreatitis. Med Clin North Am 2000; 84: 621–631.
50. Cohn J, Friedman K, Silverman L, et al. CFTR mutations predispose to chronic pancreatitis without cystic fibrosis lung disease. Gastroenterology 1997; 112 (Abstract): A434.
51. Sharer N, Schwarz M, Malone G, et al. Mutations of the cystic fibrosis gene in patients with chronic pancreatitis. N Eng J Med 1998; 339: 645–652.
52. Lowenfels A, Maisonneuve P, Palys B, et al. Mutations of cystic fibrosis gene in pantients with pancreatitis. Am J Gastroenterol 2001;96(2):614–615.
53. Knowles MR, Paradiso AM, Brocher RC. In vivo nasal potential differences: Techniques and protocols for assessing efficacy of gene transfer in cystic fibrosis. Hum Gene Ther 1995; 6: 445–455.
54. Southern KW, Noone PG, Bosworth DG, et al. A modified technique for measrument of nasal transepithelial potential difference in infants. J Pediatr 2001; 139: 353–358.
55. Applebaum-Shapiro SE, Finch R, Pfützer RH, et al. Hereditary pancreatitis in North America: the Pittsburgh-Midwest Multi-Center Pancreatic Study Group Study. Pancreatology 2001; 1 : 439–443.
56. Steer ML, Meldolesi J. Pathogenesis of acute pancreatitis. Annu Rev Med 1988; 39: 95–105.
57. Grendell JH. Acute pancreatitis. Curr Opin Gastroenterol 1997; 13: 381–385.
58. Whitcomb DC, Gorry MC, Preston RA, et al. A gene for hereditary pancreatitis maps to chromosome 7q35. Gastroenterology 1996; 110: 1975–1980.
59. Teich N, Mössner J, Keim V. Systematac overview of genetic variants of cationic trypsinogen and SLONK1 in pancreatitis patients. In: Durie P, Lerch MM, Lowenfels AB, et al., ed. Genetic Disorders of the Exocrine Pancreas: An Overview and Update. Karger, Basel, 2002: 20–22.
60. Ellis I, Lerch MM, Whitcomb DC, Committee C. Genetic testing for hereditary pancreatitis: guidelines for indications, counseling, consent and privacy issues. Pancreatology 2001; 1: 401–411.
61. Colomb E, Figarella C, Guy O. The two human trypsinogens. Evidence of complex fromation with basic pancreatic trypsin inhibitor-proteolytic activity. Biochim Biophys Acta 1979; 570: 397–405.
62. Rinderknecht H. Pancreatic Secretory Enzymes. In: Go VLW, DiMagno EP, Gardner JD, et al, ed. The Pancreas: Biology, Pathobiology, and Disease, second edition. Raven Press, New York, 1993: 219–251.
63. Ogawa M. Pancreatic secretory trypsin inhibitor as an acute phase reactant. Clin Biochem 1988; 21: 19–25.

64. Witt H, Luck W, Hennies HC, et al. Mutations in the gene encoding the serine protease inhibitor, kazal type 1 are associated with chronic pancreatitis. Nat Genet 2000; 25: 213–216.

65. Pfützer RH, Barmada MM, Brunskil APJ, et al. SPINK1/PSTI polymorphisms act as disease modifiers in familial and idiopathic chronic pancreatitis. Gastroenterology 2000; 119: 615–623.

66. Rossi L, Pfützer RL, Parvin S, et al. SPINK1/PSTI mutations are associated with tropical pancreatitis in Bangladesh: A preliminary report. Pancreatology 2001; 1: 242–245.

67. Epstein O, Chapman RW, Lake-Bakaar G, et al. The pancreas in primary biliary cirrhosis and primary sclerosing cholangitis. Gastroenterology 1982; 83: 1177–1182.

68. Ectors N, Maillet B, Aerts R, et al. Non-alcoholic duct destructive chronic pancreatitis. Gut 1997; 41: 263–268.

69. Kawaguchi K, Koike M, Tsuruta K, et al. Lymphoplasmacytic sclerosing pancreatitis with cholangitis: a variant of primary sclerosing cholangitis extensively involving pancreas. Hum Pathol 1991; 22: 387–395.

70. Takikawa H, Manabe T. Primary sclerosing cholangitis in Japan—analysis of 192 cases. J Gastroenterol 1997; 32: 134–137.

71. Schimanski U, Stiehl A, Stremmel W, Theilmann L. Low prevalence of alterations in the pancreatic duct system in patients with primary sclerosing cholangitis. Endoscopy 1996; 28: 346–349.

72. Barthet M, Hastier P, Bernard JP, et al. Chronic pancreatitis and inflammatory bowel disease: true or coincidental association? Am J Gastroenterol 1999; 94: 2141–2148.

73. Kloppel G, Maillet B. Pathology of acute and chronic pancreatitis. Pancreas 1993; 8: 659–670.

74. Furukawa N, Muranaka T, Yasumori K, et al. Autoimmune pancreatitis: radiologic findings in three histologically proven cases. J Comput Assist Tomogr 1998; 22: 880–883.

75. Irie H, Honda H, Baba S, et al. Autoimmune pancreatitis: CT and MR characteristics. Am J Roentgenol 1998; 170: 1323–1327.

76. Ito T, Nakano I, Koyanagi S, et al. Autoimmune pancreatitis as a new clinical entity. Three cases of autoimmune pancreatitis with effective steroid therapy. Dig Dis Sci 1997; 42: 1458–1468.

77. Okazaki K, Uchida K, Ohana M, et al. Autoimmune-related pancreatitis is associated with autoantibodies and a Th1/Th2-type cellular immune response. Gastroenterology 2000; 118: 573–581.

78. Ammann RW, Muellhaupt B. Progression of alcoholic acute to chronic pancreatitis. Gut 1994; 35: 552–556.

79. Kloppel G, Maillet B. A morphological analysis of 57 resection specimens and 9 autopsy pancreata. Pancreas 1991; 6: 266–274.

80. Freiburghaus AU, Redha F, Ammann RW. Does acute pancreatitis progress to chronic pancreatitis? A microvascular pancreatitis model in the rat. Pancreas 1995; 11: 374–381.

81. Seidensticker F, Otto J, Lankisch PG. Recovery of the pancreas after acute pancreatitis is not necessarily complete. Int J Pancreatol 1995; 17: 225–229.

82. Sarles H. Etiopathogenesis and definition of chronic pancreatitis. Dig Dis Sci 1986; 31: 91S–107S.

83. Bradley ELd. Chronic obstructive pancreatitis as a delayed complication of pancreatic trauma. HPB Surg 1991; 5: 49–60.

84. Lowes JR, Rode J, Lees WR, et al. Obstructive pancreatitis: unusual causes of chronic pancreatitis. Br J Surg 1988; 75: 1129–1133.
85. Odaira C, Choux R, Payan MJ, et al. Chronic obstructive pancreatitis, nesidioblastosis, and small endocrine pancreatic tumor. Dig Dis Sci 1987; 32: 770–774.
86. Tarnasky PR, Hoffman B, Aabakken L, et al. Sphincter of Oddi dysfunction is associated with chronic pancreatitis. Am J Gastroenterol 1997; 92: 1125–1129.
87. Whitcomb DC, Pogue-Geile K. Pancreatitis as a risk for pancreatic cancer. Gastroenterol Clin North Am 2002; 31: 663–678.
88. Lowenfels A, Maisonneuve P, DiMagno E, et al. Hereditary pancreatitis and the risk of pancreatic cancer. J Nat Cancer Inst 1997; 89: 442–446.
89. Neglia JP, FitzSimmons SC, Maisonneuve P, et al. The risk of cancer among patients with cystic fibrosis. Cystic Fibrosis and Cancer Study Group. N Engl J Med 1995; 332: 494–499.
90. Augustine P, Ramesh H. Is tropical pancreatitis premalignant? Am J Gastroenterol 1992; 87: 1005–1008.
91. Chari ST, Mohan V, Pitchumoni CS, et al. Risk of pancratic carcinoma in tropical calcifying pancreatitits: an epidemicologic study. Pancreas 1994; 9: 62–66.
92. Lowenfels AB, Maisonneuve P, Cavallini G, et al. Pancreatitis and the risk of pancreatic cancer. International Pancreatitis Study Group. N Eng J Med 1993; 328: 1433–1437.
93. Lowenfels AB, Maisonneuve P, Whitcomb DC, et al. Cigarette smoking as a risk factor for pancreatic cancer in patients with hereditary pancreatitis. JAMA 2001; 286: 169–170.
94. Lowenfels AB, Maisonneuve P, Whitcomb DC. Risk factors for cancer in hereditary pancreatitis. International Hereditary Pancreatitis Study Group. Med Clin North Am 2000; 84: 565–573.
95. Ulrich II CD. Pancreatic cancer in hereditary pancreatitis—Consensus guidelines for prevention, screening, and treatment. Pancreatology 2001; 1: 416–422.

11 Natural History of Chronic Pancreatitis

Supot Pongprasobchai, MD
and Jonathan E. Clain, MD

CONTENTS

INTRODUCTION
CLINICAL PRESENTATION AT ONSET OF DISEASE
CLINICAL COURSE
SPECIAL FORMS OF CHRONIC PANCREATITIS
SUMMARY
REFERENCES

INTRODUCTION

The most common form of chronic pancreatitis (CP) in the Western world is alcoholic chronic pancreatitis (ACP), which represents 70–90% of patients with CP. Nearly all of the remaining patients (10–30%) are usually designated as having idiopathic chronic pancreatitis (ICP; *1–4*).

Gene mutations have been increasingly shown to be responsible for certain forms of CP. First, hereditary pancreatitis (HP) is a rare well-characterized, dominantly inherited condition that is caused by a mutation of the cationic trypsinogen gene (protease serine 1, *PRSS1*; *5,6*). Second, CP has been associated with mutations of the cystic fibrosis transmembrane conductance regulator (*CFTR*) gene; these patients do not exhibit features of cystic fibrosis *(7–9)*. Furthermore, mutations

From: *Pancreatitis and Its Complications*
Edited by: C. E. Forsmark © Humana Press Inc., Totowa, NJ

171

of the pancreatic secretory trypsin inhibitor (*PSTI*) or serine protease inhibitor, kazal type-1 (*SPINK1*) mutations *(10,11)*, have been recently implicated as disease modifiers in other forms of CP. In the case of *CFTR*, the recognition of mutations and their precise implications, including information regarding natural history, is not yet firmly in the realm of clinical practice, and it is therefore likely that *CFTR* mutations contribute to the etiology of at least some of the patients with ICP described in this chapter. The genetics of CP are described in detail in Chapter 10.

Much of the information regarding the natural history of CP over the last two decades comes from the Ammann and Zurich group *(2,12)*, as well as the Mayo Clinic group *(4)*. In a study from Zurich *(12)*, 287 patients were followed, 205 of whom had ACP (alcohol intake ≥80 g per day for >5 years), and 82 had ICP (15 idiopathic "juvenile" CP and 49 idiopathic "senile" CP) for a median of 6.7 and 12.5 years, respectively. The study by the Mayo group *(4)* retrospectively reviewed 315 patients with CP, 249 of whom had ACP (alcohol intake ≥50 g per day) and 66 had ICP (25 early-onset ICP and 41 late-onset ICP) with median duration in observation of 14 and 18 years, respectively. Both groups found that there are three forms of CP: ACP, early-onset (or juvenile) ICP, and late-onset (or senile) ICP, and that these groups have different presentation and natural history.

Autoimmune pancreatitis (AIP) remains a rare but important cause of CP of which there has been recent interest. Although not seen frequently in North America or Europe, in some parts of the world, e.g., the southern part of India, the common form of ICP is fibrocalculous pancreatitis (FCP), previously termed "tropical pancreatitis."

This chapter reviews the natural history of ACP and ICP. Additionally, what is currently known about the natural history of AIP and FCP is discussed.

CLINICAL PRESENTATION AT ONSET OF DISEASE

Age at Onset and Gender Distribution

In the study by the Mayo group *(4)*, the median age at onset of the first symptoms of ACP was 44 years, whereas in ICP, there was a bimodal distribution of age at onset (Fig. 1). The median age at onset of early-onset ICP was 19 years and late-onset ICP was 56 years. Studies by the Mayo group *(4)*, Ammann *(12)*, and Lankisch *(3)* showed male predominance in ACP (72, 91, 89%, respectively). In contrast, patients with ICP indicated no gender difference by the Mayo group *(4)* and Lankisch *(3)*. However, male predominance (87%) was found by Ammann *(12)*.

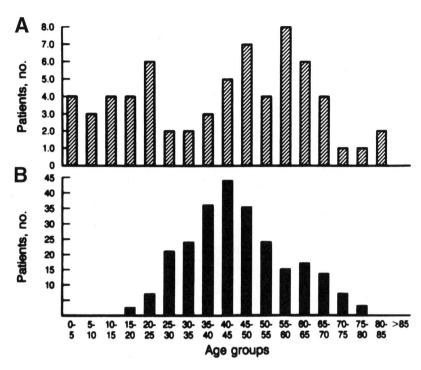

Fig. 1. Distribution of age at onset of symptoms in patients with idiopathic chronic pancreatitis (ICP) **(A)** (*n* = 66) and alcoholic chronic pancreatitis (ACP) **(B)** (*n* = 249). (Reprinted from ref. *4* with permission.)

Presenting Symptoms at Onset

Abdominal pain is the most common presenting symptom in ACP, 77% by the Mayo group *(4)* and 94% by Ammann *(2)*. In early-onset ICP, nearly all patients (96%) described by the Mayo group *(4)* and 100% by Ammann *(2)* presented with pain. In comparision, approximately half (50–55%) of late-onset ICP had no pain at presentation (primary painless CP; *2,4)*. Abdominal pain was most severe in early-onset ICP, but progressively less so in ACP and late-onset ICP (Fig. 2). Pancreatic calcifications, exocrine pancreatic insufficiency, and diabetes were rare presentations in early-onset ICP, but more common in ACP (4, 8, and 12%, respectively) and late-onset ICP (2, 22, and 22%; *4)*.

CLINICAL COURSE

Pain

Both the type and source of abdominal pain in ACP have been studied by Ammann *(13)* and divided into type A and type B. Type A are

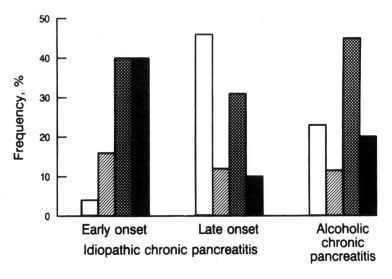

Fig. 2. Severity of pain at onset in patients with early-onset idiopathic chronic pancreatitis (ICP) ($n = 25$), late-onset ICP ($n = 41$) and alcoholic chronic pancreatitis (ACP) ($n = 249$). Pain severity: none (shaded bar), mild (hatched bar), moderate (cross-hatched bar), and severe (solid bar). (Reprinted from ref. *4* with permission.)

short-duration (usually ≤10 days) relapsing pain episodes separated by pain-free intervals (months to ≥1 year) and thought to be related to uncomplicated CP. This type of pain usually resolves spontaneously and seldom requires surgery. In contrast, type B pain is chronic persistent pain or frequent recurrent pain episodes and is likely associated with local pancreatic complications, e.g., pseudocysts, common bile duct obstruction or pancreatic ductal hypertension (dilated pancreatic duct with or without pancreatic duct stones). Type B pain is almost always improved after correction of these complications by surgery.

The frequency and severity of abdominal pain in CP usually decreases over time, and studies by the Mayo group *(4)* and Ammann *(2)* support these findings. Pain relief occurred more commonly in ACP (85% with a median time of 4.5 years *[2]* or 77% with a median time of 12 years *[4]*), but less commonly in early-onset ICP (67%, median time 25 years) and late-onset ICP (64%, median time 13 years; *4*). Ammann *(2)* demonstrated the close relationship between onset of pain relief with the development of pancreatic calcifications, exocrine insufficiency, and endocrine insufficiency (the "burning-out" pancreas hypothesis; Fig. 3). These relationships, however, were not confirmed by others studies *(4,15–17)*. Other investigators report that one fourth to one half of CP patients had significant pain attacks after

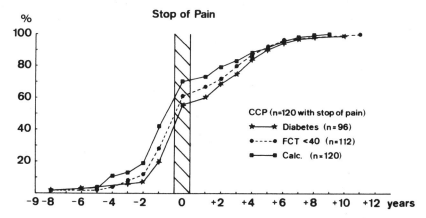

Fig. 3. Calcific alcohol-induced chronic pancreatitis. Of the 145 patients, 120 received lasting pain relief. Of the 120, 112 had marked pancreatic insufficiency (FCT <40 μg/g), and 96 had diabetes. The cumulative rate in manifestations of marked pancreatic dysfunction (with calcification) in relation (years) to onset of lasting pain relief (time 0) reveals a steep increase in pancreatic dysfunction (with calcifications) at onset (±2 years) of pain relief. FCT, fetal chymotrypsin. (Reprinted from ref. 2 with permission.)

5–10 years of observation *(3,14)*. There is also no association between pain relief and morphological changes by endoscopic retrograde cholangiopancreatography (ERCP; *15,17*). Thus, morphological changes, either pancreatic calcifications or severe ductal changes, are not always helpful to predict pain relief or the development of exocrine and endocrine insufficiency.

The effect of alcohol cessation on the natural course of pain in ACP is also an issue of debate. Some studies showed significant reduction of pain after cessation of alcohol *(18,19)*, whereas others found little or no effect *(13,17)*. It is possible that cessation may only reduce pain in early CP by reducing the episodes of attacks of pancreatitis, yet, in the advanced stage of CP with severe exocrine insufficiency, alcohol may no longer affect the pain. Abstinence should be encouraged in every patient, because patients who cease or decrease drinking have threefold lower mortality than patients who do not *(13)*, and abstinence reduces the occurrence and severity of exocrine and endocrine insufficiency (*see* below).

Pancreatic Calcification

Pancreatic calcification, which is a hallmark of CP, develops most rapidly in ACP with a median time of 5 years by Ammann *(2)* and 8.7 years by the Mayo group *(4)*, when compared to the late-onset ICP (19 years) and early-onset ICP (25 years) (*4;* Fig. 4). Smoking accelerates

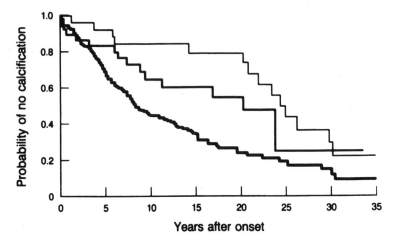

Fig. 4. Probability of remaining free of calcification in patients with early-onset chronic pancreatitis (CP) (thin solid line), late-onset CP (medium solid line), and alcoholic chronic pancreatitis (ACP) (heavy solid line). Differences were significant between early-onset idiopathic chronic pancreatitis (ICP) and ACP ($p = 0.0001$) and between late-onset ICP and ACP ($p = 0.01$). (Reprinted from ref. *4* with permission.)

the frequency and rate of calcification occurrence in late-onset ICP, but not early-onset ICP *(20)*. Pancreatic calcifications are not always progressive. In a longitudinal study of 107 patients with pancreatic calcifications by Ammann *(21)*, approximately one third showed a marked decrease and/or resolution of calcifications.

Exocrine Insufficiency

Exocrine insufficiency develops more rapidly in ACP (median time 13 years) and late-onset ICP (17 years), whereas early-onset ICP develops exocrine insufficiency significantly later in the course of disease (>26 years) (*4*; Fig. 5).

Once established, the course of exocrine insufficiency is often progressive. Ammann *(2,12)* found that in ACP, progression to severe exocrine insufficiency developed in 80% of patients within 4 years, which was more rapid than in nonalcoholic CP (80% in 8–10 years). However, subsequent studies by the same group *(22)* and others *(17)* found that pancreatic function may be stable or nonprogressive in one third to one half of patients. The effect of alcohol cessation on the natural history of exocrine function was well-demonstrated by Gullo *(23)*, who performed serial pancreatic function tests in patients that either ceased or continued drinking. Deterioration of exocrine function was significantly slower in patients who ceased drinking

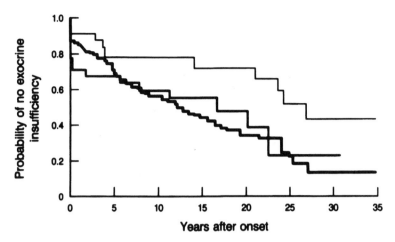

Fig. 5. Probability of remaining free of exocrine insufficiency in patients with early-onset chronic pancreatitis (CP) (thin solid line), late-onset CP (medium solid line), and alcoholic chronic pancreatitis (ACP) (heavy solid line). Differences were significant between early-onset idiopathic chronic pancreatitis (ICP) and late-onset ICP ($p = 0.024$) and between early-onset ICP and ACP ($p = 0.0008$). (Reprinted from ref. *4* with permission.)

than in patients who did not. This finding was confirmed by Lankisch *(17)*, who found that in approximately 10% of patients, pancreatic function could be reversed or improved, particularly in patients who ceased drinking and where baseline exocrine insufficiency was moderate, not severe.

Endocrine Insufficiency

The frequency of diabetes differs among studies from 38% within 14–18 years by the Mayo group *(4)*, to 74% within 5.7 years by Ammann *(2)*, or 78% within 10 years by Lankisch *(17)*, depending on the methods for diagnosis and follow-up. However, most studies found that diabetes develops earliest in ACP (median time 12 years), followed by late-onset ICP (20 years) and early-onset ICP (27 years) *(4;* Fig. 6).

Lankisch found that the frequency of patients who developed diabetes increased almost 10-fold (from 8 to 78%) within the 10-year follow-up period and 40% were insulin-dependent. Similarly, cessation of alcohol significantly reduces the occurrence and the severity of diabetes *(17)*.

Late microvascular complications of diabetes, including retinopathy and nephropathy, are found at the same rate as in patients with type 1 diabetes if corrected for disease duration *(24,25)*.

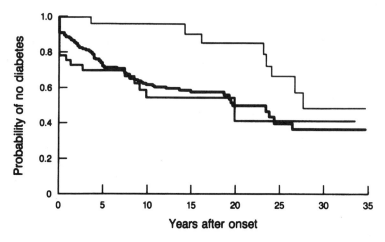

Fig. 6. Probability of remaining free of diabetes in patients with early-onset chronic pancreatitis (CP) (thin solid line), late-onset CP (medium solid line), and alcoholic chronic pancreatitis (ACP) (heavy solid line). Differences were significant between early-onset idiopathic chronic pancreatitis (ICP) and late-onset ICP ($p = 0.01$) and between early-onset ICP and ACP ($p = 0.0025$). (Reprinted from ref. *4* with permission.)

Relationship Between Calcifications, Exocrine, and Endocrine Insufficiency

The relationship between the occurrence of calcifications, exocrine insufficiency, and endocrine insufficiency, as previously mentioned remains unsettled. At present, data that support these relationships are mainly in patients with ACP. Ammann *(2,12)* showed the close relationship between the occurrence of pancreatic calcifications and development of exocrine insufficiency and diabetes (Fig. 3). Ninety percent of patients developed exocrine insufficiency within 2 years after the occurrence of calcifications, and 40% also had diabetes when exocrine insufficiency occurred. In contrast, these relationships were less evident in non-ACP, where occurrence of exocrine insufficiency and diabetes was usually delayed after calcification occurred. Sixty percent had exocrine insufficiency when calcification occurred, and only 20% had diabetes *(12)*.

Complications of Pancreatitis

Studies by both the Mayo and Zurich groups showed that CP complications, such as pseudocysts, abscesses, biliary obstruction, and fistulae, develop in 43–47% of ACP *(2,4)*, which is approximately twofold greater than in ICP (43% in ACP vs 20% and 27% in early- and late-onset ICP, respectively; *4*).

Surgery

The incidence of surgery in CP patients varies in centers from 28 to 67% *(2,4,14,17,26)*. In an international multicenter study of 2015 patients with CP *(26)*, 48% of CP patients overall underwent one or more surgical interventions. The rates of surgery were higher in ACP than ICP: 40 versus 30% by the Mayo group *(4)*, 47 versus 20% by Ammann *(12)*, 30 vs 21% by Lankisch *(17)*. However, early-onset ICP underwent surgery more frequently than late-onset ICP (60 vs 32%; *4*). The most common indication of surgery was intractable pain *(2,4,14,17)*, which was mostly related to pseudocysts (48 *[4]* and 74% *[2]* of patients who underwent surgery).

Pancreatic Cancer

CP increases the risk of pancreatic cancer 16-fold with a cumulative risk of 2% per decade *(27)*. Likely, this risk relates to the duration of CP. Thus, the risks are highest among patients with HP, which may be as high as 40% by age 70 *(28)*, and fibrocalcalus chronic pancreatitis (FCP) *(29)* because these forms of CP occur at a younger age. However, except in HP, pancreatic cancer is not the major cause of death in CP, comprising less than 3% of all deaths in patients with CP *(26)*.

Survival

Data from a multicenter cohort study of 2015 patients with CP *(26)* showed that the survival of patients with CP was significantly lower than in a normal population with a mortality ratio of 3.6. Overall, 10-year survival was 70% and 20-year survival was 45%. The etiology of CP did not significantly affect survival, although the median life expectancy was slightly shorter in ACP than ICP (72 vs 80 years; *4*). However, the main causes of death of CP patients were the complications related to smoking and alcohol use, specifically extrapancreatic cancers and cardiovascular disease (80–90% of all patients), rather than pancreatitis-related complications or pancreatic cancer (10–20%; *2,4,17,26*). Extrapancreatic cancers occurred three times more frequently than pancreatic cancer (7.9 and 2.7%, respectively; *26*). Factors associated with higher mortality in patients with CP are age at onset ($\geq$40 years), smoking, continued alcohol use, and the presence of cirrhosis *(26)*.

The impact of continued alcohol use on survival has been clearly demonstrated. Patients who ceased or reduced drinking had one third the mortality of those patients who continued drinking *(13,30)*.

SPECIAL FORMS OF CHRONIC PANCREATITIS

Autoimmune Pancreatitis

AIP has been described as a distinct entity characterized by hyper-gammaglobulinemia, positive autoantibodies, pancreatic enlargement, characteristic histology of periductal inflammation with dense infiltrations by lymphocytes and plasma cells, acinar atrophy, and severe fibrosis, and, most importantly, a response to corticosteroid treatment *(31–35)*. Although it was first reported by Sarles in 1961 as a special form of CP associated with autoimmunity *(36)*, and many sporadic case reports of pancreatitis associated with Sjögren's syndrome have been subsequently reported, it was Yoshida in 1995 *(31)* who reviewed and summarized all previously reported cases and proposed the term for AIP and diagnostic criteria.

Clinically, AIP is encountered in approximately 2% of CP patients who undergo ERCP *(34)*. Patients usually have no symptoms or only mild symptoms, including pain, enlargement of the pancreas in imaging studies, obstructive jaundice from the stenosis of distal common bile duct caused by an enlarged or fibrotic pancreatic head, recent-onset diabetes, or single or multiple pancreatic masses (mass-forming or "tumefactive" CP), leading to the suspicion of pancreatic cancer *(31,32,37)*. Episodes of acute pancreatitis are usually absent *(31,32,37)*. In the Japanese literature, clinical features of AIP in 37 reported cases have been summarized by Horiuchi *(38)* and are shown in Table 1.

Associations between AIP and autoimmune diseases have been reported in Sjögren's syndrome, primary sclerosing cholangitis, primary biliary cirrhosis, autoimmune hepatitis, inflammatory bowel disease, type 1 diabetes, and immune thrombocytopenia *(31,38–40)*. Multiple autoantibodies may be present *(41)*, including antinuclear antibodies, antilactoferrin antibodies, the rheumatoid factor, antismooth muscle antibodies, and recently proposed to be specific for AIP are anticarbonic anhydrase I and II antibodies *(42–44)* and IgG_4 *(45)*. On ultrasonography, the pancreas may have a swollen hypoechoic ("sausage-like") appearance *(32,34)*. On computed tomography, the pancreas may be diffusely enlarged with poor- or delayed-contrast enhancement or capsule-like rim enhancement *(32,35,46)*. Mass-like lesions that mimic pancreatic cancer are not uncommon *(37)*. Pancreatic calcifications and pseudocysts are usually absent, but splenic venous thrombosis may be present. Magnetic resonance imaging reveals a diffusely enlarged pancreas with hypointensity on T1-weighted *(46)*. ERCP usually shows diffuse irregular narrowing of the main pancreatic duct and, occasionally, distal common bile duct stricture within the pancreatic head. These imaging findings are in striking contrast to the common form of

Table 1
Clinical Features of 37 Reported Cases
of Suspected Autoimmune Pancreatitis *(38)*

Characteristics	Frequency (%)
Age (range)	59.6 (38–79)
Sex (M:F)	25:12 (2:1)
Jaundice	30/37 (81%)
Increased serum γ-globulin and/or IgG levels	25/33 (76%)
Presence of autoantibodies	13/22 (59%)
Diffuse enlargement of the pancreas	25/37 (68%)
Diffuse or segmental irregular narrowing of the main pancreatic duct	26/28 (93%)
Pancreatic stone	1/37 (3%)
Association with other autoimmune diseases	22/37 (60%)
Histological findings of fibrotic change and lymphocyte infiltration	30/30 (100%)
Effectiveness of steroid therapy	12/12 (100%)

IgG, immunoglobulin G.

CP, where pancreatic atrophy, dilated pancreatic duct, calcifications, and pseudocysts are usually present.

Data on the natural history of AIP are scarce. Most patients receive either corticosteroid treatment or undergo surgery from the suspicion of pancreatic cancer or lymphoma *(33,37)*. A good clinical and radiological response to oral corticosteroid treatment has been reported (i.e., 30–40 mg per day of prednisolone tapered over 1–2 months) *(31–34)*. Jaundice, diabetes, hypergammaglobulinemia, enlarged pancreas, pancreatic duct narrowing, and pancreatic insufficiency usually resolve or markedly improve after a single course of corticosteroid treatment, although some irregularities of the pancreatic duct may persist. In most patients, corticosteroids could be discontinued without recurrence, but some patients did experience relapse *(34)*.

Fibrocalculous Pancreatitis

FCP, also designated fibrocalculous pancreatic diabetes or tropical CP, is a distinct type of ICP found in the tropics and is characterized by the onset of abdominal pain early in childhood, large intraductal calculi, and early development of diabetes and exocrine insufficiency. Clinically, patients with FCP have been reported as predominantly male with a male-to-female ratio ranging from 1.6 to 2.5:1 *(47–49)*. In contrast, a population-based study showed female predominance with a male-to-female ratio of 1:1.8 *(50)*.

Most patients are lean with a mean body mass index of 18–19 because of diabetes. The body mass index before the disease is usually normal *(48)*. Severe protein–energy malnutrition is uncommon, and symptoms usually begin with abdominal pain starting during childhood or as teenagers (70–80%) *(47,48,50)*. Diabetes usually presents one or two decades later between the ages of 20 to 40, which is approximately one decade younger than ACP *(47,48)*. Overt steatorrhea is present in only one fourth to one third of patients at presentation, owing to the low-fat content in the diet, because when exocrine function is tested, or the fat content in diets is increased, exocrine insufficiency and steatorrhea are present in 80–90% of patients *(48,49,51)*.

Imaging studies usually reveal pancreatic atrophy with a dilated pancreatic duct and intraductal calculi. The calculi in FCP are present in more than 90% of patients and are typically large (>10 mm), round, dense, and discrete with well-circumscribed margins within the large ducts *(48)*. These findings are different from ACP, where the calculi are typically small, speckled with hazy margins within the pancreatic duct and also in the parenchyma *(48)*.

The natural history of abdominal pain and exocrine function in FCP has not been studied. Diabetes in FCP is mainly the result of reduced β-cell function *(52)* and is usually difficult to control, but ketosis is uncommon. Most patients require insulin treatment, but 10–20% of patients may respond to oral hypoglycemic drugs at least for the first 5–10 years *(47)*. Microvascular complications (retinopathy and nephropathy) and neuropathy occur with the same prevalence as diabetes mellitus with the same duration *(53)*. However, in contrast, macrovascular complications, such as myocardial infarction and stroke, are uncommon *(54–56)*.

The risk of pancreatic cancer in FCP is highest among all forms of chronic calcifying pancreatitis *(27,57)* with a relative risk of at least fivefold and may be up to 100-fold *(29)*. Mean age at diagnosis of pancreatic cancer in FCP is generally younger than in pancreatic cancer (47 vs 61 years; *58*), and the site of pancreatic cancer is more common in the body and tail (73% vs 37%) in other types of pancreatic cancer *(58)*.

Survival of patients with FCP is considerably lower than in the general population with a median survival of 35 years after onset of abdominal pain and 25 years after onset of diabetes *(56)*. The most common cause of death in approximately half of the patients is diabetic-related complications, especially renal failure from diabetic nephropathy (40% of causes of death), followed by pancreatic cancer (22%), malnutrition, and infections (11%; *56*).

SUMMARY

CP of all forms is generally characterized by a very prolonged but variable natural history. This chapter has described the natural history of CP in alcoholic, idiopathic, autoimmune, and fibrocalculous pancreatitis, as well as indicated the type and duration of pain, rate of development of exocrine and endocrine insufficiency and calcification, along with the occurrence of complications, which differs considerably among these groups. An understanding of the natural history of the different forms of CP is necessary to understand the approach for diagnosis and allow accurate assessments of the efficacy of therapies.

REFERENCES

1. DiMagno EP, Layer P, Clain JE. Chronic pancreatitis. In: Go VLW, DiMagno EP, Garder JD, et al., eds. The Pancreas: Biology, Pathophysiology and Disease. Raven Press, New York, 1993: 665–706.
2. Ammann RW, Akovbiantz A, Largiader F, Schueler G. Course and outcome of chronic pancreatitis. Longitudinal study of a mixed medical-surgical series of 245 patients. Gastroenterology 1984; 86: 820–828.
3. Lankisch PG, Seidensticker F, Lohr-Happe A, et al. The course of pain is the same in alcohol- and nonalcohol-induced chronic pancreatitis. Pancreas 1995; 10: 338–341.
4. Layer P, Yamamoto H, Kalthoff L, et al. The different courses of early- and late-onset idiopathic and alcoholic chronic pancreatitis. Gastroenterology 1994; 107: 1481–1487.
5. Whitcomb DC, Gorry MC, Preston RA, et al. Hereditary pancreatitis is caused by a mutation in the cationic trypsinogen gene. Nat Genet 1996; 14: 141–145.
6. Whitcomb DC, Preston RA, Aston CE, et al. A gene for hereditary pancreatitis maps to chromosome 7q35. Gastroenterology 1996; 110: 1975–1980.
7. Sharer N, Schwarz M, Malone G, et al. Mutations of the cystic fibrosis gene in patients with chronic pancreatitis. N Engl J Med 1998; 339: 645–652.
8. Cohn JA, Friedman KJ, Noone PG, et al. Relation between mutations of the cystic fibrosis gene and idiopathic pancreatitis. N Engl J Med 1998; 339: 653–658.
9. Noone PG, Zhou ZC, Silverman LM, et al. Cystic fibrosis gene mutations and pancreatic risks: relation to epithelial ion transport and trypsin inhibitor gene mutations. Gastroenterology 2001; 121: 1310–1319.
10. Witt H, Luck W, Hennies HC, et al. Mutations in the gene encoding the serine protease inhibitor, Kazal type 1 are associated with chronic pancreatitis. Nat Genet 2000; 25: 213–216.
11. Pfutzer RH, Barmada MM, Brunskill AP, et al. SPINK1/PSTI polymorphisms act as disease modifiers in familial and idiopathic chronic pancreatitis. Gastroenterology 2000; 119: 615–623.
12. Ammann RW, Buehler H, Muench R, et al. Differences in the natural history of idiopathic (nonalcoholic) and alcoholic chronic pancreatitis. A comparative long-term study of 287 patients. Pancreas 1987; 2: 368–377.
13. Ammann RW, Muellhaupt B. The natural history of pain in alcoholic chronic pancreatitis. Gastroenterology 1999; 116: 1132–1140.
14. Miyake H, Harada H, Kunichika K, et al. Clinical course and prognosis of chronic pancreatitis. Pancreas 1987; 2: 378–385.

15. Malfertheiner P, Buchler M, Stanescu A, Ditschuneit H. Pancreatic morphology and function in relationship to pain in chronic pancreatitis. Int J Pancreatol 1987; 2: 59–66.
16. Thorsgaard Pedersen N, Nyboe Andersen B, Pedersen G, Worning H. Chronic pancreatitis in Copenhagen. A retrospective study of 64 consecutive patients. Scand J Gastroenterol 1982; 17: 925–931.
17. Lankisch PG, Lohr-Happe A, Otto J, Creutzfeldt W. Natural course in chronic pancreatitis. Pain, exocrine and endocrine pancreatic insufficiency and prognosis of the disease. Digestion 1993; 54: 148–155.
18. Trapnell JE. Chronic relapsing pancreatitis: a review of 64 cases. Br J Surg 1979; 66: 471–475.
19. Marks IN, Girdwood AH, Bank S, Louw JH. The prognosis of alcohol-induced calcific pancreatitis. S Afr Med J 1980; 57: 640–643.
20. Imoto M, DiMagno EP. Cigarette smoking increases the risk of pancreatic calcification in late-onset but not early-onset idiopathic chronic pancreatitis. Pancreas 2000; 21: 115–119.
21. Ammann RW, Muench R, Otto R, et al. Evolution and regression of pancreatic calcification in chronic pancreatitis. A prospective long-term study of 107 patients. Gastroenterology 1988; 95: 1018–1028.
22. Ammann RW, Buehler H, Bruehlmann W, et al. Acute (nonprogressive) alcoholic pancreatitis: prospective longitudinal study of 144 patients with recurrent alcoholic pancreatitis. Pancreas 1986; 1: 195–203.
23. Gullo L, Barbara L, Labo G. Effect of cessation of alcohol use on the course of pancreatic dysfunction in alcoholic pancreatitis. Gastroenterology 1988; 95: 1063–1068.
24. Gullo L, Parenti M, Monti L, et al. Diabetic retinopathy in chronic pancreatitis. Gastroenterology 1990; 98: 1577–1581.
25. Levitt NS, Adams G, Salmon J, et al. The prevalence and severity of microvascular complications in pancreatic diabetes and IDDM. Diabetes Care 1995; 18: 971–974.
26. Lowenfels AB, Maisonneuve P, Cavallini G, et al. Prognosis of chronic pancreatitis: an international multicenter study. International Pancreatitis Study Group. Am J Gastroenterol 1994; 89: 1467–1471.
27. Lowenfels AB, Maisonneuve P, Cavallini G, et al. Pancreatitis and the risk of pancreatic cancer. International Pancreatitis Study Group. N Engl J Med 1993; 328: 1433–1437.
28. Lowenfels AB, Maisonneuve P, DiMagno EP, et al. Hereditary pancreatitis and the risk of pancreatic cancer. International Hereditary Pancreatitis Study Group. J Natl Cancer Inst 1997; 89: 442–446.
29. Chari ST, Mohan V, Pitchumoni CS, et al. Risk of pancreatic carcinoma in tropical calcifying pancreatitis: an epidemiologic study. Pancreas 1994; 9: 62–66.
30. Miyake H, Harada H, Ochi K, et al. Prognosis and prognostic factors in chronic pancreatitis. Dig Dis Sci 1989; 34: 449–455.
31. Yoshida K, Toki F, Takeuchi T, et al. Chronic pancreatitis caused by an autoimmune abnormality. Proposal of the concept of autoimmune pancreatitis. Dig Dis Sci 1995; 40: 1561–1568.
32. Furukawa N, Muranaka T, Yasumori K, et al. Autoimmune pancreatitis: radiologic findings in three histologically proven cases. J Comput Assist Tomogr 1998; 22: 880–883.
33. Horiuchi A, Kaneko T, Yamamura N, et al. Autoimmune chronic pancreatitis simulating pancreatic lymphoma. Am J Gastroenterol 1996; 91: 2607–2609.

34. Ito T, Nakano I, Koyanagi S, et al. Autoimmune pancreatitis as a new clinical entity. Three cases of autoimmune pancreatitis with effective steroid therapy. Dig Dis Sci 1997; 42: 1458–1468.

35. Procacci C, Carbognin G, Biasiutti C, et al. Autoimmune pancreatitis: possibilities of CT characterization. Pancreatology 2001; 1: 246–253.

36. Sarles H, Sarles JC, Muratore R, Guien C. Chronic inflammatory sclerosis of the pancreas: an autoimmune pancreatitis? Am J Dig Dis 1961; 6: 688–698.

37. Ohana M, Okazaki K, Hajiro K, Kobashi Y. Multiple pancreatic masses associated with autoimmunity. Am J Gastroenterol 1998; 93: 99–102.

38. Horiuchi A, Kawa S, Akamatsu T, et al. Characteristic pancreatic duct appearance in autoimmune chronic pancreatitis: a case report and review of the Japanese literature. Am J Gastroenterol 1998; 93: 260–263.

39. Seko S, Taniguchi T, Nishikawa H, et al. A case of autoimmune pancreatitis associated with immune thrombocytopenia. Gastrointest Endosc 2000; 42: 192–197.

40. Taniguchi T, Seko S, Okamoto M, et al. Association of autoimmune pancreatitis and type 1 diabetes: autoimmune exocrinopathy and endocrinopathy of the pancreas. Diabetes Care 2000; 23: 1592–1594.

41. Okazaki K, Uchida K, Ohana M, et al. Autoimmune-related pancreatitis is associated with autoantibodies and a Th1/Th2-type cellular immune response. Gastroenterology 2000; 118: 573–581.

42. Kino-Ohsaki J, Nishimori I, Morita M, et al. Serum antibodies to carbonic anhydrase I and II in patients with idiopathic chronic pancreatitis and Sjogren's syndrome. Gastroenterology 1996; 110: 1579–1586.

43. Cavallini G, Frulloni L, Bovo P, et al. Carbonic anhydrase and primary chronic pancreatitis. Gastroenterology 1997; 112: 1054–1056.

44. Frulloni L, Bovo P, Brunelli S, et al. Elevated serum levels of antibodies to carbonic anhydrase I and II in patients with chronic pancreatitis. Pancreas 2000; 20: 382–388.

45. Hamano H, Kawa S, Horiuchi A, et al. High serum IgG4 concentrations in patients with sclerosing pancreatitis. N Engl J Med 2001; 344: 732–8.

46. Irie H, Honda H, Baba S, et al. Autoimmune pancreatitis: CT and MR characteristics. AJR Am J Roentgenol 1998; 170: 1323–1327.

47. Mohan V, Nagalotimath SJ, Yajnik CS, Tripathy BB. Fibrocalculous pancreatic diabetes. Diabetes Metab Rev 1998; 14: 153–170.

48. Chari ST, Mohan V, Jayanthi V, et al. Comparative study of the clinical profiles of alcoholic chronic pancreatitis and tropical chronic pancreatitis in Tamil Nadu, south India. Pancreas 1992; 7: 52–58.

49. Balakrishanan V. Tropical pancreatitis (pancreatic tropicale). In: Bernades P, Hugier M, eds. Maladies du Pancreas Exocrine. Doin, Paris, 1987: 207–227.

50. Balaji LN. The problem of chronic calcific pancreatitis. PhD thesis. All India Institute of Medical Sciences, New Delhi 1988.

51. Ramachandran M, Pai KN. Clinical features and management of pancreatic diabetes. In: Rao B, ed. Diabetes Mellitus. New Delhi, Arnold Heinemann, 1977: 239–246.

52. Mehrotra RN, Bhatia E, Choudhuri G. Beta-cell function and insulin sensitivity in tropical calcific pancreatitis from north India. Metabolism 1997; 46: 441–444.

53. Mohan V, Mohan R, Susheela L, et al. Tropical pancreatic diabetes in South India: heterogeneity in clinical and biochemical profile. Diabetologia 1985; 28: 229–232.

54. Mohan V, Ramachandran A, Viswanathan M. Two case reports of macrovascular complications in fibrocalculous pancreatic diabetes. Acta Diabetol Lat 1989; 26: 345–349.

55. Sastry NG, Mohan V. Hemiplegia in a patient with fibrocalculous pancreatic diabetes. J Assoc Physicians India 2000; 48: 1129.
56. Mohan V, Premalatha G, Padma A, et al. Fibrocalculous pancreatic diabetes. Long-term survival analysis. Diabetes Care 1996; 19: 1274–1278.
57. Lowenfels AB, Patel VP, Pitchumoni CS. Chronic calcific pancreatitis and pancreatic cancer. Dig Dis Sci 1985; 30: 982.
58. Augustine P, Ramesh H. Is tropical pancreatitis premalignant? Am J Gastroenterol 1992; 87: 1005–1008.

12 Diagnosis of Chronic Pancreatitis

Chris E. Forsmark, MD

CONTENTS

INTRODUCTION
TESTS OF PANCREATIC FUNCTION
TESTS OF PANCREATIC STRUCTURE
DIAGNOSTIC STRATEGY
REFERENCES

INTRODUCTION

The diagnosis of chronic pancreatitis (CP) is usually suspected on the basis of suggestive signs and symptoms, but the clinical presentation alone is rarely specific enough to reach a diagnosis. The diagnosis requires confirmation by diagnostic tests that measure perturbations of either pancreatic structure or pancreatic function. In the majority of patients, the disease is suspected based on the presence of abdominal pain. Although not universal, the vast majority of patients with CP develop pain *(1–3)*. The pain may be episodic or constant and continuous. In those patients who present with acute attacks, they may be initially labeled as having acute pancreatitis (AP), until the disease progresses to a point at which the diagnosis of CP is possible. Pain is most commonly felt in the epigastrium with radiation to the back and is usually associated with nausea and vomiting. Some patients may present with more gradual onset of constant abdominal pain, and a small minority may not have pain. In other patients, the disease may be suspected based on the development of exocrine insufficiency (steatorrhea, weight

From: *Pancreatitis and Its Complications*
Edited by: C. E. Forsmark © Humana Press Inc., Totowa, NJ

Table 1
Diagnostic Tests for Chronic Pancreatitis

Tests of structure	Tests of function
Endoscopic ultrasonography	Direct hormonal stimulation test (secretin or secretin-CCK test)
Endoscopic retrograde pancreatography	Fecal elastase
Computed tomography	Serum trypsin
Magnetic resonance imaging/magnetic resonance cholangiopancreatography	Fecal fat
Abdominal ultrasound	Serum glucose
Plain abdominal radiograph	

Ranked in approximate order of decreasing sensitivity. CCK, cholecystokinin.

loss, and malnutrition), endocrine insufficiency (diabetes mellitus), or by findings on an abdominal imaging test (e.g., computed tomography [CT]).

The signs and symptoms previously outlined are not generally specific for CP. Diagnosis requires confirmatory tests, and a bewildering variety of diagnostic tests have been developed over the years. It is useful to remember that the gold-standard for diagnosis is pancreatic histology. The histological features are characteristic with chronic inflammation, fibrosis, necrosis, and destruction of acinar, islet, and ductal tissue (4). Unfortunately, the disease may affect the gland nonuniformly, such that a small biopsy specimen may not adequately reflect the presence of disease. Even more importantly, the pancreas is difficult to biopsy and relatively unforgiving in that severe pancreatitis can develop as a consequence of pancreatic biopsy. Hence, clinicians rely on tests that substitute for the gold standard. The fact that no single test is favored in all circumstances is a testament that no single test is an adequate substitute for the true gold standard—histology. Clinicians must therefore choose a diagnostic test or series of tests based on knowledge of the strengths and weaknesses of individual tests, as well as their cost, risk, and availability.

Diagnostic tests are traditionally separated into tests that detect abnormalities of pancreatic function and those that detect abnormalities of pancreatic structure (Table 1). CP is a slowly progressive disease, and these abnormalities may take years to develop or may never develop at all. Hence, all of these tests are most accurate in far-advanced disease when obvious structural or functional abnormalities have developed. Structural abnormalities that can be diagnostic include changes within the main pancreatic duct (dilation, strictures, irregularity, and pancreatic ductal stones), side branches of the pancreatic duct (dilation, irregularity), or pancreatic parenchyma (diffuse pancreatic calcifications). These findings can be visualized utilizing the diagnostic tests that evaluate pancreatic structure. Functional abnormalities in CP include a decrease in stimulated secretory capacity, exocrine insufficiency (malabsorption and steatorrhea), and endocrine insufficiency (diabetes mellitus). The rate at which these structural and functional abnormalities develop is variable and influenced by the etiology of the disease (*see* Chapter 11). Patients with alcoholic chronic pancreatitis (ACP), hereditary CP, and late-onset idiopathic chronic pancreatitis (ICP) are most prone to develop these abnormalities, although it may still take many years. Patients with early-onset ICP may not develop them at all.

In one large natural history study *(2)*, those with ACP developed exocrine insufficiency, endocrine insufficiency, and diffuse pancreatic calcifications at a median of 13.1, 19.8, and 8.7 years, respectively. In the same study, those with early-onset ICP developed the same features at median times of 26.3, 27.5, and 24.9 years, respectively. If a diagnostic test is based on documenting these functional or structural abnormalities, it might take many years of disease before the diagnostic test was highly accurate.

This concept has led to a general classification of CP as either "big-duct" or "small-duct" disease *(1,5,6)*. Big-duct disease implies substantial abnormalities of the pancreatic duct or gland that are visible on routinely performed imaging studies. This could include main pancreatic duct dilation, pancreatic atrophy or diffuse calcifications visible on ultrasound (US), CT, or endoscopic retrograde cholangiopancreatography (ERCP). Small-duct disease implies the absence of these findings (e.g., a normal or near normal US, CT, or ERCP) (Figs. 1 and 2). This distinction has both diagnostic and therapeutic implications. Those with big-duct disease obviously have progressed to the point that they have advanced structural abnormalities and also often have associated exocrine or endocrine insufficiency. The diagnosis of big-duct disease is therefore much simpler as both advanced structural and functional abnormalities are present, and these can be easily detected on a wide variety of diagnostic tests. The diagnosis of small-duct disease is much more difficult, as imaging studies may be normal, and functional abnormalities are usually absent. In these patients, many of the widely available diagnostic tests are inaccurate, and only tests of maximum sensitivity have a chance of making the diagnosis. The available diagnostic tests vary in their sensitivity, specificity, cost, and risk. Choosing the most useful diagnostic test for an individual patient requires an understanding of not only sensitivity and specificity, but also an appreciation of how the stage of the disease (i.e., big-duct or small-duct disease) influences

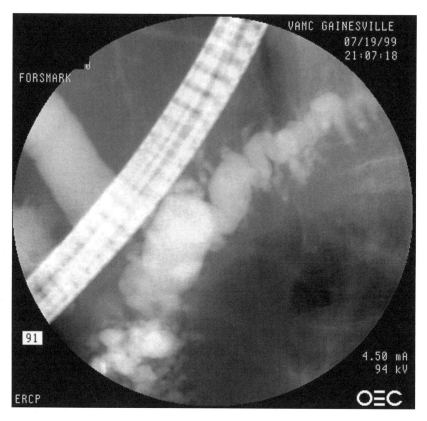

Fig. 1. An endoscopic retrograde cholangiopancreatography (ERCP) demonstrating massive pancreatic duct dilation in a patient with "big-duct" chronic pancreatitis.

sensitivity and specificity. In addition to the traditional separation of diagnostic tests into those which measure functional abnormalities and those which measure structural abnormalities, tests of pancreatic function have been further subdivided into direct and indirect tests. The distinction between direct and indirect is somewhat vague, but in general tests that measure pancreatic secretion or measure a pancreatic enzyme in blood or stool are direct tests. Those tests that measure the effect of a secreted enzyme (or lack of effect in the case of CP) are indirect tests. Generally, diagnostic tests have also been divided into invasive and noninvasive tests. Invasive tests are those that require a tube or endoscope to be inserted, whereas noninvasive tests require a collection of blood, stool, or exhaled breath. We begin with a description of the diagnostic tests and then discuss the appropriate choice and order of tests to maximize yield and minimize cost and risk.

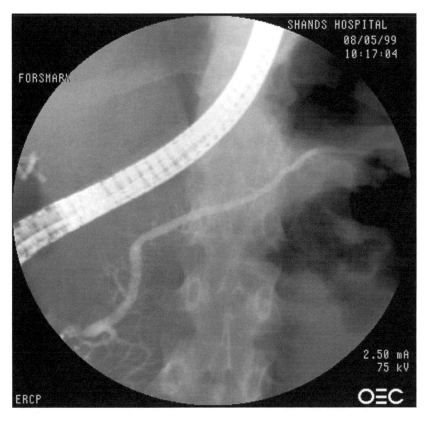

Fig. 2. An endoscopic retrograde cholangiopancreatography (ERCP) demonstrating minimal pancreatic duct abnormalities in a patient with painful "small-duct" chronic pancreatitis.

TESTS OF PANCREATIC FUNCTION

Routine Laboratory Tests

Many pancreatic enzymes can be measured in serum. Serum levels of amylase or lipase may become elevated during acute flares of pancreatitis superimposed on pre-existing CP. These elevations are often only modest and not routinely present. They cannot be used for the diagnosis of CP, as the majority of patients with CP have a normal serum level of these enzymes. Serum trypsinogen (often called "serum trypsin") can be also measured in serum, and it is the only enzyme measured that has certain diagnostic value. Serum levels of trypsinogen may be low in patients with advanced CP. Low levels of serum trypsinogen (<20 ng/mL) are highly specific for CP *(7)* but only reach this low level in advanced disease (as defined by exocrine insufficiency or steatorrhea). Overall, the sensitivity of serum trypsin is only approximately 50% *(7,8)*. A very low level is consequently a marker of severely deranged pancreatic function with exocrine insufficiency. Very low levels may also be occasionally seen in patients with pancreatic adenocarcinoma, where the tumor obstruction of the pancreatic duct is causing CP in the upstream gland. Serum trypsinogen levels are in the normal range in many patients with less advanced CP. The test is widely available, inexpensive (about $100), and risk-free.

Stool Tests

Analysis of stool may be considered either to document the presence of steatorrhea (exocrine insufficiency) or to diagnose CP. Among other things, fat digestion requires adequate pancreatic lipolytic enzymes delivered to the intestine during the prandial and postprandial period. The pancreas has substantial exocrine reserve. Steatorrhea only occurs when 90% or more of the lipolytic secretory capacity is lost *(9)*. As might be suspected, this only occurs when the disease is advanced and long-standing. In one large natural history study, steatorrhea occurred after a median disease duration of 13.1 years in those with ACP, 16.9 years in those with late-onset ICP, and 26.3 years in those with early-onset ICP *(2)*. Ultimately, about 50–80% of patients with CP will eventually develop exocrine insufficiency and steatorrhea *(1)*. A 72-hour stool collection for fat is the gold standard to detect steatorrhea. Levels of stool fat greater than 7% of the daily ingested dietary fat are abnormal. An accurate 72-hour fecal fat collection is difficult to perform. The patient needs to be on a diet high in fat (typically 100 g/day), but more importantly, the fat content of the diet needs to be precisely known. Otherwise, it will be impossible to determine if more than 7% of the ingested fat reaches the stool. The patient needs to be on this high-fat diet for at least 3 days before the test is performed. Therefore, the test is not generally possible to perform accurately outside of a clinical research center with a nutritional research kitchen. Fat in the stool may also be assessed by qualitative stool stains using a Sudan III stain. This qualitative test is obviously not as accurate or precise as a 72-hour fecal fat collection, but it is easier to perform. More than 6 globules of fat per high power field is generally considered abnormal. For this test to be somewhat reliable, the test should be performed while the patient is on a high-fat diet. A positive 72-hour fecal fat or positive Sudan III stain of stool do not prove that steatorrhea is the result of pancreatic exocrine insufficiency, but merely confirm that steatorrhea is present.

An entirely different way to utilize stool measurements is as a diagnostic test by measuring pancreatic digestive enzyme concentrations in stool. In theory, reduced output of enzymes from the pancreas would be reflected in reduced concentrations of these enzymes in stool. Several enzymes have been measured, including trypsin, chymotrypsin, and elastase. Trypsin activity is not a reliable predictor of pancreatic insufficiency, probably because of proteolytic and autocatalytic digestion of the protease during intestinal transit. Chymotrypsin is more stable during intestinal transit, and fecal chymotrypsin has been used for many years (primarily in Europe) as a diagnostic test for CP. Fecal levels of chymotrypsin are usually decreased in patients with ACP and exocrine insufficiency. The overall sensitivity of this test varies with the degree and severity of CP. In those with advanced disease (big-duct disease and/or pancreatic exocrine insufficiency), the sensitivity is about 80–90%, which drops to 50% for patients with moderate disease and only 25% for those with mild disease (8,10). Fecal chymotrypsin is a reliable diagnostic test in those with advanced CP but is insensitive in early or less-advanced disease. Fecal chymotrypsin can also be used to assess the compliance with and response to pancreatic enzyme therapy as it is contained in commercially available pancreatic enzyme products. Fecal pancreatic elastase-1 can also be measured in stool. Fecal elastase levels can also be easily measured with commercially available tests, and it correlates well with levels of pancreatic enzymes present in the duodenum. Numerous studies have evaluated fecal elastase as a diagnostic test (10–13). Generally, these studies show fecal elastase to be somewhat more sensitive than fecal chymotrypsin. Still, fecal elastase is most accurate in those with advanced CP (90–95% sensitivity) in comparison to those with less-advanced disease (sensitivity about 60%). Fecal elastase is becoming more widely available at reference laboratories. Unlike chymotrypsin, elastase is not contained in commercially available pancreatic enzyme supplements; hence, its level cannot be used to gauge compliance with prescribed enzyme therapy. This disadvantage may also be an advantage, as levels of pancreatic fecal elastase in stool can still be used as a diagnostic test in patients already on enzyme therapy. The sensitivity of these stool tests is very high in advanced disease but less so in patients without steatorrhea. However, the tests are simple, inexpensive, risk-free, and widely available.

Urine Tests

Two tests of historical interest measure the level of metabolites in urine. The bentiromide test (NBT-PABA) and pancreolauryl test both utilize the measurement of a metabolite that can only be produced by the action of pancreatic enzymes upon an orally administered substrate. In those patients with reduced levels of pancreatic enzymes in the duodenum, inadequate digestion of the test substrate occurs, and less metabolite can be measured. There is substantial functional reserve in the pancreas, such that only small amounts of digestive enzymes need to be present in the duodenum and jejunum for normal digestion. These tests become abnormal only when levels of pancreatic enzymes within the intestine are inadequate for normal digestion, which only occurs in those with advanced CP *(8,9)*. The bentiromide test uses an orally administered substrate that can only be metabolized by pancreatic chymotrypsin, causing P-aminobenzoic acid (PABA) to be liberated from the substrate. PABA is absorbed in the intestine, conjugated in the liver, and excreted in the urine. A 6-hour urine collection is performed to determine the excretion of PABA conjugates. A collection of less than 50% of the administered dose is abnormal. The pancreolauryl test administers a substrate that can only be metabolized by pancreatic arylesterases. Digestion liberates fluorescein and is absorbed, conjugated in the liver, and excreted in the urine. The test is repeated with free fluorescein to provide a baseline for comparison. The sensitivity of these tests is good for patients with advanced CP but is only about 40–50% for those with less advanced CP *(8)*. The tests are relatively inexpensive and risk-free. The bentiromide test is no longer available in the United States, and the pancreolauryl test has never been available for clinical use in the United States but continues to be used in Europe.

Breath Tests

Several variations of breath tests have been developed as diagnostic tests for CP. Generally, these variations involve the labeling of the carbon atoms in a triglyceride with radioactive carbon (^{14}C) or with a stable nonradioactive isotope (^{13}C). The triglyceride is given orally, digested by pancreatic lipase, and the liberated carbon atoms are incorporated into CO_2. The labeled CO_2 ($^{14}CO_2$ or $^{13}CO_2$) can then be measured in the breath. Numerous different triglycerides have been used; triolein is the most well-studied and has the best diagnostic accuracy. The tests are designed to document the presence of inadequate lipid digestion (exocrine insufficiency or steatorrhea). In several studies, these tests are accurate in patients with pancreatic exocrine insufficiency *(1,8,14,15)*. Yet an abnormal breath test does not distinguish pancreatic steatorrhea from other forms of steatorrhea because metabolism of triglyceride to CO_2 requires not only hydrolysis by lipases but also subsequent intestinal absorption, hepatic metabolism, and ventilation. Various modifications have been developed using combined triglycerides and fatty acids and by various alterations of triglyceride used and type and intensity of carbon labeling *(16)*. Breath tests are accurate in advanced CP (80–90% sensitivity) but not in less-advanced disease (only ~50–60% sensitivity). Breath tests are not widely available ouside of ongoing research protocols.

Direct Pancreatic Function Tests

Tests that involve placing a tube into the duodenum or pancreatic duct to collect pancreatic secretions are direct pancreatic function tests. The goal of this type of testing is to directly measure the pancreatic output of enzymes or bicarbonate after stimulation with a secretagogue (secretin or cholecystokinin [CCK] , its analog, or both). If secretin is used as the secretagogue, it will stimulate pancreatic ductal cells to secrete a bicarbonate-rich fluid. If CCK or one of its analogs is used, pancreatic acinar cells are stimulated to secrete digestive enzymes. The bicarbonate or enzyme content of pancreatic secretions can be measured. Because basal pancreatic secretion is so variable, it is necessary to measure stimulated secretory capacity. The concept of direct pancreatic function testing is more than 60 years old, and since that time, a number of variations and modifications have been made *(1,17)*. Unfortunately, there is no uniformly accepted protocol, and each center performing this type of test has its own protocol. These tests are only performed at a few referral centers in the United States. Regardless of the specific protocol, every test of this kind requires an ability to collect pancreatic secretions. The most commonly used method utilizes an oroduodenal tube placed into the duodenum. This tube must be positioned so that it can adequately collect pancreatic juice, and methods must be in place to minimize contamination from gastric contents. Different methods have been used to maximize the collection of pancreatic secretions. The tube is usually placed fluoroscopically for the aspiration ports to be in the descending duodenum, and these ports are kept under continuous low-negative pressure suction. The tube also has aspiration ports in the stomach, which are likewise kept under low-negative pressure suction to maximize the removal of all gastric secretions and minimize any contamination by gastric juice. It is possible to measure the adequacy of collection and degree of contamination by using a nonabsorbable perfusion marker, such as polyethylene glycol. This marker can be perfused into the stomach, and the amount can be recovered in the duodenal port as a measure of the degree of contamination. Similarly, a perfusion marker can be perfused into the proximal duodenum as well with the collection of this marker from a more distal duodenal aspiration port to gauge the adequacy of collection of pancreatic secretions. It is accepted that a collection of more than 85% of pancreatic secretions is necessary for an accurate test. In many studies that use a nonabsorbable marker, recovery of marker is at or above this level *(18)*, but some studies have documented only 40% recovery of marker

(19). Proper positioning of the tube is therefore critical for an accuracy. One way to attempt to minimize the error induced by inadequate collections of pancreatic secretions is to measure concentrations rather than the total quantitative output. For example, if peak bicarbonate concentration instead of total bicarbonate output is measured, no perfusion markers are thought to be necessary, as concentrations, should not vary tremendously depending on which part of the pancreatic secretions is collected. In this situation, a double-lumen port with one port in the stomach and another in the descending duodenum is adequate. When total output of enzymes or bicarbonate is used as the diagnostic parameter, the use of a nonabsorbable marker is advised.

Some centers use secretin alone as the secretagogue, whereas others use CCK (or its analog, cerulein), and some use both. The dosage and method of administration differs, as do the timing of collections and the normal ranges. If secretin alone is used as the secretagogue, the output of bicarbonate is measured. If CCK or one of its analogs is used, the output of enzymes (amylase, lipase, or others) is used as the diagnostic parameter. These tests usually last 60–90 minutes, over which time pancreatic secretions are suctioned from the duodenum and subsequently analyzed. It can be difficult for some patients to tolerate either having this oroduodenal tube initially placed or in leaving it in place for that period of time. Several variations of the test have been developed or proposed utilizing endoscopy under conscious sedation. These variations include placing the oroduodenal tube with endoscopic assistance or over an endoscopically placed guide wire *(20)*, collecting pancreatic secretions directly through the suction channel of an endoscope *(21)*, and collecting pure pancreatic secretions through a tube placed into the pancreatic duct at the time of ERCP *(22)*. These methods have not been as well-studied as the traditionally used techniques.

It has been generally agreed that direct pancreatic function tests are the most sensitive tests available to detect CP in its earlier stages, before the development of exocrine and endocrine insufficiency and before the development of advanced structural abnormalities. In a few studies, the results of direct pancreatic function testing have been compared to the gold standard—histology. In one particular study *(23)*, there was a nearly linear relationship between maximum bicarbonate concentration in pancreatic secretions and the degree of histological damage. In this study, the sensitivity of a direct pancreatic function test using both secretin and CCK for the diagnosis of moderate-to-severe CP was 79%, when compared to 66% for ERCP. In other words, this direct pancreatic function test was able to detect CP in a group of patients who had not yet developed structural abnormalities seen on ERCP (i.e., patients with small-duct CP). This result has been confirmed in other studies comparing direct pancreatic function testing to histology (6,7,24,25). There are also numerous studies that compare direct pancreatic function testing to other diagnostic tests, particularly ERCP. The two tests (direct pancreatic function testing and ERCP) reach similar conclusions in more than three-quarters of patients. In 3–20% of patients, the two tests disagree (6,7,26–30). Two small studies have followed such patients with discordant test results. In those patients with an abnormal direct pancreatic function test and a normal ERCP, CP ultimately develops in 90% (28,31). In those with a normal direct pancreatic function test and an abnormal ERCP, chronic pancreatitis develops in 0–26% patients (28,31). These data suggest that direct pancreatic function testing is somewhat more sensitive and specific than ERCP. Although, like all diagnostic tests, direct pancreatic function tests are most accurate in more severe and advanced disease. The degree of damage necessary to affect stimulated pancreatic secretion is unknown; some experts suggested that 50% of the gland must be affected before direct pancreatic function tests are reliably positive, despite the lack of evidence to confirm this opinion.

Even if direct pancreatic function tests appear to be the most sensitive diagnostic test available, these tests suffer from important limitations. First and foremost is the lack of availability. The tests are only performed at a few centers, and although this number is slowly growing, they are still unavailable to most clinicians. The test is not standardized, cumbersome to perform, and unpleasant for patients. Nonetheless, the test is safe, relatively inexpensive, and better able to detect CP in its earlier stages than other available diagnostic tests. Direct pancreatic function tests are particularly useful to diagnose those patients with small-duct CP, in whom alternative diagnostic tests are likely to miss the diagnosis. Almost by definition, those with small-duct CP do not have structural abnormalities visible on imaging procedures or ERCP and do not usually have exocrine or endocrine insufficiency detectable on most tests of pancreatic function. Making a diagnosis in patients with small-duct CP may be difficult or impossible if direct tests of pancreatic function are not available.

Several modifications of direct pancreatic function tests have been developed to make the procedure more widely accessible. One such method has been to place the oroduodenal tube via endoscopy, which bypasses one of the most difficult components of the standard test—the unpleasant process of placing the tube without sedation. This method is feasible and, in small studies, appears to provide accurate data (20), Yet concern still arises on the potential effect of sedation on pancreatic secretion. A second method is to administer the secretagogue 30 minutes before endoscopy, then use an endoscope to collect pancreatic secretions for a brief period of time *(21)*. Standard pancreatic function tests utilize a 60- to 90-minute collection period. The peak in pancreatic secretion may, in fact, be delayed for up to 90 minutes after injection of the secretagogue. Whether shorter collection periods maintain adequate sensitivity and specificity is still unknown. In one study of 633 subjects undergoing standard 60-minute direct pancreatic function testing, but only using data from the first 15-minute collection period, the specificity of the test was only 35% *(32)*. In other words, two thirds of patients with normal overall test results would have been labeled as having CP if only the first 15-minute collection was used instead of the full 60-minute collection period. Thus, tests that use short periods of collection may not give an adequate perspective of the pancreatic secretory capacity, although they may allow this type of testing to be more widely available.

One of the problems that can make traditional direct pancreatic function tests inaccurate is inadequate collection of pancreatic secretions. One method to prevent inaccuracy is to collect pure pancreatic secretions at the time of ERCP. This involves placing a catheter into the pancreatic duct, administering a secretagogue (typically secretin), and collecting pancreatic secretions directly. To minimize the risk of causing pancreatitis, the catheter cannot be left in place for prolonged periods of time. This test uses only two 5-minute collection periods, but pancreatitis can still occur. This test is not well-studied, and the accuracy of this method remains unknown. Preliminary data suggest rather poor sensitivity and specificity *(22,33)*. Recently, pancreatic function testing has been extensively reviewed *(34)*.

TESTS OF PANCREATIC STRUCTURE

Plain Abdominal Radiographs

A standard abdominal radiograph (KUB) may detect diffuse pancreatic calcification in very far-advanced CP. The finding of diffuse calcification is specific for CP but is quite insensitive. Diffuse calcification may take up to 20 years to develop. Focal calcification is not specific for CP, and calcifications may appear and disappear over time in patients with CP.

Abdominal Ultrasonography

The primary diagnostic findings of CP on abdominal US include pancreatic calcifications, a dilated pancreatic duct, gland atrophy or enlargement, irregular gland margins, pseudocysts, and changes in gland echotexture. A consensus conference defined the features of ultrasonography in CP (Table 2; *34a*). Although this conference occurred

Table 2
Diagnosis and Grading of Chronic Pancreatitis on Ultrasound
and Computed Tomography

Grade of chronic pancreatitis	US or CT findings
Normal–no evidence of chronic pancreatitis	Study of good-quality visualizing entire gland with no abnormal findings
Equivocal evidence of chronic pancreatitis	One of the following: Mild enlargement of the pancreatic duct (2–4 mm) Overall gland enlargement ≤ twofold normal
Mild-to-moderate chronic pancreatitis	One of the above plus at least one of the following: Pancreatic duct dilation >4 mm Pancreatic duct irregularity Cavities <10-mm diameter Parenchymal heterogeneity Increased echogenicity of duct wall Irregular contour of gland in head or body Focal necrosis of parenchyma
Severe chronic pancreatitis	Mild-to-moderate plus one or more of the following: Cavity >10-mm diameter Intraductal filling defects Calculi or pancreatic calcifications Ductal stricture or obstruction Severe duct dilation or irregularity Contiguous organ involvement

Adapted from ref. *34a*. US, ultrasound; CT, computed tomography.

25 years ago, and the criteria developed are a mixture of both diagnosis and grading of severity, these features continue to be used. Overall, the sensitivity of US is approximately 60% *(1,8)*. The low sensitivity is partly a result of the difficulty of visualizing the pancreas from overlying bowel gas. One additional problem that can make the interpretation of abdominal ultrasonograpy challenging is the tremendous spectrum of changes that can occur in the pancreas as a consequence of aging. Changes in echotexture, pancreatic duct dilation, cystic cavities, and even ductal calcifications may develop with aging *(35,36)*. These findings mimic those in CP. It can be difficult or impossible in some patients to differentiate age-related changes from pathological CP. These age-related changes are rare before the age of 60 but become increasingly common after that age. Nonetheless, transabdominal ultrasonography remains a very useful diagnostic test for CP and is

often able to identify other diseases that might mimic CP (e.g., pancreatic cancer and biliary disease), as well as complications of CP (e.g., pseudocyst or biliary obstruction). Abdominal ultrasonography is widely available, inexpensive, and risk-free.

Computed Tomography

CT, particularly state-of-the-art multidetector CT, is much more sensitive than ultrasonography (75–90%) because of its improved capacity to detect more focal abnormalities, such as calcification, a dilated pancreatic duct, fluid collections, or focal enlargements (1). In addition, CT images of the pancreas are not obscured by intestinal gas, and CT can image the pancreas in essentially every patient. The same consensus panel that developed criteria for ultrasonography defined the abnormalities that might be detected by CT in patients with CP (Table 2). CT, like all diagnostic tests, is most accurate in more advanced disease. Recently available multidetector rapid-sequence CT provides images of much better detail and resolution than previous technologies, which it could be assumed will result in improved sensitivity and specificity. The test is widely available and reasonably safe, but substantially more expensive than US.

Magnetic Resonance Imaging

In recent years, an improvement in magnetic resonance technology has also allowed more accurate imaging of both the pancreatic parenchyma and pancreatic duct (with so-called magnetic resonance cholangiopancreatography [MRCP]). It is not clear that magnetic resonance imaging (MRI) and MRCP are superior to CT but do appear to be at least equivalent in overall accuracy. MRCP is becoming much more widely used in the evaluation of pancreatic and biliary diseases (37). MRCP is particularly good at imaging the pancreatic duct when it is dilated. When compared to ERCP, the sensitivity of MRCP for CP is about 70–80% (1,37). Agreement is best when significant pancreatic ductal abnormalities are present, and when the pancreatic duct is dilated. MRI is currently widely available, generally risk-free, and moderately expensive, but not all centers have the capacity to perform MRCP.

Endoscopic Retrograde Cholangiopancreatography

ERCP is generally considered the most sensitive and specific method of detecting structural abnormalities of the pancreatic duct. During ERCP, radiographic contrast is injected into the pancreatic duct and good-quality radiographs can provide a highly detailed view of the pancreatic duct. Changes in the pancreatic duct consistent with CP include ductal dilation, strictures, irregularity, and filling defects (stones) with-

Table 3
Grading of Chronic Pancreatitis by Endoscopic
Retrograde Cholangiopancreatography

Grade of chronic pancreatitis	Main pancreatic duct	Side branches of duct
Normal– no evidence of chronic pancreatitis	Normal	Normal
Equivocal evidence of chronic pancreatitis	Normal	<3 Abnormal
Mild chronic pancreatitis	Normal	≥3 Abnormal
Moderate chronic pancreatitis	Abnormal	≥3 Abnormal
Severe chronic pancreatitis	Abnormal with at least one of the following: Large cavity (>10 mm) Duct stricture or obstruction Intraductal filling defects or stones Severe duct irregularity or dilation	≥3 Abnormal

Adapted from ref. *37a.*

in the pancreatic duct (Fig. 1). ERCP only detects abnormalities of the pancreatic ductal system, and unlike US or CT, it is unable to visualize any changes within the parenchyma of the gland. Like US and CT, a consensus panel developed criteria that can be used for both the diagnosis and staging of disease (Table 3; *37a*). Given the high sensitivity and widespread accessibility of ERCP, it is often considered the defacto gold standard. The estimated sensitivity of the test is 70–90% *(1,5,6,8)* with a specificity of 80–90%. ERCP is highly accurate in those with advanced or big-duct CP and has the advantage over other diagnostic tests in that therapy (stenting of a ductal stricture, removal of a pancreatic duct stone) may also be administered. At its most advanced, CP can produce significant duct abnormalities with alternating areas of stricture and dilation. This "chain-of-lakes" appearance is a pathognomonic form of advanced CP. Less dramatic changes can also be visualized. Accurate interpretation of these less dramatic changes can be difficult. One of the problems is related to the fact that these more subtle pancreatic ductal changes can occur in other diseases and conditions, which can produce changes within the pancreatic duct that mimic those seen in CP. These conditions include underfilling of the pancreatic duct with contrast, pancreatic carcinoma, normal aging effects, a recent attack of AP, and the effect of placing a stent in the pancreatic duct at the time of ERCP *(5,6)*. Underfilling of the pancreatic duct can occur in up to 30% of pancreatograms, and this is usually done intentionally to try to minimize the chance of causing pancreatitis from the procedure (which can occur in about 5–10% of patients who undergo ERCP). Although a reasonable goal, it does limit the ability to interpret the pancreatogram. An underfilled ductal system may appear to have irregularities of the main ductal margin that disappear with additional ductal filling, possibly leading to diagnostic errors.

Several specific conditions can also produce changes within the pancreatic duct that mimic those seen in CP, and the most common is the effect of aging. Despite that pancreatic function is generally maintained throughout life, aging can produce significant abnormalities of the pancreatic duct, including focal or diffuse dilation, cystic cavities, and even ductal calculi *(35)*. In one large study of screening ultrasonography performed in Japan, more than one half of all pancreatic calcification and more than 80% of all ductal dilation and cystic lesions were considered to be a result of aging, not CP *(36)*. This US study is not strictly a study of ERCP, but does relate to the changes that can occur with aging. Changes within the pancreatic duct can also follow an attack of AP, including duct irregularity, cavities, and ductal strictures. Although these changes resolve in the vast majority of patients, it may take several months after the attack to do so. Pancreatic carcinoma may also mimic the changes viewed in CP, particularly carcinoma of the pancreatic head, which can produce significant dilation and irregularity of the pancreatic duct usptream from the malignant stricture. The finding of a dominant stricture with upstream dilation should lead to the immediate suspicion of pancreatic carcinoma, not CP. Finally, pancreatic duct stents can produce changes within the pancreatic duct and parenchyma in up to one half of patients, and these may not resolve *(38,39)*.

A second difficulty relates to the issue of small-duct CP (Fig. 2). CP can exist in the absence of any changes in the pancreatic duct, in which case ERCP, by definition, will miss the diagnosis. CP can also exist with minimal or subtle abnormalities within the pancreatic duct. This is related to the difficulty of interpretation of these subtle changes and the fact that this interpretation is subjective and prone to interobserver and intraobserver variation. In one study of 69 postmortem pancreatograms submitted to six experienced endoscopists, between 2 and 58% of these pancreatograms were interpreted as normal, depending on the endoscopist *(40)*. In another study, pancreatograms were shown to four expert endoscopists on three separate occasions *(41)*. The four endoscopists were unanimous in their own three reports between 47 and 95% of the time. This problem with interobserver and intraobserver

Table 4
Diagnosis of Chronic Pancreatitis by Endoscopic Ultrasound

Parenchmyal abnormalities	Ductal abnormalities
Hyperechoic foci	Dilation of main pancreatic duct
Hyperechoic strands	Irregularity of ductal margin
Lobularity of contour of gland	Hyperechoic ductal margins
Cystic collections	Dilated ductal side branches
	Ductal stones

variation is not surprising if one recalls that the changes can be subtle and interpretation is subjective. Astute clinicians should be aware of these issues and not give inordinate diagnostic weight to slight changes within the pancreatic duct.

ERCP is widely available and is a powerful diagnostic and therapeutic tool. Overall, it is accurate provided that subtle ductal changes are not overinterpreted. However, it does pose the highest risk of all the diagnostic tests with complications occurring in 5–10% of patients who undergo ERCP. It is also one of the most expensive of all diagnostic tests. For these reasons, ERCP is usually not used as the first diagnostic test and is reserved for those situations that arise when other tests are not diagnostic or when therapy (rather than diagnosis) is contemplated.

Endoscopic Ultrasound

Endoscopic ultrasound (EUS) uses a high-frequency US probe mounted on the end of a flexible endoscope. It allows the pancreas to be imaged through the gastric and duodenal wall with highly detailed images of the pancreatic parenchyma and pancreatic duct. The diagnosis is usually based on the finding of numerous features (Table 4). A positive test is arbitrarily chosen, in most cases a range of more than 3–5 criteria. Higher cut-offs produce improved test specificity but worsen sensitivity. When compared to ERCP, the two tests reach the same diagnosis in about 80% of patients *(42)*. EUS has also been compared with direct pancreatic function testing and intraductal pancreatic function testing (at the time of ERCP), and the two types of tests reach a similar finding about 75% of patients *(6,42)*. EUS is continuing to be intensively studied. When EUS and ERCP or pancreatic function tests reach different conclusions (i.e., one test is abnormal and the other test is normal), it is usually EUS that is abnormal. Part of the explanation may be from the fact that the EUS features of CP do not appear to be entirely specific for CP and can be seen in association with other conditions

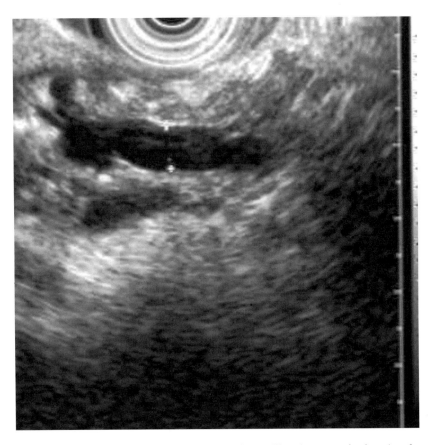

Fig. 3. An endoscopic ultrasound demonstrating a dilated pancreatic duct (markers) in a patient with advanced chronic pancreatitis.

(43) or as a consequence of aging. A normal EUS essentially eliminates the diagnosis of CP. Abnormalities are routinely seen at EUS in patients with advanced or big-duct CP (Fig. 3). Additionally, EUS is an accurate method of detecting pancreatic cancer that might mimic CP (Fig. 4). The test appears to be most useful when normal or dramatically abnormal, but the sensitivity and specificity of the test for moderate or mild CP requires further study. EUS, like ERCP, is relatively expensive, but unlike ERCP, EUS is not universally available. However, it is safer than ERCP.

DIAGNOSTIC STRATEGY

The diagnostic approach should begin with tests that are safe, inexpensive, and able to detect relatively far-advanced or big-duct disease. Diagnostic tests that fit in this category include serum trypsin, fecal

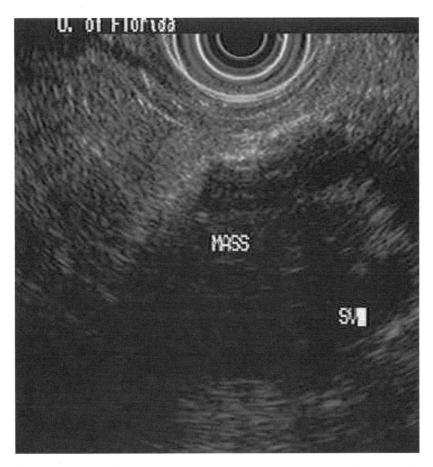

Fig. 4. An endoscopic ultrasound demonstrating a mass in a patient with pancreatic carcinoma.

elastase, or abdominal ultrasonography. If these do not lead to a diagnosis, more risky or expensive tests will generally need to be employed (e.g., MRI/MRCP, CT, ERCP, or EUS). Direct pancreatic function testing, if available, should logically be used after the initial tests and prior to these more expensive or invasive tests, as these pancreatic function tests are the most sensitive tests available and are neither as costly nor as risky as the second echelon tests noted previously. If pancreatic function testing is unavailable, as is often the case, these second echelon tests should be used, usually starting with a good-quality multidetector CT. If ERCP or EUS is used, clinicians need to be aware of both the strengths and weaknesses of these techniques in diagnosing CP.

REFERENCES

1. Forsmark CE. Chronic pancreatitis. In: Feldman M, Friedman LS, Sleisenger MH, eds. Gastrointestinal and Liver Disease. Pathophysiology, Diagnosis, Management, 7th edition. WB Saunders, Philadelphia, PA, 2002: 943–969.
2. Layer P, Yamamoto H, Kalthoff L, et al. The different courses of early- and late-onset idiopathic and alcoholic chronic pancreatitis. Gastroenterology 1994; 107: 1481–1487.
3. Ammann RW, Akovbiantz A, Largiarder F, et al. Course and outcome of chronic pancreatitis. Gastroenterology 1984; 86: 820–828.
4. Kloppel G, Maillet B. Pathology of chronic pancreatitis. In: Beger HG, Warshaw AL, Buchler MW, et al., eds. The Pancreas. Blackwell Science, Malden, MA, 1998: 720–723.
5. Forsmark CE, Toskes PP. What does an abnormal pancreatogram mean? Gastrointest Endosc Clin North Am 1995; 5: 105–123.
6. Forsmark CE. The diagnosis of chronic pancreatitis. Gastrointest Endosc 2000; 52: 293–295.
7. Jacobsen DG, Currington C, Connery K, et al. Trypsin-like immunoreactivity as a test for pancreatic insufficiency. N Engl J Med 1984; 310: 1307–1309.
8. Niederau C, Grendell JH. Diagnosis of chronic pancreatitis. Gastroenterology 1985; 88: 1973–95.
9. DiMagno EP, Go VLW, Summerskill WHJ. Relations between pancreatic enzyme outputs and malabsorption in severe pancreatic insufficiency. N Engl J Med 1973; 288: 813–815.
10. Loser C, Mollgaard A, Folsch UR. Fecal elastase 1. A novel, highly sensitive and specific tubeless pancreatic function tests. Gut 1996; 39:580–586.
11. Lüth S, Teyssen K, Forssmann K, et al. Fecal elastase-1 determination: "Gold Standard" of indirect pancreatic function tests? Scand J Gastroenterol 2001; 10: 1092–1099.
12. Gullo L. Fecal elastase-1 in chronic pancreatitis. Gut 1999; 44: 291–292.
13. Amann ST, Bishop M, Curington C, Toskes PP. Fecal pancreatic elastase-1 is inaccurate in the diagnosis of chronic pancreatitis. Pancreas 1996; 13: 226–230.
14. Lembeke B, Braden B, Caspary WF. Exocrine pancreatic insufficiency: accuracy and clinical value of the uniformly labeled 13C-hiolein-breath test. Gut 1996; 39: 668–674.
15. Goff JS. Two-stage triolein breath test differentiates pancreatic insufficiency from other causes of malabsorption. Gastroenterology 1982; 83: 44–46.
16. Loser CHR, Brauser C, Aygen S, et al. Comparative clinical evaluation of the 13C-mixed triglyceride breath test as an indirect pancreatic function test. Scand J Gastroenterol 1998; 33: 327–334.
17. Ochi K, Mizushima T, Harada H, et al. Chronic pancreatitis: Functional testing. Pancreas 1998; 16: 343–348.
18. Lankisch PG, Creutzfeldt W. Effects of synthetic and natural secretin on the function of the exocrine pancreas in man. Digestion 1981; 22: 61–65.
19. Tympner F, Domschke S, Domschke W, et al. Reproducibility of the response to secretin and secretin plus pancreozymin in man. Scand J Gastroenterol 1974; 9: 377–381.
20. Waxman I, Steere ML, Freedman SD. Endoscopically assisted direct pancreatic function testing: A simplified technique. Gastrointest Endosc 1996; 44: 630.
21. Conwell DL, Zuccaro G, Vargo JJ, et al. An endoscopic pancreatic function test for the diagnosis of chronic pancreatitis: A case-control study. Pancreas 2002 (Abstract); 25: 423.

22. Pollack BJ, Forsmark CE. Adjunct diagnosis of pancreatic disease and pancreatic physiology. In: Michael V. Sivak, Jr, ed. Gastroenterologic Endoscopy. WB Saunders, Philadelphia, PA, 2000: 1116–1125.
23. Hayakawa T, Kondo T, Shibata T, et al. Relationship between pancreatic exocrine function and histological changes in chronic pancreatitis. Am J Gastroenterol 1992; 87: 1170–1174.
24. Heij HA, Obertop H, van Blankenstein M, et al. Relationship between functional and histological changes in chronic pancreatitis. Dig Dis Sci 1986; 31: 1009–1113.
25. Waye JD, Adler M, Dreiling DA. The pancreas. A correlation of function and structure. Am L Gastroenterol 1978; 69: 176–181.
26. Rolny P, Lukes PJ, Gamklou R, et al. A comparative evaluation of endoscopic retrograde pancreatography and secretin-CCK test in the diagnosis of pancreatic disease. Scand J Gastroenterol 1978; 13: 777–781.
27. Bozkurt T, Braun U, Leferink S, et al. Comparison of pancreatic morphology and exocrine functional impairment in patients with chronic pancreatitis. Gut 1994; 35: 1132–1136.
28. Lankisch PG, Seidensticker F, Otto J, et al. Secretin-pancreozymin test (SPT) and endoscopic retrograde cholangiopancreatography (ERCP): Both are necessary for diagnosing or excluding chronic pancreatitis. Pancreas 1996; 12: 149–152.
29. Malfertheiner P, Büchler M, Stanescu A, Ditschuneit H. Exocrine pancreatic function in correlation to ductal and parenchymal morphology in chronic pancreatitis. Hepato-Gastroenterol 1986; 33: 110–114.
30. Girdwood AH, Hatfield ARW, Bornman PC, et al. Structure and function in non-calcific pancreatitis. Dig Dis Sci 1984; 29: 721–726.
31. Lambiase L, Forsmark CE, Toskes PP. Secretin test diagnoses chronic pancreatitis earlier than ERCP. Gastroenterology 1993; 104 (Abstract): A315.
32. Amann S, Newman MB, Toskes PP. Relationship of the etiology of chronic pancreatitis to the time to reach peak bicarbonate secretion in duodenal aspirates after secretin stimulation. Gastroenterology 1999; 116 (Abstract): G4811.
33. Josephson SA, Amann ST, Toskes PP, Forsmark CE. Utility of the intraductal secretin test prospectively compared to the standard secretin test. Pancreas 1996; 13 (Abstract): 441.
34. Chowdhury RS, Forsmark CE. Review article: Pancreatic function testing. Aliment Pharmacol Ther 2003; 17: 733–750.
34a. Sarner M, Cotton PB. Classification of Pancreatitis. Gut 1984; 25: 756–759.
35. Ross SO, Forsmark CE. Pancreatic and biliary diseases in the elderly. Gastrointerol Clin North Am 2001; 30: 531–546.
36. Ikeda M, Sato T, Morozumi A. Morphologic changes in the pancreas detected by screening ultrasonography in a mass survey, with special reference to main duct dilation, cyst formation, and calcification. Pancreas 1994; 9: 508–512.
37. MacEneaney P, Mitchell MT, McDermott R. Update on magnetic resonance cholangiopancreatography. Gastrointerol Clin North Am 2002; 31: 731–746.
37a. Axon ATR, Classen M, Cotton PB, et al. Pancreatography in chronic pancreatitis: Internal definations. gut 1984; 25: 1107–1112.
38. Smith MT, Sherman S, Ikenberry SO, et al. Alterations in pancreatic duct morphology following polyethylene stent therapy. Gastrointest Endosc 1996; 44: 268–275.
39. Sherman S, Hawes RH, Savides TJ, et al. Stent-induced pancreatic ductal and parenchymal changes: correlation of endoscopic ultrasound with ERCP. Gastrointest Endosc 1996; 44: 276–282.
40. Schmitz-Moormann P, Himmelmann GW, Brandes JW, et al. Comparative radiological and morphological study of human pancreas. Pancreatitis-like changes in

postmortem ductograms and their morphological pattern. Possible implication for ERCP. Gut 1985; 26: 406–414.

41. Cotton PB. Progress report: ERCP. Gut 1977; 18: 316–341.
42. Wallace MB, Hawes RH. Endoscopic ultrasound in the diagnosis and treatment of chronic pancreatitis. Pancreas 2001; 23: 26–35.
43. Sahai AV, Mishra G, Penman ID, et al. EUS to detect evidence of pancreatic disease in patients with persistent or nonspecific dyspepsia. Gastrointest Endosc 2000; 52: 293–298.

13 Treatment of Chronic Pancreatitis Pain

Overview and Medical Management

Phillip P. Toskes, MD

CONTENTS

INTRODUCTION

Patients with chronic pancreatitis (CP) come to medical attention because of abdominal pain or symptoms of maldigestion or diabetes.

From: *Pancreatitis and Its Complications*
Edited by: C. E. Forsmark © Humana Press Inc., Totowa, NJ

Abdominal pain is clearly the most common and most significant of symptoms and is the most difficult to treat and generally interferes with quality of life. The abdominal pain is quite variable in location, severity, and frequency. Patients with acute pancreatitis (AP) experience mid-epigastric pain that radiates to the back. The pain of CP often does not follow this classical pattern. Indeed, many variations of abdominal pain may be caused by CP. The pain can be constant or intermittent, and there may be frequent pain-free intervals. Eating may exacerbate the pain, leading to fear of eating and weight loss. The spectrum of abdominal pain ranges from mild to severe, often with narcotic dependence as a consequence.

The natural history of abdominal pain in patients with CP is also quite variable. Some patients may suffer from continuous pain, whereas others have prolonged pain-free intervals, and still others gradually become pain-free. The evolution of pain does not always follow the progressive downhill course that some patients may experience with the late development of exocrine and endocrine pancreatic insufficiency. In these latter stages of disease (discussed in Chapters 11 and 16), some patients will actually lose their pain. Approximately 20% of patients initially present with symptoms of maldigestion and never experience abdominal pain. The extremely diverse nature and evolution of abdominal pain make judgments of therapeutic efficacy difficult. To account for this variability, large randomized trials are required. No large randomized trial yet exists in this field, and the following insights and recommendations are therefore based on imperfect data and reflect the opinion and experience of the author based on years of experience managing these patients. What is quite clear is that the management of pain and management of this progression to end-stage pancreatitis is associated with significant morbidity, mortality, and utilization of societal resources (1,2).

Any management strategy of CP must be based on an accurate diagnosis and understanding of the difference between "big duct" disease and "small duct" disease. CP is not one disease, and clinicians have made the mistake of trying to treat all patients with CP as if they were all the same. Many patients with CP suffer injury to acinar cells and small ducts without obvious abnormalities in the main pancreatic duct. These patients with small duct disease can be exceedingly difficult to diagnose, as standard diagnostic tests are insensitive to small duct disease. Most of the literature has focused on severe CP secondary to alcohol, because this is generally a big duct disease and easy to diagnose. As such, it is likely that the prevalence of CP has been largely underestimated. An appreciable percentage of patients suffering from unexplained chronic abdominal pain may be suffering from small duct pancreatitis, and the diagnosis may be missed by standard radiographic evaluation (3). Numerous studies have described patients with painful CP and normal findings on

Table 1
Etiology of Chronic Pancreatitis Pain

Neural inflammation
Ductal hypertension
Parenchymal hypertension
Stenosis of common bile duct
Pseudocyst
Acute inflammation

ultrasound, computed tomography (CT), and endoscopic retrograde cholangiopancreatography (ERCP). When such patients have been brought to surgery, histological abnormalities of inflammation, fibrosis, and small duct abnormalities were detected within the pancreas. Similarly, there are a group of patients with chronic abdominal pain and negative radiographic evaluation who have been labeled as having CP based on minimal abnormalities of serum lipase or amylase. The pitfalls in accurate diagnosis are discussed in Chapter 12. It is worth re-emphasizing within the context of this chapter that therapy directed at CP pain (whether it is medical, endoscopic, or surgical therapy) is inappropriate if the patient does not have a secure diagnosis of CP.

PATHOPHYSIOLOGY

The pathophysiology of pain in CP remains uncertain. All known causes of CP appear to result in a common group of histopathological changes, which include inflammatory acinar and ductal cell injury and fibrosis with damage to the intrapancreatic nerves. The exact molecular events leading to CP remain undefined. Recent research has identified specific genetic abnormalities that may provide insight into the pathophysiology of CP. This is discussed more fully in Chapter 10.

The cause of pain in CP is multifactorial, and therein is the difficulty in management (Table 1). Pain may be caused by an associated anatomic problem, such as duodenal or biliary obstruction or an associated pseudocyst. In those without these anatomic abnormalities, the currently favored theories as to why patients with CP have pain include perineural inflammation, elevated pressures in both big and small ducts and in the pancreatic parenchyma, ischemia of the gland, and abnormal negative feedback mechanisms involving hormone mediators, such as cholecystokinin (CCK; 4). It may be difficult to determine the contribution of each of these potential causes in an individual patient. Several observations have pointed to the existence of neuroimmune interactions as a mechanism in the pain of CP. These interactions

Table 2
Features of Large Duct and Small Duct Chronic Pancreatitis

Feature	Large duct	Small duct
Sex predominance	Male	Female
Diagnostic findings		
Secretin test	Abnormal	Abnormal
Serum trypsinogen	Often abnormal	Typically normal
Diffuse pancreatic calcifications on imaging	Frequent	Infrequent
ERCP	Often markedly abnormal	Minimally abnormal to normal
Natural history		
Progression to steatorrhea	Frequent	Rare
Pain therapy		
Pancreatic enzymes	Poor-to-fair response	Good-to-excellent response
Surgical Procedures	Often helpful	Usually not indicated

ERCP, endoscopic retrograde cholangiopancreatography.

include overexpression of fibroblast and other growth factors in the tissue of patients of CP, increased interleukin-8 expression, high levels of transforming growth factor-α and its receptor, and increased expression of epidermal growth factor. The importance of these interacting factors still needs to be fully clarified.

DIAGNOSIS

The diagnosis of CP is thoroughly reviewed in Chapter 12. It is important to point out that it is easy to make a diagnosis in patients with big duct CP. Table 2 describes the features of big duct and small duct CP.

Any of the various diagnostic tests will likely be abnormal in patients with big duct CP. The challenge in the diagnosis of patients with CP is in evaluating the subgroup of patients with abdominal pain and negative radiographic studies who may have small duct CP. All referral centers focusing on CP pain recognize that there is a subset of patients thought to have painful CP but who are not able to be diagnosed with radiographic procedures, such as conventional abdominal ultrasound, CT, magnetic resonance imaging, and ERCP. The percentage of patients with CP within this subset remains controversial, but may be as high as 40% in some centers. It appears that some combination of a direct hormone stimulation test, such as the secretin test and/or endoscopic ultrasound (EUS) is apt to give the best detection rate in these patients. Many referral centers (including my own) see two groups of patients in approximately equal numbers. The first is a group with chronic abdominal pain and negative imaging studies labeled as having CP who do not have CP. Many in this group have undergone multiple risky therapies (often multiple ERCPs with various interventions) without relief. The second is a group of patients with similar symptoms labeled as having functional abdominal pain, but who actually have CP. Distinguishing between these groups of patients is difficult but necessary for proper management.

GENERAL PRINCIPLES OF PAIN MANAGEMENT

Appropriate pain management in patients with CP continues to be a frustrating undertaking for both patients and physicians. First, in a patient suspected to have CP pain, it is important that other causes of abdominal pain that can mimic CP pain be eliminated, such as peptic ulcer disease, gallbladder-related causes, gastrointestinal motility disorders, and other complications associated with CP (e.g., pseudocyst, duodenal obstruction, and common bile duct obstruction). Abdominal pain caused by motility disturbances of the gastrointestinal tract, particularly the stomach or small intestine, may mimic the abdominal pain associated with CP, such that even seasoned consultants cannot distinguish the pain of dysmotility from the pain of CP. Patients with these dysmotility syndromes may even manifest a mild elevation of serum amylase and/or lipase. It is understood that these enzymes may come from the inflammation of other tissues rather than just the pancreas. These mild to moderate elevation of pancreatic enzymes in the blood more often reflect nonpancreatic causes of pain.

A recent study at our medical center (5) presented preliminary data on 74 patients referring to our pancreatitis clinic, who were suspected by the referring gastroenterologist and surgeons as having radiographic-negative CP or small duct CP. The evaluation of these patients with unexplained pain of presumed pancreatic origin revealed that 40% actually had CP diagnosed by the secretin hormone stimulation test, 50% had dysmotility (most commonly of the stomach), and 10% had no cause that could be found. Pancreatic enzyme therapy decreased abdominal pain in those patients with small duct CP and prokinetic therapy (Erythromycin ethyl succinate suspension orally administered at 100 mg, four times a day or 200 mg intravenously four times a day) remarkably decreased abdominal pain in patients with gastroparesis. Even retrospectively, the CP pain could not be distinguished in any accurate manner from the pain that was caused by dysmotility.

Recently, it has also been recognized by our group that the interaction of motility disturbances with CP is even more complex than previously thought, because we have recently reported that the prevalence of gastroparesis is increased in patients with abdominal pain and small duct CP *(6)*. In 56 patients with small duct CP documented by hormone stimulation test, 25 of the 56 patients (44%) had gastroparesis. The etiology of this gastroparesis in such patients is unclear but may be related to high levels of CCK that some patients with CP manifest to the concomitant use of narcotic analgesics or to other unknown causes. High CCK levels can lead to a decrease in gastric emptying. Medical treatment of the pain of CP involves, among other therapies, the administration of nonenteric-coated pancreatic enzymes. In the experience of this author, the presence of gastroparesis greatly diminishes the effectiveness of enzymes. Administration of a prokinetic agent enhances delivery of these enzymes from the stomach into the proximal small intestine. It is within this segment of the small intestine where feedback control of pancreatic secretion is operative, that pancreatic enzyme therapy may effect pancreatic feedback control. The proximal small intestine is the sole site for this process and this process is mediated by the action of serine proteases (trypsin, chymotrypsin, and elastase) on CCK-releasing peptide. Because of this association between gastroparesis and CP, which is quite striking in our experience, we try to use anodynes that do not affect gastrointestinal motility such as acetaminophen, propopxyphene, or tramadol. Narcotics will decrease gastrointestinal motility and thus impair the delivery of enzymes from the stomach to the proximal small intestine. The initial approach in patients with CP pain is generally conservative management, including analgesics, abstinence from alcohol, if that appears to be involved in the pathogenesis of the disease, and suppression of pancreatic secretion.

ANALGESIC AGENTS

Narcotic addition is an unfortunate and very common result of the use of narcotic analgesics in patients with CP pain. The rate of narcotic addiction is not precisely known, but most experts agree it occurs in one fourth of patients or more. It is best to start with non-narcotic or low-potency narcotics initially using agents like acetaminophen, nonsteroidal anti-inflammatory drugs, propopxyphene, or tramadol. Adding a tricyclic antidepressant or selective serotonin reuptake inhibitor is also often useful to minimize the need for high-potency narcotics. Despite these approaches, many patients remain on narcotics for prolonged periods of time.

ABSTINENCE FROM ALCOHOL

Abstinence from alcohol appears to slow the progression of CP, yet it does not prevent progression. The effect of abstinence on pain is not clear-cut, but some patients may experience a reduction in pain. Apart from a possible beneficial effect on pain, abstinence is appropriate to slow the development of CP and prevent other alcohol-induced complications.

PANCREATIC ENZYME PREPARATIONS

The use of nonenteric-coated pancreatic enzyme preparations to decrease abdominal pain in patients with CP is based on the concept of feedback control of pancreatic exocrine secretion (7). Pancreatic enzyme preparations appear to inhibit pancreatic secretion by a negative feedback mechanism involving intraduodenal serine proteases. These serine proteases modulate pancreactic secretion by regulating CCK release. Because patients with CP often have decreased intraduodenal proteases activity owing to a damaged gland, they may not be capable of inactivating the CCK-releasing peptide, a peptide that exists in the proximal small bowel and is largely responsible for stimulating CCK-release. In these patients, high levels of CCK releasing peptide are constantly present, and high levels of CCK persist, producing overstimulation of the pancreas. In these patients, pain may occur because of this hyperstimulation. Hence, in a subset of patients, the gland is under constant stimulation by CCK. CCK-releasing peptides can be denatured by serine proteases delivered to the duodenum, decreasing CCK release, which then decreases pancreatic stimulation and may decrease pain. Because this is a proximal small intestine phenomenon, the pancreatic proteases must be delivered to the upper small intestine. This can only be done consistently by the administration of nonenteric-coated pancreatic enzyme preparations. It is important to know that these preparations are not protected against the destruction of gastric acid as they pass through the stomach; therefore, it is recommended that an acid-reducing agent, such as an H_2- receptor antagonist or a proton pump inhibitor, be given along with the pancreatic enzymes. We have found the most consistent preparation that affords control of feedback inhibition and relieves abdominal pain is the preparation of Viokase-16® (Axcan Scandipharm, Birmingham, AL). This preparation should be orally given in a dose of four tablets four times a day along with an acid-reducing agent. These pancreatic enzyme preparations are remarkably devoid of side effects. Occasionally, patients complain of dyspepsia, diarrhea, bloating, and very rarely a patient may have an allergic reaction to the pork preparation. One side effect of pancreatic enzyme therapy that has recently received much attention is colonic strictures. However, this complication has been largely seen in patients with cystic fibrosis who were overdosed with an incredibly high amount of pancreatic enzymes. These patients with cystic fibrosis had severe pancreatic insuffiency and did not respond to normal doses of pancreatic enzyme preparations. Rather than receiving from 9 to 12 capsules per day, these children were receiving as much as 60 or 90 capsules per day. Such colonic strictures have not been noted in adult patients with CP. Our extensive experience with this Viokase 16® preparation in a very large group of patients with CP pain has not led to any observation of colonic strictures in such patients.

Six randomized trials have evaluated the effectiveness of pancreatic enzymes and the reduction of pain associated with CP. Of these trials, two used nonenteric coat enzymes and were effective in reducing pain, whereas the four studies using the enteric coat preparation showed no statistical improvement in pain relief *(8)*. In the studies demonstrating efficacy, patients with big duct disease had, at best, a 25% response rate in decreasing abdominal pain, whereas the response rate was approximately 70% in those with small duct disease. Previous work in our laboratory has demonstrated that once patients with big duct disease developed severe pancreatic insufficiency (steatorrhea), feedback control of pancreatic secretion cannot be restored. Information now exists both from randomized trials and extensive clinical experience that nonenteric-coated enzyme preparations are preferable to enteric-coated enzymes for relieving abdominal pain in patients with CP. When a nonenteric-coated enzyme preparation was given, the proteases that escape destruction by gastric acid are delivered directly into the proximal small bowel. In contrast, enteric-coated enzyme preparations often do not open their enteric coat and deliver enzymes until the preparation reaches the jejunum or ileum. Evidence suggests that the feedback mechanism is not operative in the distal small bowel. Thus, optimal results are obtained with pancreatic enzymes when a nonenteric-coated enzyme preparation is utilized along with a proton pump inhibitor and given to the appropriate patient (i.e., one with small duct disease who has not developed pancreatic steatorrhea). Despite the lack of uniform results from randomized trials of enzyme therapy, practice guidelines continue to recommend a trial of enzyme therapy for painful CP *(8)*.

OCTREOTIDE

Following the concept of feedback inhibition, it was proposed that octreotide, an analog of the native hormone somatostatin, might be effective in the control of CP pain. Octreotide holds promise as a potent therapeutic agent, because it markedly inhibits pancreactic secretion as it significantly lowers CCK levels. Several small short-term studies resulted in variable findings regarding the efficiency of octreotide in this area.

Results of a multicenter double-blind placebo-controlled dose-ranging pilot study suggested a dosage of 200 mcg subcutaneously adminis-tered three times a day was superior to placebo *(9)*. Our own extensive clinical experience with octreotide demonstrates that this compound can dramatically relieve pain in some patients with severe CP who do not respond to any other medical treatment. However, not all patients respond to octreotide therapy. What determines a response is not fully defined. The decrement in CCK blood levels found after octreotide therapy may be the determining factor. In some preliminary pilot studies, it appears that patients who experience at least a 50% decrement in the CCK blood levels have responded well to octreotide in respect to pain relief. Studies are currently being carried out with a long-acting form of octreotide, which can be intramuscularly administered by depot injec-tion every 28 days. This form of compound should remarkably increase compliance. It should be stressed that the current studies with octreotide have utilized the compound in patients with big duct disease who have very severe CP and often pancreatic insufficiency. Such patients did not respond to pancreatic enzymes.

ANTIOXIDANTS

Experimental studies have demonstrated that free-oxygen radicals accumulate in the tissue of patients with CP. One study where 10 patients were treated for 1 year with a complex containing antioxidants, including L-methionine, β carotene, vitamin C, vitamin E, and selenium, demonstrated a significant decrease in the intensity of pain in these patients with CP *(10)*. Another study reported on the beneficial effect of micronutrients and antioxidants in decreasing oxidative stress in patients with CP *(11)*. Clearly, further study is needed to determine the efficiency, if any in the treatment of CP pain.

CHOLECYSTOKININ ANTAGONISTS

CCK antagonists may have a role in the treatment of painful CP. A double-blind placebo-controlled study evaluated the effect of orally administered MK 329, a CCK antagonist, versus placebo on liquid meal-stimulated and phenylalanine-stimulated enzyme output in four CP patients with protease-specific responsive abdominal pain *(12)*. Each patient served as his or her own control and received the CCK antagonist and placebo. In three of the four patients, the CCK antagonist suppressed meal-stimulated output of amylase and trypsin by 75–80%. Remarkably, a fivefold increase was observed in the plasma CCK levels following the administration of this CCK antagonist. Two of two patients demonstrated 70–80% suppression of phenylalanine-stimulated output of lipase amylase and trypsin. This potent CCK antagonist had no appreciable effect on the volume of secretions produced by either stimulus. CCK antagonists might reduce pain by the same mechanism proposed for enzymes and octreotide.

A recent multicenter dose–response control trial was conducted in Japan to evaluate the therapeutic efficiency of the CCK-A receptor antagonist, loxiglumide, in patients with abdominal pain induced by CP *(13)*. In this study, 207 patients were randomly assigned to oral treatment with 300 mg, 600 mg, and 1200 mg loxiglumide a day or placebo for 4 weeks. The overall improvement rate was 46% in the 300-mg dose group, 58% in the 600-mg group, and 52% in the 1200-mg group versus 34% in the placebo group.

These studies again underscore the potential importance of CCK in feedback control of pancreatic secretion. The possibility of CCK antagonists in the treatment of CP pain needs to be further explored.

NONSPECIFIC SUPPORT TREATMENT

Various other modalities have been used to treat the pain of CP, including tricyclic antidepressants, gabapentin and selective serotonin, reuptake inhibitors, such as paroxetine *(14)*. These agents are utilized empirically based on the premise that modifying neural transmission alters the perception of pain. The overall effectiveness of these agents is poorly studied, but they may have benefit. Avoidance of alcohol ingestion and moderation of fat intake are lifestyle changes that may benefit the patient.

CELIAC PLEXUS BLOCKADE

Chemical destruction of the nerve plexus has proved disappointing in most clinical experiences, particularly in patients who have previously undergone surgery. EUS or CT-guided celiac plexus block is an alternative way of treating patients who have failed medical treatment with constant intractable pain of CP. In a recent study utilizing EUS-guided celiac blockade in 90 patients, a combination of bupivacaine and triamcinolone on each side of the celiac plexus was utilized *(15)*. Significant improvement was reported in 55% of the patients, but the benefits appeared to be short-lived, and the average duration of pain relief was 10 weeks. In patients younger than 45 years old and those who had previous surgery, CP pain did not appear to benefit from the procedure. Celiac plexus blockade can also be performed under CT guidance. It appears that when CT plexus block is compared with EUS-guided blockade, the EUS-guided blockade provides more persistent pain relief than the CT-guided blockade. Long-term follow-up data in the use of EUS-guided blockade is not available; therefore, this treatment should be limited to patients with CP whose pain is not responding to any other treatment.

THORACOSCOPIC SPLANCHNICECTOMY

This is a minimally invasive approach in which nociceptive fibers originating from the pancreatic area are transected at the thoracic level. Recent studies indicate pain scores 6 months after this procedure were significantly lower than preoperative scores, and the need for pain medication seemed to decrease as well *(16)*. Pain eventually recurred in approximately 50% of patients. To date, the evidence indicates that this procedure is, at best, a temporizing measure for the relief of CP pain.

ENDOSCOPIC AND SURGICAL TREATMENT

Endoscopic therapy used in patients with CP include sphincterotomy, stricture dilation, stone extraction, and stent placement. Although there have been no double-blind placebo-controlled trials in endoscopic therapy in such patients, encouraging results have been reported in individual patients with pancreatitis pain. It is important to point out that pancreatic ductal stenting may also damage the pancreatic duct and pancreactic parenchyma. (This is discussed in detail in Chapter 14.) There are no trials that compare endoscopic and medical therapy. A recent randomized trial comparing endoscopic to surgical therapy found surgical therapy superior *(17)*.

In the United States, the most common surgical procedure performed for treatment of CP pain is a modified Peustow procedure, which is a longitudinal pancreaticojejunostomy *(18)*. Surgical therapy is discussed in Chapter 15. Most studies report that immediate pain relief occurs in about 80% of patients, and long-term relief occurs in only 30–50% of patients. The ductal decompression surgery has largely been performed in patients with big duct disease. Many surgeons require at least 6-mm dilation of the main pancreatic duct before such a surgical procedure is performed. The surgical approach for small duct disease is much more controversial and includes various procedures (e.g., including pancreaticoduodenectomy and other modified resections that preserve the duodenum and pylorus). Such resections lead to significant metabolic derangements of both the exocrine and endocrine pancreas. There are no comparisons of surgical therapy with medical therapy.

INDICATIONS FOR CONSULTING THE SUBSPECIALIST

Patients with chronic abdominal pain are quite common and often present to their primary care physician for evaluation and management. If the cause of the abdominal pain is not obvious by radiographic evaluation, then the gastroenterologist should be consulted for further sophisticated diagnostic testing. What should not be done is an expedient referral to a pain clinic without proper diagnosis. A clinical diagnosis of CP based on scant evidence leads to the administration of narcotics for an indefinite period by such pain clinics. With the new knowledge of how frequent coexisting motility problems are in such patients, and the observation that narcotics commonly used by physicians that direct pain clinics make such motility patients worse, it is very important that a proper diagnosis be made, and consideration of the pathophysiology of the pain be considered rather than just treating the symptoms. If the patient has well-documented CP by examination such as CT, then the gastroenterologist should be consulted in helping to define what subset of CP the patient in question is into and what the appropriate therapy should be. Evaluation of whether a patient has small duct or big duct disease must be made, and consideration of dysmotility of the stomach and small bowel must be ascertained.

SUMMARY

CP should be considered in all patients with unexplained abdominal pain. Management of the pain associated with CP remains a source of frustration for physicians and patients. It is important to recognize that CP is not one disease, and all patients with CP cannot be treated the same. The importance of small duct versus big duct disease must be emphasized. If radiographic tests do not provide a secure diagnosis of CP, then other more sophisticated testing should be employed, such as a direct hormone stimulation test. Nonenteric-coated pancreatic enzyme preparations are quite useful for the treatment in a subset of patients who have small duct disease. Octreotide is being used more increasingly for abdominal pain that is unresponsive to pancreatic enzyme therapy. If medical therapy fails, then expertise must be sought to attempt endoscopic therapy, EUS-guided celiac plexus block, and thorascopic splanchnicectomy in highly selected patients. Surgical duct compression is appropriate in patients who have considerable dilation of the main pancreatic duct. Future efforts will be directed to testing highly concentrated enzyme preparations that contain very large doses of pancreatic proteases, CCK receptor antagonists, and antioxidants.

REFERENCES

1. Toskes PP, Greenberger NJ. Approach to the patient with pancreatic disease. In: Braunwald E, Fauci AS, Kasper DL, et al., eds. Harrison's Principles of Internal Medicine, ed. 15. McGraw Hill, New York, 2001: 1788–1792.
2. Greenberger NJ, Toskes PP. Acute and chronic pancreatitis. In: Braunwald E, Fauci AS, Kasper DL, et al., eds. Harrison's Principles of Internal Medicine, ed. 15. McGraw Hill, New York, 2001: 1792–1804.
3. Toskes PP. Update on diagnosis and management of chronic pancreatitis. Curr Gastroenterol Rep 1999; 1: 145–153.
4. Draganov R, Toskes PP. Chronic pancratitis. Curr Opin Gastroenterol 2002; 18: 558–562.
5. Chowdhury R, Forsmark CE, Toskes PP, et al. The evaluation of unexplained pain of presumed pancreatic origin. Gastroenterology 2001; A-760(Abstract): 120.
6. Chowdhury R, Forsmark C, Toskes PP, et al. Prevalence of gastroparesis in patients with small duct chronic pancreatitis. Pancreas 2003; 26: 235–238.
7. Slaff J, Jacobson D, Tillman CR, et al. Protease-specific suppression of pancreatic exocrine secretion. Gastroenterology 1984; 87: 44–52.
8. Warshaw AL, Banks PA, Fernandez-Del Castillo CAG. A technical review: treatment of pain in chronic pancreatitis. Gastroenterology 1998; 115: 765–776.
9. Toskes PP, Forsmark CE, DeMeo Mt, et al. A multi-center controlled trial of octreotide for the pain of chronic pancreatitis. Pancreas 1993; 8(abstract): 774.
10. De las Heras Castano G, Garcia de la Paz A, Fernandez MD, Fernandez Forcelledo JL. Use of antioxidants to treat pain in chronic pancreatitis. Rev Esp Enferm Dig 2000; 92: 375–385.
11. Uden S, Bilton D, Guyan PM, et al. Rational for antioxidant therapy in pancreatitis and cystic fibrosis. Adv Exp Med Biol 1990; 264: 555–572.
12. Toskes PP, Currington C, Cintron M, et al. Oral administration of the CCK-antagonist MK329. substantiates feedback control of pancreatic secretion in chronic pancreatitis patients. Gastroenterology 1990; 98(abstract): 237.
13. Shiratori K, Takeuchi T, Satake K, Matsuno S. Clinical evaluation of oral administration of a cholecystokinin-a receptor antagonist (loxiglumide) to patients with acute, painful attacks of chronic pancreatitis: a multicenter dose-response study in Japan. Pancreas 2002; 25: E1–E5.
14. Mitchell RMS, Byrne MF, Baillie J. Pancreatitis. Lancet 2003; 361: 1447–1455.
15. Gress F, Schmitt C, Sherman S, et al. Endoscopic ultrasound guided celiac plexus block for managing abdominal pain associated with chronic pancreatitis: a prospective single center experience. Am J Gastroenterol 2001; 96: 409–416.
16. Buscher HC, Jansen JB, van Dongen R, et al. Results of bilateral thoracoscopic splanchnicectomy in patients with chronic pancreatitis. Br J Surg 2002; 89: 158–162.
17. Dite P, Ruzicka M, Zboril V, et al. Randomized trial comparing endoscopic with surgical therapy for chronic pancreatitis. Endoscopy 2003; 35: 553–558.
18. Howell JG, Johnson LW, Sehon JK, Lee WC. Surgical management for chronic pancreatitis. Am Surg 2001; 67: 487–490.

14 Endoscopic Approach to Chronic Pancreatitis

Lee McHenry, MD, Glen Lehman, MD, and Stuart Sherman, MD

CONTENTS

CHRONIC PANCREATITIS
PANCREATIC DUCTAL STRICTURES
PANCREATIC DUCTAL STONES
PANCREATIC PSEUDOCYSTS
BILIARY OBSTRUCTION IN CHRONIC PANCREATITIS
SPHINCTER OF ODDI DYSFUNCTION
PANCREAS DIVISUM
CONCLUSION
REFERENCES

CHRONIC PANCREATITIS

Chronic pancreatitis (CP) is an inflammatory process of the pancreas that may result in chronic disabling abdominal pain, maldigestion of protein and fat, and diabetes mellitus. The histologic hallmarks of CP are irreversible destruction of the pancreatic parenchyma and ductal architecture associated with fibrosis, protein plugs, and ductal calculi *(1)*. Pain, with a multifactorial pathogenesis, is the predominant symptom of CP and may be caused by pancreatic or extrapancreatic processes (Table 1; *2,3*). Pancreatic duct and parenchymal pressures are generally increased in CP whether the main pancreatic duct is

From: *Pancreatitis and Its Complications*
Edited by: C. E. Forsmark © Humana Press Inc., Totowa, NJ

Table 1
Abdominal Pain in Chronic Pancreatitis

Pancreatic causes	Extrapancreatic causes
Acute inflammation	Common bile duct obstruction
Increased intrapancreatic pressure	Descending duodenal
Ducts	obstruction
Pseudocysts	Colonic obstruction
Parenchyma	Duodenal/gastric ulcer
Perineural inflammation	
Pancreatic ischemia	

dilated or normal in diameter *(4)*. Such elevated parenchymal and duct pressures contribute to pancreatic ischemia, which appears to have a significant role in the pain of CP *(5,6)*. Therapeutic efforts are directed at reducing pancreatic parenchymal and ductal hypertension. Pharmacological agents, endoscopic techniques, and surgical procedures (resective, drainage, and denervative) have been employed to reduce pain with variable results. The complexity and multiplicity of the causes of pain in CP may explain the mixed results achieved by current therapeutic methods.

Most of these efforts in the treatment of CP are directed toward relief of obstruction and control of the chronic pain symptoms. Medical therapy that consists of analgesics, dietary alterations, nerve blocks, enzyme supplements, intervals of pancreatic rest, and suppression of pancreatic secretion (octreotide) is variably effective in relieving pain. Surgical therapy has been the main therapeutic recourse for patients with disabling symptoms that fail to improve with standard medical therapy. A surgical drainage procedure is usually performed in the setting of a dilated main pancreatic duct, whereas pancreatic resection and/or denervation are reserved for those patients with normal or small-diameter ducts. Immediate pain relief is seen in 70–90% of patients following surgical drainage procedures. However, pain recurs in 20–50% of patients during long-term follow-up. Surgical drainage procedures are associated with a morbidity of 20–40% and a mortality that averages 4%.

Since its inception and initial application in the early 1970s, endoscopic therapy has revolutionized the approach to a variety of biliary tract disorders. Within the past 15 years, similar endoscopic techniques have been applied and adopted to diseases of the pancreas *(8)*. However, these techniques have not been widely utilized because of the concern of prohibitive morbidity and difficulty in achieving technical success. It was not until the relative safety was recognized of endoscopic retrograde cholangiopancreatography (ERCP) and endoscopic sphincterotomy in acute gallstone pancreatitis that the indications for endoscopic therapy in pancreatic disorders were expanded *(8–10)*. Pharmacological agents, such as gabexate and interleukin-10, have shown promise in reducing the incidence and severity of pancreatitis in patients undergoing therapeutic ERCP and may further the safety of endoscopic interventions of the pancreas *(11,12)*. Endoscopic therapy is now being applied in the CP setting for patients who present with pain and/or clinical episodes of acute pancreatitis *(13,14)*. One aim of endoscopic therapy is to alleviate the obstruction to exocrine juice flow. Certain pathological alterations of the pancreatic duct, bile duct, and/or sphincter are targeted in endoscopic therapy. Outflow obstruction may be caused by ductal strictures (biliary or pancreatic), pancreatic stones, pseudocysts, and minor or major papilla stenosis. Although the endoscopic approach has never been directly compared with surgery, endoscopic drainage is appealing because it may offer an alternative to surgical drainage procedures with generally less morbidity and mortality. Furthermore, endoscopic procedures do not preclude subsequent surgery if it was necessary. Moreover, the outcome in reducing the intraductal pressure by endoscopic methods could be a predictor for the success of surgical drainage *(15)*.

Outcome data following endoscopic therapy in CP are rapidly accumulating. But, the data in this area are often difficult to interpret because of the heterogeneous populations with one or more pathological process being treated (e.g., pancreatic duct stones, strictures, and pseudocysts) and because of the multiple therapies performed in a given patient (e.g., stricture dilation, stone extraction, biliary and/or pancreatic sphincterotomy).

Table 2 lists the currently available endoscopic techniques for the treatment of acute pancreatitis and CP along with their complications. This table is (intentionally) all inclusive because differentiating acute recurrent pancreatitis from exacerbations of CP may be clinically difficult *(16)*. This chapter analyzes the current state of some of these exciting new applications of endoscopy in the treatment of CP.

PANCREATIC DUCTAL STRICTURES

Benign strictures of the main pancreatic duct may be a consequence of generalized or focal inflammation or necrosis around the main pancreatic duct. Given the putative role of ductal hypertension in the genesis of symptoms (at least in a subpopulation of patients), the utility of pancreatic duct stents for the treatment of dominant pancreatic duct strictures

Table 2
Endoscopic Interventions for Pancreatic Diseases

Clinical condition	Endoscopic therapy
Acute pancreatitis	Endoscopic sphincterotomy (bile duct and/or pancreatic duct), sphincter dilation, bile duct or pancreatic duct stent, nasobiliary/nasopancreatic drain, gallstone removal, Ascaris parasite removal
Chronic pancreatitis	Endoscopic sphincterotomy (bile duct and/or pancreatic duct), stricture dilation, bile duct or pancreatic duct stents, pancreatic stone extraction +/– extracorporeal shock wave lithotripsy, endoscopic ultrasound-guided celiac plexus block
Pancreatic pseudocysts Duct disruption Pancreatic ascites	Endoscopic cystgastrostomy or cystduodenostomy, transpapillary stents, or nasopancreatic drainage
Pancreas divisum	Minor papilla sphincterotomy, stent, sphincter dilation
Ampullary tumors	Endoscopic ampullectomy, stenting, thermal ablation
Pancreatic cancer	Bile duct plastic or metallic stent, pancreatic duct plastic stent, endoscopic ultrasound-guided celiac plexus block

is being evaluated *(17–26)*. In experimental models, pancreatic duct stents have been shown to significantly reduce elevated ductal pressures, but not as effectively as surgical measures *(27)*. The best candidates for stenting are those patients with a distal stricture (in the pancreatic head) and upstream dilation (type IV lesion; *17*). Most patients with a stricture have associated calcified pancreatic duct stones. For optimal results, the therapy must address both the stones and stricture. Underlying malignancy must be excluded by noninvasive and tissue sampling means *(28–30)*.

Pancreatic Stent Placement Techniques

Most pancreatic stents are simply standard polyethylene biliary stents with extra side holes at approximately 1-cm intervals to permit improved side branch juice flow (Fig. 1). Stents made of other materials have received limited evaluation. The technique for placing a stent in the pancreatic duct is similar to that used for inserting a biliary stent. In most patients, a pancreatic sphincterotomy (with or without a biliary sphincterotomy) via the major or minor papilla is performed to facilitate

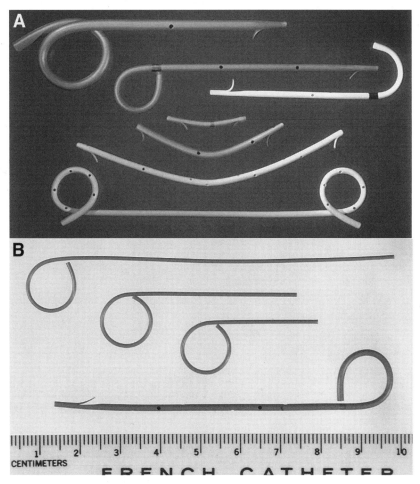

Fig. 1. (A) Pancreatic stents: Various sized pancreatic stents are commercially available. Note the external pigtail will prevent proximal migration of the stent into the pancreatic duct and the single flange for anchoring the stent in the pancreatic duct **(B)**. Comparison of (top three): 3-Fr protective pancreatic stents with external pigtail and without internal flange to allow for spontaneous dislodgement; and (bottom): 5-Fr flanged pancreatic stent with three fourths external pigtail used for longer term stenting.

placement of accessories and stents. A guidewire must be maneuvered upstream to the narrowing. Hydrophilic flexible tip wires are especially helpful for bypassing strictures. Torqueable wires are occasionally necessary to achieve this goal. High-grade strictures require dilation prior to the insertion of the endoprosthesis, which may be performed with hydrostatic balloon dilating catheters or graduated dilating catheters (Fig. 2). Extremely tight strictures may permit the passage of only a

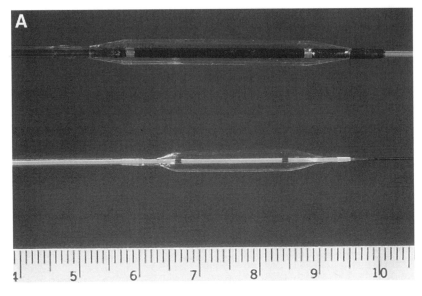

Fig. 2.(A)

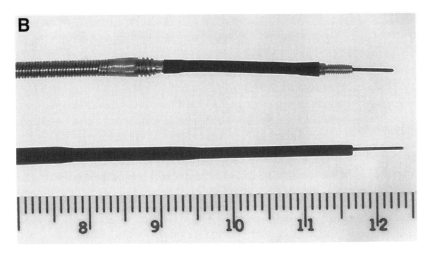

Fig. 2. (A) Hydrostatic dilation balloons for pancreatic stricture dilation:
(Top): 5-Fr catheter with 3 × 6-mm outer diameter balloon. Accepts an 0.035-
inch diameter guidewire. (Bottom): 3-Fr angioplasty catheter 2 cm in length by
4-mm outer diameter balloon. Accepts an 0.018-inch diameter guidewire. **(B)**
Catheter dilation devices for pancreatic strictures. (Top): Soehendra stent
extraction device utilized for stricture dilation with 7-Fr screw at tip and 10-Fr
screw located 2.5-cm proximal. This device is rarely used owing to concern of
excessive pancreatic ductal trauma. (Bottom): Graduated dilation catheter pictured
with 5 × 7 × 8.5-Fr outer diameter that accomodates a 0.035-inch diameter
guidewire.

small-caliber guidewire. Such wires may be left *in situ* overnight and usually permit dilator passage the next day. Alternatively, 3-Fr angioplasty balloons or the Soehendra stent retriever may be helpful *(31)*. The Soehendra stent retriever is rarely used owing to the concern of excessive duct damage from the device *(32,33)*. Although one preliminary report *(34)* suggested that luminal patency of the duct persisted at a mean time of 5 months following balloon dilation alone, most authorities have observed recurrence of strictures after dilation once and therefore advocate stenting *(15)*. As a rule, the diameter of the stent should not exceed the size of the downstream duct. Therefore, 5-, 7-, or 8.5-Fr stents are commonly used in smaller ducts, whereas 10–11.5-Fr stents or dual side-by-side 5–7-Fr stents may be inserted in patients with severe CP and a dilated main pancreatic duct. The tip of the stent must extend upstream to the narrowed ductal segment and into a straight portion of the pancreatic duct to avoid stent tip erosion through the duct wall. For diagnostic trials of pancreatic stenting in patients with nearly daily pain, most stents are left in place for 3–4 weeks. When long-term pancreatic stents are placed for therapy, stents have remained in place for 3–116 months *(17,24)*. Stents are known to occlude within the first several weeks *(35)*; yet, clinical improvement may persist much longer possibly because of the siphoning of pancreatic juice along the stent. At this time, self-expanding metallic stents have no role in the management of refractory pancreatic strictures owing to the high-occlusion rate from mucosal hyperplasia *(36)*.

Efficacy of Pancreatic Duct Stenting

The results of pancreatic duct stent placement (usually with ancillary procedures) are detailed in Table 3 *(17–26)*. Successful stent placement was achieved in 82–100% of patients. Of patients with successful stent placement, 66% were reported to benefit from therapy during a mean follow-up of 8–39 months (many patients still had their stent in place during the follow-up period).

Cremer and colleagues *(17)* reported their experience with pancreatic duct stenting in 76 patients with severe CP (primarily alcohol-related) complicated by a distal pancreatic duct stricture and upstream dilation. A 10-Fr stent was successfully placed in 75 patients (98.7%) through the major ($n = 54$) or minor papilla ($n = 21$). Patients had undergone biliary and pancreatic sphincterotomy, stricture dilation, and extracorporeal shock wave lithotripsy (ESWL; most patients) to fragment pancreatic duct stones. A dramatic decrease or complete relief of pain was initially observed in 94% of patients, associated with a decrease in the main pancreatic duct diameter. Clinically, stents were thought to remain patent for a mean time of 12 months (range: 2–38 months).

Table 3
Selected Series Reporting the Results of Pancreatic Duct Stenting
for Dominant Strictures

Authors/ref.	No. of patients	Technical success[a]	Mean follow-up (months)	No. of patients symptomatically improved	Major complications	Deaths
McCarthy et al. (21)	5	5	14	4	2[b]	0
Grimm et al. (18)	63	55	19	31[b]	20[b]	1
Cremer et al. (17)	76	75	37	41	12	1
Kozarek et al. (20)	N/A	17	8	13	3	0
Binmoeller et al. (23)	93	84	39	61	6	0
Ponchon et al. (25)	28	23	26	12	10	0
Smits et al. (24)	51	49	34	40	8	0
Total	311[c]	308	34[b]	202[d] (66%)	61[b] (19%)	2 (1%)

[a]Technical success refers to the number of patients successfully stented.
[b]Estimate.
[c]Does not include the studies from which the number of patients attempted is not available.
[d]Percentage improved refers to the number of patients who benefited (during the follow-up period) of the total number of patients successfully stented.
N/A, not available.

Disappearance of the stricture was observed in only 7 of 64 nonoperated patients after 13 months (range: 2–30 months). Eleven patients underwent pancreaticojejunostomy after confirmation of pain reduction with main pancreatic duct decompression. The remainder required repeated stent changes. Fifty-five percent of nonoperated patients remained symptom-free at a mean 3-year follow-up (19). Early complications were related to pancreatic and/or biliary sphincterotomy (cholangitis in 3 patients, hemobilia in 10). Intraductal infection caused by stent clogging developed in 8 patients, and 3 had their stent migrate inwardly. Stent therapy was believed by the authors to be an acceptable medium-term treatment of pain associated with main pancreatic duct stricture. Unfortunately, because the stricture persists in the majority of patients, compliance with long-term use of plastic stents (i.e., requirement of multiple stent changes) would be difficult. Consequently, the expandable stents (18-Fr diameter, 23-mm long) have been tried in 29 patients *(19)*. Early follow-up to 6 months was encouraging, because stent clogging did not occur during this short follow-up interval. However, during longer-term follow-up, mucosal hyperplasia (i.e., tissue ingrowth) resulted in stent occlusion in the majority of patients *(36)*. Because these stents are not removable by endoscopic techniques, their use should perhaps be limited to patients in whom resective therapy (during which the pancreatic stent and head would both be removed) is the next step. Evaluation of the covered metal stents is in progress.

Ponchon et al. *(25)* successfully placed 10-Fr multi-sidehole stents after biliary and pancreatic sphincterotomy and balloon dilation of strictures in 28 of 33 patients (85%) with a distal pancreatic duct stricture and upstream dilation. This was a highly selected subgroup, because patients with multiple sites of strictures, pancreatic duct stones, pancreas divisum, common bile duct narrowing with cholestasis, duodenal impingement, or the presence of a pseudocyst larger than 1 cm were excluded. The stents were exchanged at 2-month intervals for a total stenting duration of 6 months. Twenty-three patients were observed for at least 1 year after removal of the stent, comprising the basis of this report. During the stenting period, 21 patients (91%) had resolution or reduction in pain usually within days of stent insertion, and 17 patients (74%) discontinued analgesic medications. Initial relief of symptoms correlated with a decreased diameter (2 mm; $p < 0.01$) of the main pancreatic duct. Twelve patients (52%) had a persistent beneficial outcome for at least 1 year after stent removal. Disappearance of the stenosis on pancreatography at stent removal ($p < 0.05$) and 1 year later ($p < 0.005$) as well as reduction in the pancreatic duct diameter (2 mm) were significantly associated with pain relief. Complications of therapy occurred in 10 patients (30%) and included mild pancreatitis (resolved within 48 hours) in 9 and development of a communicating pseudocyst in 1 pateints.

Smits and colleagues *(24)* evaluated the long-term efficacy of pancreatic duct stenting (5 or 7 Fr in 9 patients, 10 Fr in 40) in a heterogeneous group of 51 patients with pancreatic duct strictures (44 dominant, 7 multiple) located in the head ($n = 38$), body ($n = 14$), or tail ($n = 6$) and upstream dilation. Associated pancreatic pathology treated at the time of stenting included pancreatic duct stones ($n = 17$), pseudocysts ($n = 10$), common bile duct strictures with concomitant cholestasis ($n = 12$), and pancreas divisum ($n = 3$). Stents were successfully placed in 49 patients (96%) after pancreatic sphincterotomy ($n = 31$) and stricture dilation ($n = 9$). Patients were re-evaluated within 3 months of stent placement and were followed for a median duration of 34 months. Responders underwent stent exchanges (approximately every 3 months) until such time that the stricture patency was improved. Clinical benefit was noted in 40 of 49 patients (82%) during the stenting period. In 16 of these 40 patients, the stents were still *in situ* at the time of the report and offered continued clinical improvement over periods ranging from 6 to 116 months. In 22 of these 40 patients, the stents were electively removed. All 22 experienced persistent clinical improvement during periods ranging between 6 and 41 months (median: 28.5 months) after stent removal. There were no demographic (age, sex, duration of pancreatitis, alcohol abuse), ERCP findings (single or multiple strictures, presence of pancreatic duct stones, pseudocyst, or biliary stricture), or additional interventions (stricture dilation, removal of stones, drainage of pseudocyst, stenting of bile duct stricture) that predicted the clinical outcome.

From the United States, Ashby and Lo *(40)* reported results of pancreatic stenting for strictures that was different from the European experience. Although symptom relief was common (86% had significant improvement in their symptom score), this was usually not evident until day 7. More disappointing, there was a lack of long-term benefit, with the recurrence of symptoms within 1 month of stenting. This study was relatively small (21 successfully stented patients) and included five patients with pancreatic cancer. Possible explanations for the less favorable results were that sphincterotomy was not performed and strictures were not dilated routinely before stent placement (to improve pancreatic duct drainage).

Pancreatic endotherapy was evaluated in patients with hereditary pancreatitis and idiopathic early-onset CP. In a report by Choudari et al., 27 consecutive patients with hereditary CP underwent endoscopic or surgical therapy of the pancreatic duct. Nineteen (70%) underwent endoscopic therapy and 8 patients (30%) underwent surgery as their primary treatment. After a mean 32-month follow-up, 50% of patients undergoing endoscopic therapy were symptom-free, 38% were improved, and 12% were unchanged with respect to pain. After surgery, 38% were symptom-free, 25% were improved, and 37% were unchanged *(38)*. In a cohort of patients with painful early-onset idiopathic chronic pancreatitis (ICP) (age 16–34 years) and a dilated pancreatic duct, 11 patients underwent endoscopic therapy and were followed for over 6 years. Median interval between onset of symptoms and endoscopic therapy was 5 years (3–10 years). Pancreatic sphincterotomy and stent insertion provided short-term relief in 11 patients (100%). Complications included fever in 3 patients and cholecystitis in 1 patient. Four patients (37%) developed recurrent pain considered because of recurrent pancreatic strictures or stones and underwent further endo-scopic therapy. These two patient populations of hereditary CP and early-onset ICP indicate the value of endoscopic therapy in providing short- and medium-term pain relief. Repeat endoscopic therapy is not uncommon (39).

There are few studies designed to identify subgroups of patients with CP who were most likely to benefit from stenting. In a preliminary report, 65 CP patients with duct dilation (≥6 mm), obstruction (usually a stricture with a diameter 1 mm or less), obstruction and dilation, or no obstruction or dilation underwent pancreatic duct stenting for 3–6 months (37). The presence of both obstruction and dilation was a sig-nificant predictor of improvement. Figure 3 depicts a patient treated with stent therapy.

The appropriate duration of pancreatic stent placement and the interval from placement to change of the pancreatic stent is unknown. Two options are available (15): the stent can be left in place until symptoms or com-plications occur; or the stent can be left in place for a predetermined interval (e.g., 3 months). If the patient fails to improve, the stent should be removed because ductal hypertension is unlikely to be the cause of pain. If the patient has benefited from stenting, the stent can be removed and the patient followed clinically, stenting continued for a more pro-longed period, or a surgical drainage procedure can be perfomed. (The last option assumes that the results of endoscopic stenting will predict the surgical outcome.) Limited data exists to support any of these options.

In a recent preliminary report, Borel et al. evaluated the effect of definitive pancreatic duct stent placement only exchanged on demand when symptoms recurred. In 42 patients, a single 10-Fr stent was inserted into the main pancreatic duct following pancreatic sphinctero-tomy. The patients were followed for a median of 33 months regarding pain reduction, weight gain or loss, and recurrence of symptoms. With recurrence of symptoms, the stent was exchanged. Of the 42 patients, 72% had pain relief with pancreatic stenting (pain score reduced >50%) and 69% gained weight. Two thirds of the patients ($n = 28$) required only the single pancreatic stent placement, and 12 patients required a stent exchange after a 15-month median. Two patients required repeated stent exchanges for recurrence of pain. Persistence or recurrence of pain was significantly associated with the development of cholestasis and continued alcohol abuse. These authors conclude that long-term pancreatic stenting appears to be an effective, and possibly superior, option when compared to temporary stenting (42).

The question may be posed: In patients with CP and a dilated pan-creatic duct, will the response to pancreatic stent placement predict the response to surgical duct decompression? In a preliminary report

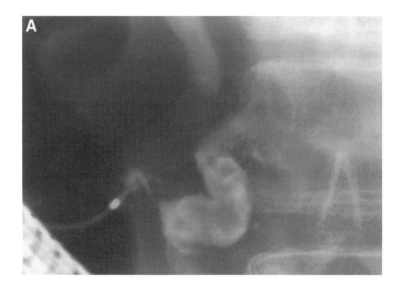

Fig. 3. (A)

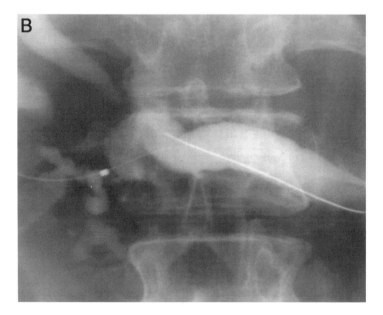

Fig. 3. (B)

Fig. 3. A 57-year-old male with chronic calcific pancreatitis with recurrent bouts of pancreatitis and pain. The patient underwent extracorporeal shock wave lithotripsy (ESWL) of pancreatic stones in the head of the pancreas 1 day prior to endoscopic retrograde cholangiopancreatography (ERCP). **(A)** High-grade stricture of the head of pancreatic duct with upstream dilation and stones in the

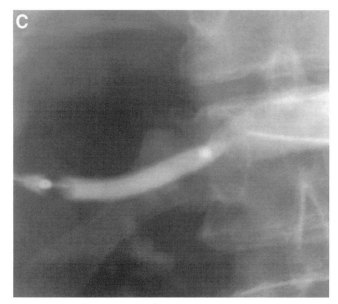

Fig. 3. (C)

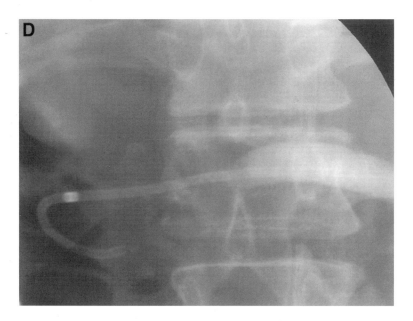

Fig. 3. (D)

dilated segment. **(B)** 5-Fr catheter and 0.025-inch diameter wire traversing stricture to the dilated pancreatic duct segment **(C)**. Dilation of the stricture with a 4-mm diameter hydrostatic balloon with waist from stricture completely ablated **(D)**. 7-Fr × 8-cm multiside hole, single internal flanged pancreatic stent placed to upstream dilated segment.

of a randomized controlled trial ($n = 8$), McHenry and associates evaluated the utility of short-term (12 weeks) pancreatic duct stenting to relieve pain and predict the response to surgical decompression in patients with CP and a dilated main pancreatic duct *(43)*. Four of eight patients benefited from stenting, whereas no control patient improved. Among five patients who underwent a Puestow procedure following stent therapy, four had pain relief. Improvement with the pancreatic stent was seen in two of four patients responding to surgery; one patient benefited from the stent but did not improve with surgery. In another preliminary series reported by DuVall and colleagues *(44)*, endoscopic therapy predicted the outcome from surgical decompression in 9 of 11 patients (82%; positive and negative predictive values were 80% and 83%, respectively) during a 2-year postoperative follow-up interval.

Several institutions have recently reported that symptomatic improvement may persist after pancreatic stent removal despite stricture persistence *(17,23–25)*. When summarizing the results of two studies ($n = 54$) that evaluated the efficacy of pancreatic duct stenting for dominant strictures, 65% of patients had persistent symptom improvement after stent removal, although the stricture resolved in only 33% (Table 4). Although these data indicate that complete stricture resolution is not a prerequisite for symptom improvement, several other factors may account for this outcome. First, other therapies performed at the time of stenting (e.g., pancreatic stone removal and pancreatic sphincterotomy) may contribute to patient benefit. Second, many of the unresolved strictures had improved luminal patency (but without return of lumen diameter to normal). Third, the pain of CP tends to decrease with time and may resolve when marked deterioration of pancreatic function occurs *(40)*.

Long-term follow-up of more than 1000 patients with CP undergoing initial endoscopic therapy during the period of 1989–1995 was recently reported by Rosch et al. *(26)*. From eight centers in Europe, 1211 patients with pain and obstructive CP underwent endoscopic therapy, including endoscopic pancreatic sphincterotomy, pancreatic stricture dilation, pancreatic stone removal, pancreatic stent placement, or a combination of these methods. In this study, 1018 patients (84%) were followed for symptomatic improvement and the need for pancreatic surgery over a mean of 4.9 years (range: 2–12 years). Successful endoscopic therapy was defined as a significant reduction or elimination of pain and reduction in pain medication. Partial success was defined as reduction in pain, but further interventions were necessary for pain relief. Failure of endoscopic therapy was defined as requiring pancreatic decompressive surgery or patients that were lost to follow-up. Over long-term follow-up, 69% of patients were successfully treated with

Table 4
Pancreatic Duct Stenting for Dominant Strictures:
Clinical Outcome and Stricture Resolution After Stent Removal

Author/ref.	Persistent improvement after stent removal	Median follow-up after stent removal (months)	Stricture resolution
Smits et al. (24)	23/33 (70%)	29	10/33 (20%)
Ponchon et al. (25)	12/21 (57%)	14	8/21 (38%)
Total	35/54 (65%)	23	18/54 (33%)

endoscopic therapy, and 15% experienced a partial success. Twenty percent of patients required surgery with a 55% significant reduction in pain, and 5% of patients were lost to follow-up. The group of patients with the highest frequency of completed treatment were patients with stones alone (76%) in comparison to patients with strictures alone (57%) and patients with strictures and stones (57%; $p < 0.001$). Interestingly, the percent of patients with no or minimal residual pain at follow-up was similar in all groups (strictures alone, 84%, stones alone, 84%, and strictures plus stones, 87%; $p = 0.677$). In conclusion, endoscopic therapy of CP in experienced centers is effective in most patients, and the beneficial response to successful endoscopic therapy in CP is durable and long-term (26).

Only randomized controlled studies comparing surgical, medical, and endoscopic techniques will allow the true long-term efficacy of pancreatic duct stenting for stricture therapy to be determined. There remain many unanswered questions: Which patients are the best candidates? Is proximal pancreatic ductal dilation a prerequisite? Does the response to stenting depend on the etiology of the CP? Finally, as noted, how does endoscopic therapy compare with medical and surgical management?

Complications Associated With Pancreatic Stents

True complication rates are difficult to decipher owing to the (1) simultaneous performance of other procedures (e.g., pancreatic sphincterotomy, and stricture dilation), (2) heterogeneous patient populations treated (i.e., patients with acute pancreatitis or CP), and (3) lack of uniform definitions of complications and a grading system of their severity (47). Complications related directly to stent therapy are listed in Table 5 (47,49). The rate of pancreatic stent occlusion appears to be similar to that for biliary stents (33). The pathogenesis of pancreatic stent occlusion on scanning electron microscopy also mirrors biliary stent blockage with typical biofilm and microcolonies of bacteria

Table 5
Complications Directly Related to Pancreatic Duct Stents

Occlusion, which may result in pain and/or pancreatitis
Migration into or out of duct
Duodenal erosions
Pancreatic infection
Ductal perforation
Ductal and parenchymal changes
Stone formation

mixed with crystals, resembling biliary sludge. We found that 50% of pancreatic stents (primarily 5–7 Fr) were occluded within 8 weeks of placement when carefully evaluated by water flow methods (35). More than 80% of these early occlusions were not associated with adverse clinical events. In such circumstances, the stent perhaps serves as a dilator or wick. Similarly, stents reported to be patent for as long as 38 months (17) are clinically patent but would presumably be occluded by water flow testing.

Stent migration may be upstream (into the duct) or downstream (into the duodenum). Migration in either direction may be heralded by return of pain or pancreatitis. Johanson and associates (50) reported inward migration in 5.2% of patients and duodenal migration in 7.5%. These events occurred with single intraductal and single duodenal stent flanges. Rarely, surgery is necessary to remove a proximally migrated stent. Modifications in pancreatic stent design have largely reduced the frequency of such occurrences. Dean and associates (51) reported no inward migration in 112 patients stented with a four-barbed (two internal and two external) stent. We have had no inward migration in greater than 3000 stents with a duodenal pigtail.

Although therapeutic benefit has been reported for pancreatic stenting, it is evident that morphologic changes of the pancreatic duct directly related to this therapy occur in the majority of patients. In assessing the results of seven published series (52–55,57–59), new ductal changes were seen in 54% (range: 33–83%) of 297 patients. Limited observations to date indicate a tendency of these ductal changes to improve with time following stent change and/or removal (44,45,47,49,50,52,53,55,57,58). The long-term consequences of these stent-induced ductal changes remain uncertain. Moreover, the long-term parenchymal effects have not been studied in humans. In a pilot study, six mongrel dogs underwent pancreatic duct stenting for 2–4 months (49). Radiographic, gross, and histologic abnormalities developed in all dogs. The radiographic findings (stenosis in the stented region with upstream dilation) were associated with gross evidence of fibrosis, which increased proportionally with the duration of the stenting period. Histologic changes of obstructive pancreatitis were present in most experimental dogs. Although the follow-up after stent removal was short, the atrophy and fibrosis seen were not likely to be reversible. Sherman and colleagues *(59)* reported that parenchymal changes (hypoechoic area around the stent, heterogeneity, and cystic changes) were seen on endoscopic ultrasound in 17 of 25 patients undergoing short-term pancreatic duct stenting. Four patients with parenchymal changes at stent removal had a follow-up study at a mean time of 16 months. Two patients had (new) changes suggestive of CP (heterogeneous echotexture, echogenic foci in the parenchyma, and a thickened hyperechoic irregular pancreatic duct) in the stented region. Although such damage in a normal pancreas may have significant long-term consequences, the outcome in patients with advanced CP may be inconsequential.

If brief interval stenting is needed, such as for pancreatitis prophylaxis, now commonly used are small diameter stents (3 or 4 Fr) with no intra-ductal barb. *(83)* (Fig. 1). Depending on their length, 80–90% of these stents migrate out of the duct spontaneously. Further studies addressing issues of stent diameter, as well as composition and duration of therapy as they relate to safety and efficacy are needed. Additionally, further evaluation of expandable stents, particularly the coated models, is forthcoming.

PANCREATIC DUCTAL STONES

Worldwide, alcohol consumption appears to be the most important factor associated with chronic calcifying pancreatitis. Although the exact mechanism of intraductal stone formation has not been clearly elucidated, considerable progress in this area has been made *(60)*. Alcohol appears to be directly toxic to the pancreas and produces a dysregulation of secretion of pancreatic enzymes (including zymogens), citrate (a potent calcium chelator), lithostathine (pancreatic stone protein), and calcium. These changes favor the formation of a nidus (a protein plug) followed by precipitation of calcium carbonate to form a stone *(60,61)*. The rationale for intervention is based on the premise that pancreatic stones increase the intraductal pressure (and likely the parenchymal pressure with resultant pancreatic ischemia) proximal to the obstructed focus. Reports indicating that endoscopic (with or without ESWL) or surgical removal of pancreatic calculi results in improvement of symptoms support this notion *(15)*. Moreover, stone impaction may cause further trauma to the pancreatic duct with epithelial destruction and stricture formation *(53,55)*. Thus, identification of pancreatic ductal stones in a symptomatic patient warrants consideration of removal. Figures 4 and 5 depict two such patients. Large stone(s) in the head with upstream asymptomatic parenchymal atrophy likely also warrant therapy.

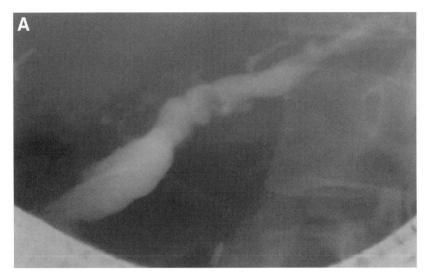

Fig. 4. (A)

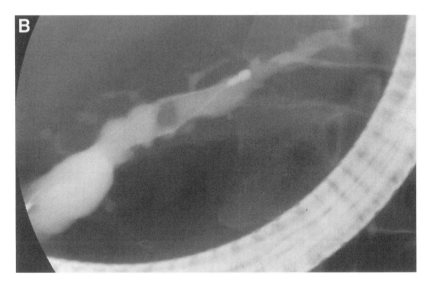

Fig. 4. (B)

Endoscopic Techniques

A major papilla pancreatic sphincterotomy (in patients with normal anatomy, i.e., no pancreas divisum) is usually performed to facilitate access to the duct prior to attempts at stone removal. There are two methods to cut the major pancreatic sphincter *(63,64)*. A standard pull-type sphincterotome (with or without a wire guide) is inserted

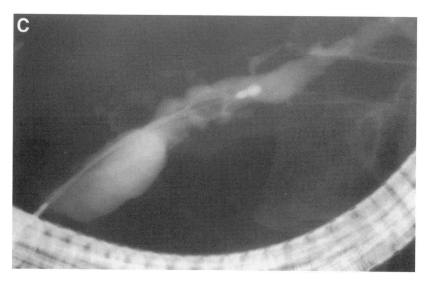

Fig. 4. (C)

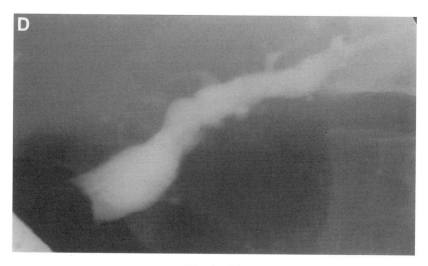

Fig. 4. (D)

Fig. 4. A 40-year-old female with alcohol-induced chronic pancreatitis (CP) complicated by main pancreatic duct stones. **(A)** Pancreatogram revealing dilated pancreatic duct with 5-mm diameter filling defect consistent with a pancreatic stone. **(B)** After pancreatic sphincterotomy, a nonwire-guided stone extraction basket was utilized. The basket is opened fully in the dilated pancreatic duct, and the stone is engaged. **(C)** Basket is slowly closed on the stone. **(D)** Stone is extracted and follow-up pancreatogram with a balloon catheter reveals no residual filling defects. No further stenting was performed.

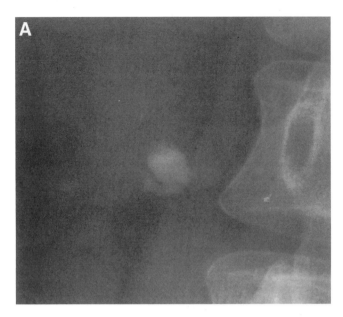

Fig. 5. (A)

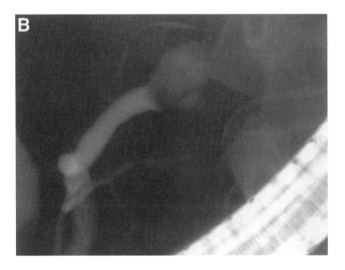

Fig. 5. (B)

into the pancreatic duct and oriented along its axis (usually in the 12 to 1 o'clock position). Although the landmarks to determine the length of incision are imprecise, authorities recommend cutting 5–10 mm *(63)* (Fig. 6A). The cutting wire should not extend more than 6–7 mm up the duct when applying electrocautery to prevent deep

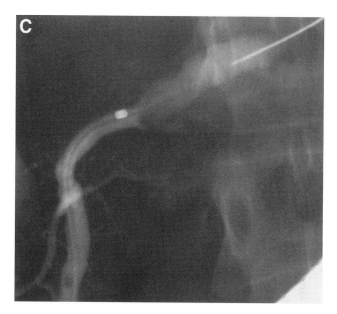

Fig. 5. (C)

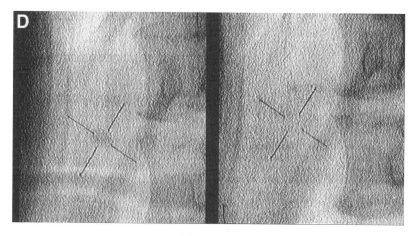

Fig. 5. (D)

ductal injury. Alternatively, a needle knife can be used to perform the sphincterotomy over a previously placed pancreatic stent *(63,64)*. Some authorities prefer performing a biliary sphincterotomy before the pancreatic sphincterotomy because of the high incidence of cholangitis if this is not done *(64)*. Patients with alkaline phosphatase elevation from CP-induced biliary strictures are especially at risk for cholangitis (if no biliary sphincterotomy is performed; *65*). Such complications were not found by others *(23,24,64,65)*. However,

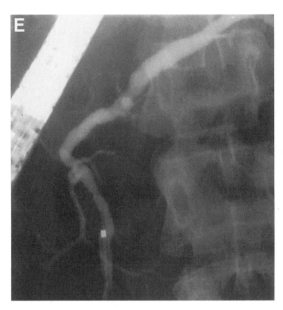

Fig. 5. A 41-year-old woman with a history of abdominal pain, pancreatitis, and pancreatic calcification on computed tomography (CT) scan. **(A)** Abdominal radiograph reveals solitary radioopaque stone in head/body region. **(B)** Pancreatogram reveals an 8-mm obstructing stone in body of pancreas pancreatic duct. **(C)** A 0.018-inch diameter guidewire was advanced beyond the stone. Further contrast filling of duct demonstrating upstream dilation. Following pancreatic sphincterotomy, stone extraction with basket was unsuccessful. **(D)** extracorporeal shock wave lithotripsy (ESWL) performed with Healthronics Lithotron spark-gap lithotriptor at a setting of 26 kV for a total of 2500 shocks. Fragmentation of the stone demonstrated post-ESWL. **(E)** Pancreatogram 1 week post-ESWL. Mild duct irregularity in body of pancreas duct with minimal upstream dilation. Stone fragments were removed. No pancreatic stent was placed.

performing a biliary sphincterotomy first can expose the pancreaticobiliary septum and allow the length of the cut to be gauged more accurately. In patients with pancreas divisum, a minor papilla sphincterotomy is usually necessary. The technique is similar to that of major papilla sphincterotomy, except that the incision direction is usually in the 10 to 12 o'clock position, and the length of the sphincterotomy is limited to 4–8 mm (Fig. 6B). The ability to remove a stone by endoscopic methods alone is dependent on the stone size and number, duct location, presence of downstream stricture, and the degree of impaction *(67,68)*. Downstream strictures usually require dilation with either catheters or hydrostatic balloons. Standard stone retrieval balloons and baskets are the most common accessories used to remove stones. Passage of these instruments around a tortuous duct

A

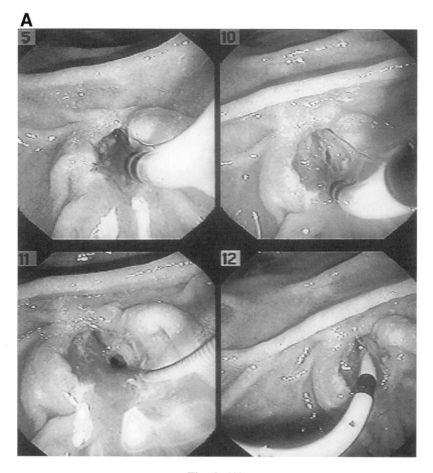

Fig. 6. (A)

can be difficult, but use of over-the-wire accessories are often help-ful. Stone removal is then performed in a similar manner to bile duct stone extraction (Fig. 6). Occasionally, mechanical lithotripsy is nec-essary, particularly when the stone is larger in diameter than the downstream duct, or the stone is proximal to a stricture. Rat tooth forceps may be helpful when a stone is located in the head of the pancreas close to the pancreatic orifice.

Endoscopic Results

Sherman and associates attempted to identify those patients with predominately main pancreatic duct stones most amenable to endo-scopic removal and determine the effects of such removal on the patients' clinical course *(67)*. Thirty-two patients with ductographic

B

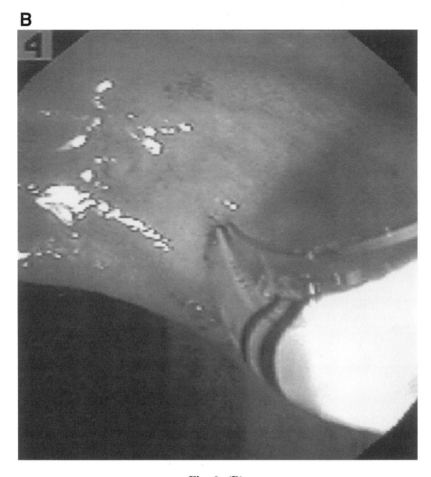

Fig. 6. (B)

evidence of CP and pancreatic duct stones underwent attempted endoscopic removal using various techniques, including bile duct and/or
pancreatic duct sphincterotomy, stricture dilation, pancreatic duct
stenting, stone basketing, balloon extraction, and/or flushing. Of these
patients, 72% had complete or partial stone removal, and 68% had
significant symptomatic improvement after endoscopic therapy.
Symptomatic improvement was most evident in the group of patients
with chronic relapsing pancreatitis (versus those presenting with chronic
continuous pain alone; 83 versus 46%). Factors that favor complete stone
removal included three or fewer stones, stones confined to the pancreatic
head or body, absence of a downstream stricture, stone diameter less than
or equal to 10 mm, and absence of impacted stones. After successful
stone removal, 25% of patients had regression of the ductographic

C

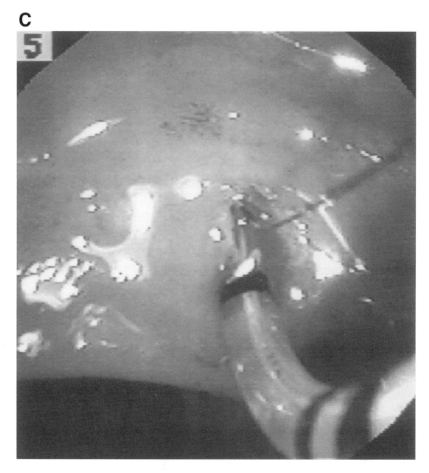

Fig. 6. (C)

changes of CP, and 42% had a decrease in the main pancreatic duct diameter. The only complication from therapy was mild pancreatitis, which occurred in 8%.

Smits and colleagues reported *(68)* results of 53 patients with pancreatic duct stones primarily treated by endoscopic methods alone (8 pateints had ESWL). Stone removal was successful in 42 patients (79%; complete in 39 and partial in 3), with initial relief of symptoms in 38 (90%). Similar to the results reported by Sherman et al. *(67)* in this series, 3 of 11 patients (27%) with failed stone removal had improvement in symptoms, suggesting that some of the clinical response may be related to other therapies performed at the time of attempted stone removal (e.g., pancreatic sphincterotomy). During a median follow-up of 33 months, 13 patients had recurrent symptoms owing to stone recurrence.

D

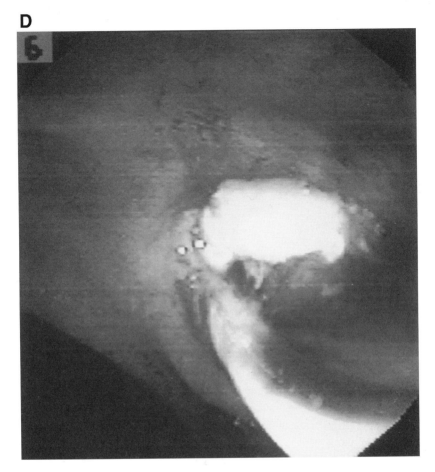

Fig. 6. (D)

The stones were successfully removed in 10 (77%). No factor evaluated (etiology of pancreatitis, presentation with pain or pancreatitis, presence of single or multiple stones, location of stones, and presence or absence of a stricture) was shown to predict successful stone treatment (defined as complete or partial removal of stones, resulting in relief of symptoms).

Cremer and colleagues *(37)* reported the findings of 40 patients with pancreatic duct stones treated by endoscopic methods alone. Complete stone clearance was achieved in only 18 (45%). However, immediate resolution of pain occurred in 77%. During a 3-year follow-up, 63% remained symptom-free. Clinical steatorrhea improved in 11 of 15 patients (73%).

Table 6 summarizes six selected series *(37,67–71)* describing the results of pancreatic stone removal by endoscopic methods alone.

E

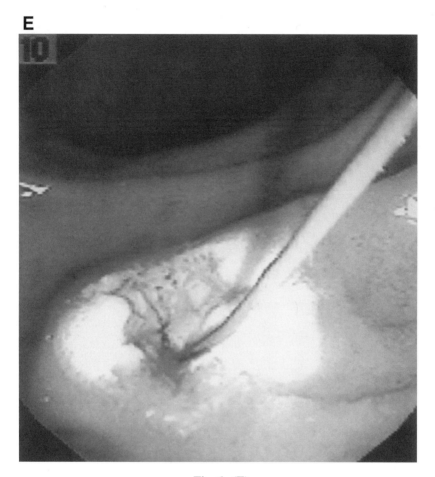

Fig. 6. (E)

Complete stone clearance was achieved in 93 of 147 patients (63%). The major complication rate was 9% (primarily pancreatitis), and the mortality rate was 0%. Cremer et al. *(37)* reported bleeding in 3% and retroperitoneal perforation in 1.4%. Sepsis was an infrequent complication. During an approximate 2.5-year follow-up, 74% of patients had improvement in their symptoms.

Endoscopic Results With Lithotripsy

As noted previously, endoscopic methods alone will likely fail in the presence of large or impacted stones along with stones proximal to a stricture. ESWL can be used to fragment stones and facilitate their removal (Fig. 5). Thus, this procedure is complementary to endoscopic techniques and improves the success of nonsurgical ductal decompression.

F

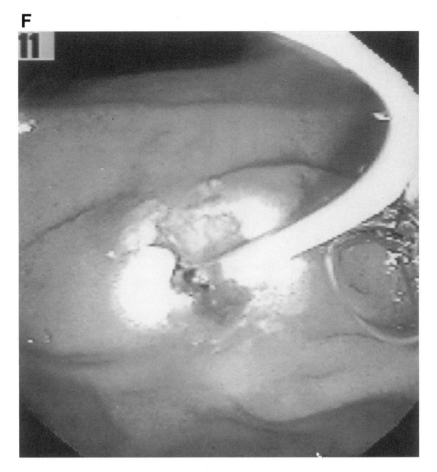

Fig. 6. (A) Technique of major papilla pancreatic sphincterotomy using a pull-type sphincterotome. (Left top) Biliary sphincterotomy is performed using a standard pull-type sphincterotome. (Right top) Pancreatic spincterotomy performed with a pull-type sphincterotome cutting in the 1 o'clock direction. (Left bottom) Completed biliary and pancreatic sphincterotomy. A guidewire is in the pancreatic duct. (Right bottom) A 6-Fr pancreatic stent is placed following performance of the pancreatic sphincterotomy. **(B)** Technique of minor papilla pancreatic sphincterotomy using a pull type sphincterotome. Traction sphincterotome positioned in minor papilla. The mound of the minor papilla can be seen extending for a few millimeters above the flexed wire. Duodenal juice at the minor papilla orifice is aspirated away before cutting to prevent heat dissipation to juice and boiling the adjacent tissues during the sphincterotomy. **(C)** Wire is bowed taught and cut is performed rapidly with minimal coagulation. The optimal cut length in this setting is unknown. The 5-mm length minor papilla sphincterotomy is complete without white tissue coagulum. **(D)** White pancreatic stone removed through patent sphincterotomy orifice with balloon catheter. **(E)** Excessive white coagulum at the cut edge of the sphincterotomy in a patient who underwent minor papilla sphincterotomy. This may potentially lead to restenosis of the sphincterotomy orifice. **(F)** Placement of a pancreatic duct stent to try to reduce the chance of pancreatitis and possibly stenosis of the pancreatic duct orifice in the same patient as **E**.

Table 6
Selected Series Reporting the Results of Endoscopic Therapy
of Pancreatic Ductal Stones

Author/ref.	N	Complete stone clearance (%)	Major complications(%)	Mortality (%)	Mean follow-up (months)	Symptom improvement (%)
Schneider et al. *(69)*	3	100	0	0	N/A	N/A
Fuji et al. *(70)*	11	55	0	0	N/A	N/A
Sherman et al. *(67)*	32	59	8	0	26	68
Kozarek et al. *(71)*	8	88	13	0	17	88
Cremer et al. *(37)*	40	45	10	0	36	63
Smits et al. *(68)*	53[b]	74	9	0	33	81
Total	147	63	9	0	31[a]	74

[a]Estimate.
[b]Eight patients also had extracorporeal shock wave lithotripsy.
N/A, Not available
This study reports results using endoscopic retrograde cholangiopancreatography alone.

In 1987, Sauerbruch and associates *(76)* were the first to report the successful use of ESWL in the treatment of pancreatic duct stones. Since that time, more than 400 patients have been reported in the literature *(66,74–81)*. Patients with obstructing prepapillary concrement and upstream ductal dilation appear to be the best candidates for ESWL. In this large series, 123 patients with main pancreatic duct stones and proximal dilation were treated with an electromagnetic lithotriptor usually before pancreatic duct sphincterotomy *(66)*. Stones were successfully fragmented in 99%, resulting in a decrease of duct dilation in 90%. The main pancreatic duct was completely cleared of all stones in 59%. Eighty-five percent of patients noted pain improvement during a mean 14-month follow-up. However, 41% of patients had a clinical relapse caused by stone migration into the main pancreatic duct, progressive stricture, or stent occlusion.

This same center compared their results of pancreatic stone removal prior to the availability of ESWL and after the introduction of adjunctive ESWL therapy *(37)*. Stones were successfully cleared in 18 of 40 patients (45%) by endoscopic methods alone when compared with 22 of 28 (78.6%) with ESWL. Table 7 summarizes the results of nine selected series that report the efficacy and safety of adjunctive ESWL *(66,67,74,75,77–81)*. Complications in these series were primarily related to the endoscopic procedure.

Although ultrasound-focused ESWL has been shown to achieve stone fragmentation, such focusing is clearly more difficult. In the series reported by Schneider and associates *(77)* stone localization was achieved in 17 of 119 sessions (14%) when only ultrasonography was used to monitor the position of the stone.

The Brussels group *(79)* studied 70 pancreatic stone patients who underwent attempts at endoscopic removal with adjunctive ESWL used in 41 (59%). This was a fairly homogeneous group of patients in that those with strictures, previous pancreatic surgery, and failed pancreatic sphincterotomy were excluded. The authors evaluated the immediate technical and clinical results and reviewed the long-term outcome in patients followed for more than 2 years. Complete ($n = 35$) or partial ($n = 20$) stone removal was achieved in 79% and was more frequently observed when ESWL was performed ($p < 0.005$) and in the absence of a nonpapillary ductal stenosis or complete main duct obstruction ($p < 0.05$). Complete stone clearance was most often observed with single stones or stones confined to the head ($p < 0.05$). In the multivariate analysis, ESWL was the only independent factor influencing the technical results of endoscopic management. In this series, the number of ERCPs performed per patient was reduced from 3.4 to 2.7 after the introduction of ESWL ($p < 0.01$). Of the 56 patients with pain on admission, 53 (95%) were pain-free ($n = 41$) or had a reduction in pain ($n = 12$).

In both the univariate and multivariate analyses, a significant association was found between immediate disappearance of pain and complete or partial main pancreatic duct clearance. During the first 2 years of follow-up after therapy, 25 of 46 (54%) patients were totally pain-free, whereas the frequency of pain attacks in the remaining 21 decreased by half. This frequency of recurrent symptoms (46%) is comparable to that of surgical series *(82)*. Long-term pain relief was associated with earlier treatment after disease onset ($p < 0.005$), a low frequency of pain attacks before therapy ($p < 0.05$), and absence of nonpapillary stenosis of the main pancreatic duct ($p < 0.05$). Interestingly, outcome was not associated with prior or continued alcohol intake. In the multivariate analysis, pain recurrence was independently associated with the frequency of pain attacks before therapy, the duration of disease, and presence of nonpapillary stenosis of the main pancreatic duct. It was suggested that such substenosis can induce ductal hypertension by blocking migration of fragmented stones or by progressing to higher grade stenosis.

Table 7
Selected Series Reporting the Results of Endoscopic Therapy of Pancreatic Ductal Stones Using Adjunctive Extracorporeal Shock Wave Lithotripsy

Author/ref.	N	Mean no. ESWL sessions	Complete stone clearance (%)	Major complications (%)	Mortality (%)	Mean follow-up (months)	Symptom improvement (%)
Neuhaus et al. (74)	12	1.6	67	0	0	8	91
Soehendra et al. (73)	8	N/A	100	0	0	6	75
Delhaye et al. (66)	123	1.8	59	36	0	14	63
Sauerbruch et al. (76)	24	1.5	42	0	0	24	83
Schneider et al. (77)	50	2.4	60	0	0	20	90
Van der Hul et al. (78)	17	1.9	41	6	0	30	65
Sherman et al. (67)	26	1.2	61	12	0	26	81
Kozarek et al. (80)	40	1.1	100	20	0	29	80
Farnbacher et al. (81)	125	2.5	51	0	0	29	93
Total	425	2.0	60	9	0	21*	80

*Estimate.
ESWL, extracorporeal shock wave lithotripsy; N/A, Not available.

253

In a recent retrospective review pertaining to the efficacy of ESWL as an adjunct to endoscopic therapy, Kozarek et al. evaluated 40 patients who underwent a total of 46 ESWL sessions (average 1.15 sessions/pateint). Eighty percent (80%) of patients did not require surgery and had significant pain relief, reduced number of hospitalizations, and reduced narcotic use when compared to the pre-ESWL period over a mean 2.4-year follow-up *(80)*. In an even larger quantity of patients, Farnbacher et al. retrospectively reviewed the efficacy of pancreatic stone clearance with endoscopic and ESWL therapy. Technical success as defined by stone clearance from the duct was achieved in 85% of the 125 patients. Most patients (111 of 125) required piezoelectric ESWL for stone fragmentation. ESWL was safe without any serious complications. Middle-aged patients in the early stages of CP with stones in a prepapillary location were the best candidates for successful treatment and required the least number of ESWL treatment sessions *(81)*. These aforementioned studies reaffirm that ESWL as an adjunct to endoscopic pancreatic therapy is effective, and the results of the combined modality may obviate the need for surgery. The results of endoscopic therapy in conjunction with ESWL for pancreatic stone disease compares favorably to the outcomes in surgically treated patients.

Intraductal lithotripsy via "mother–baby" scope systems has largely failed because of the inability to maneuver within the relatively narrow ductal system. Results with fluoroscopy-guided laser lithotripsy were similarly poor *(71)*. Pancreatoscopy (via a mother–baby scope system) can be used to directly visualize laser fiber contact with the stone and fragmentation. To date, experience is limited *(70,84)*.

Stone dissolution via ductal irrigation (contact dissolution) or oral agent is an appealing endoscopic adjunct for stone removal. Sahel and Sarles found that intraduodenal infusion of citrate in dogs significantly increased the citrate concentration in pancreatic juice *(85)*. This finding led to a nonrandomized study of oral citrate in 18 patients with CP, 17 of whom had pancreatic duct stones. Seven patients responded during a mean duration of 9.5-month therapy, with a mean stone size reduction of 21% and an improvement in symptoms *(61)*. Berger et al. *(86)* performed nasopancreatic drainage in six patients with main pancreatic duct stones. The pancreatic duct was perfused with a mixture of isotonic citrate and saline at 3 mL/minute for 4 days, and a stone-free state was achieved in all cases. Pancreatic pain disappeared during the perfusion, and four patients remained pain-free during the follow-up period (1–12 months). The remaining two patients had repeat therapy, which resulted in pain resolution. Pancreatic exocrine function was evaluated by the Lundh test in five patients before and after therapy. An increase of 50–360% was observed in enzyme output in three patients, whereas no improvement was noted in the remaining two patients. Trimethadione, an epileptic agent and a weak organic acid, has been shown in vitro to induce a concentration-dependent increase in calcium solubility *(61)*.

Noda et al. *(87)* showed promising results for trimethadione in a dog model of pancreatic stones. Unfortunately, if extrapolated to humans, the doses used in the dogs could be potentially toxic. At the present time, no rapidly effective solvent for human use is available to treat pancreatic stones. Further trials in humans are necessary to establish a role for medical therapy (either alone or as an aid to endoscopic measures) in treating patients with symptomatic pancreatic duct stones. These data suggest that removal of pancreatic duct stones may result in symptomatic benefit. Longer follow-up is necessary to determine the stone recurrence rate and whether endoscopic success results in long-standing clinical improvement or permanent regression of the morphological changes. Overall, endoscopists are encouraged to remove pancreatic duct stones in symptomatic patients when the stones are located in the main duct (in the head, body, or both) and are therefore readily accessible. Currently available data suggest that the clinical outcome after successful endoscopic removal is similar to surgical outcome with lower morbidity and mortality *(88)*. Moreover, recurrence of symptoms from migrated stone fragments can be treated again by endoscopy with or without ESWL. On the other hand, reoperation rates for recurrent pain after surgery are as high as 20% with a striking increase in morbidity and mortality after repeated surgery *(82)*.

PANCREATIC PSEUDOCYSTS

Pancreatic pseudocysts may complicate the course of CP in 20–40% of cases *(89,90)*. Traditionally, surgery has been the treatment of choice for such patients. The introduction of the ultrasound and computed tomography (CT)-guided needle and catheter drainage techniques provided a nonoperative alternative for managing patients with pseudocysts. More recently, an endoscopic approach has been applied for this indication. The aim of endoscopic therapy is to create a communication between the pseudocyst cavity and the bowel lumen and can be done by a transpapillary and/or a transmural approach. The method taken depends on the location of the pseudocyst and whether it communicates with the pancreatic duct or compresses the gut lumen. More than 400 cases of endoscopically managed pseudocysts have been reported (Table 8; *91–100*). The results indicate that endoscopic therapy is associated with a high technical success rate

Table 8
Selected Series Reporting the Results of Endoscopic Therapy of Pseudocysts

| Author/ref. | Technical success | Method of pseudocyst decompression | | | Complications | Deaths |
		No. trans-papillary	No. ECG	No. ECD		
Grimm et al. *(18)*	14/16	5	1	8	5	1
Cremer et al. *(99)*	32/33	0	11	21	3	0
Kozarek et al. *(100)*	12/14	12	0	0	5	0
Sahel et al. *(98)*	58/67[a]	26	1	31	9	1
Catalano et al. *(93)*	17/21	17	0	0	1	0
Smits et al. *(91)*	31/37[a]	16	8	7	6	0
Binmoeller et al. *(94)*	47/53	31	6	10	6	0
Barth et al. *(92)*	30/30[a]	30	10	0	13	0
Howell et al. *(96)*	100/108	37	38	25	25	0
Baron et al. *(140)*	113/138	NS	NS	NS	33	2
Total	454/517 (88%)	174	75	102	106 (20%)	4 (1%)

[a]Estimate.

ECG, endoscopic cystgastrostomy; ECD, endoscopic cystduodenostomy; NS, not stated.

(80–95%), acceptably low complication rates (equal to or less than surgical rates), and a pseudocyst recurrence rate of 10–20% *(95)*. In the largest series reported *(97)*, 100 of 108 patients (93%) had their pseudocysts successfully drained, and pseudocysts recurred in 13 (13%). The presence of CP, obstructed pancreatic duct, ductal stricture, necrosis on CT scan, and a pseudocyst greater than 10 cm in size were not predictive of recurrent pseudocyst disease. Also, endoscopic therapy has proven to be effective in the management of partial *(100)* and complete pancreatic ductal disruptions *(101)*, pancreaticocutaneous fistulas, infected fluid collections *(102)*, pancreatic ascites, pancreatic pleural effusions *(9,103)*, and traumatic duct disruptions *(103–104)*. Costamagna confirmed the relative safety of endoscopic intervention in peripancreatic fluid collections *(105)*.

Baron et al. retrospectively evaluated the efficacy and safety of endoscopic drainage of pancreatic fluid collections, including acute pseudocysts (31 patients), chronic pseudocysts (64 patients), and organized necrosis (43 patients) in 138 consecutive patients. Pseudoscysts resolved completely in 113 patients (82%), and resolution occurred more often in chronic pseudocysts (92%) than in those with acute pseudocysts (74%; $p = 0.02$) or necrosis (72%; $p = 0.006$). Complications were more frequent in patients with necrosis (37%) than in those with chronic (17%) or acute (19%) pseudocysts This study is the largest to date and adds to the growing body of literature that supports the efficacy of endoscopic therapy in pancreatic pseudocysts, although caution must be exercised in the setting of pancreatic necrosis. Because of the high-risk nature of the endoscopic intervention, these therapeutic approaches should be performed by highly experienced endoscopists in collaboration with pancreatic surgeons and interventional radiologists who are skilled in the management of pancreatic fluid collections *(140)*.

BILIARY OBSTRUCTION IN CHRONIC PANCREATITIS

Intrapancreatic common bile duct strictures have been reported to occur in 2.7–45.6% of patients with CP (Fig. 7). Such strictures are a result of fibrotic inflammatory restriction or compression by a pseudocyst *(107)*. In one ERCP series, a common bile duct stricture was seen in 30% of patients and was associated with persistent cholestasis, jaundice, or cholangitis in 9% *(108)*. Because long-standing biliary obstruction can lead to secondary biliary cirrhosis and/or recurrent cholangitis, biliary decompression has been recommended. Surgical therapy has been the traditional approach. Yet, based on the excellent outcome (with low morbidity) from endoscopic biliary stenting in postoperative stricture *(109)*, evaluation of similar techniques for bile duct strictures that complicate CP was undertaken.

Deviere and colleagues *(108)* evaluated the use of biliary stenting (one or two plastic 10-Fr C-shaped stents) in 25 CP patients with bile duct obstruction and significant cholestasis (alkaline phosphatase at least two times above the upper limits of normal). Nineteen patients had jaundice, and seven presented with cholangitis. Following stent placement, cholestasis, hyperbilirubinemia, and cholangitis resolved in all patients. Late follow-up (mean: 14 months; range: 4–72 months) of 22 patients was much less satisfactory. One patient died of acute cholecystitis and postsurgical complications, whereas a second died 10

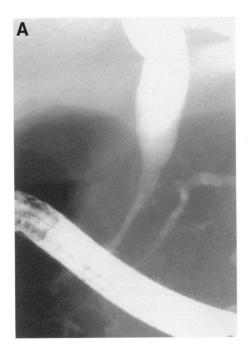

Fig. 7. (A)

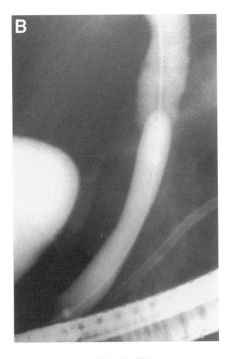

Fig. 7. (B)

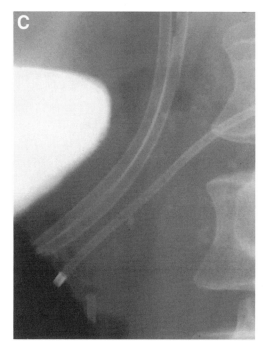

Fig. 7. (C)

months following stenting of sepsis, which was thought to be a result of stent blockage or dislodgment. Stent migration occurred in 10 patients and stent occlusion in 8, resulting in cholestasis with or without jaundice (n = 12), cholangitis (n = 4), or no symptoms (n = 2). These patients were treated with stent replacement, surgery, or both (n = 7). Ten patients continued to have a stent in place (8-month mean follow-up) and remained asymptomatic. Because of the resolution of their biliary stricture, only three patients did not require further stents. The initial observation of this study is that biliary drainage is an effective therapy for resolving cholangitis or jaundice in patients with CP and a biliary stricture. The long-term efficacy of this treatment, however, is much less satisfactory, because stricture resolution rarely occurs.

Barthet and colleagues *(110)* also found that biliary stenting is not a definitive therapy for CP patients with a distal common bile duct stricture. In their series of 19 patients (mean duration of stenting: 10 months) only two had complete clinical (resolution of symptoms), biological (normalization of cholestatic liver tests), and radiological (resolution of biliary stricture and upstream dilation) recovery. Six of 10 (60%) possible clinical successes, 8 of 19 (42%) possible biologic successes, and 3 of 19 (16%) possible radiological successes were obtained.

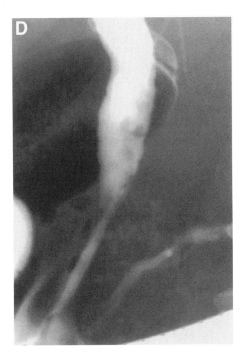

Fig. 7. A 38-year-old male with alcohol-induced chronic pancreatitis (CP) with recurrent bouts of pain, cholestatic serum liver chemistries, and elevated serum amylase. Computed tomography scan revealed enlarged head of pancreas, calcifications, and new biliary dilation. **(A)** Cholangiogram revealed smooth, 3-cm long narrowing of the distal common bile duct within the head of the pancreas with upstream dilation typical of benign biliary stricture complicating CP. Biliary intraductal brush cytology was negative. Pancreatogram revealed narrowing of the head of pancreas pancreatic duct, dilated secondary branches and calcifications. **(B)** 7-Fr multiple side hole pancreatic stent in place. Balloon dilation of the bile duct stricture was performed with 10-mm hydrostatic balloon. **(C)** Placement of two 10-Fr polyethylene stents into bile duct and 7-Fr multiple side hole pancreatic stent into pancreatic duct. Serum liver chemistries normalized and abdominal pain improved. **(D)** Six months later, the patient's pain was moderately improved and endoscopic retrograde cholangiopancreatography was performed for possible bile duct and pancreatic stent removal. Cholangiogram revealed persistent bile duct narrowing, requiring further bile duct stenting. Pancreatic ductal sticture in the head was improved and did not require further pancreatic stenting.

Because of the disappointing results with plastic stents and concern for the high morbidity associated with surgically performed biliary drainage procedures in alcoholic (frequently debilitated) patients, the group from Brussels evaluated the use of uncoated expandable metal stents for this indication *(112)*. Twenty patients were treated with a 34-mm-long metal stent, which becomes 10 mm in diameter when fully expanded. The short length of the stent was chosen so surgical bypass (e.g., choledochoduodenostomy) would still be possible if necessary. Cholestasis ($n = 20$), jaundice ($n = 7$), and cholangitis ($n = 3$) resolved in all patients. Eighteen patients had no further biliary problems during a 33-month follow-up period (range: 24–42 months). Two patients (10%) developed epithelial hyperplasia within the stent, resulting in recurrent cholestasis in one and jaundice in the other. These patients were treated endoscopically with standard plastic stents with one of these patients ultimately requiring surgical drainage. The authors concluded that this therapy could be an effective alternative to surgical biliary diversion, but longer follow-up and controlled trials are needed to confirm these results. In a recent abstract report, the Amsterdam group reported the long-term follow-up (50-month mean) of a cohort of 13 patients with CP-induced biliary strictures who had undergone uncovered biliary Wallstent (Boston Scientific, Natick, MA) placement. The Wallstent was successfully placed in all patients between 1994 and 1999. In follow-up, nine patients (69%) were successfully treated and four patients failed Wallstent therapy. Of the nine patients treated successfully, four (44%) patients required repeated endoscopic intervention (three with second Wallstent and one patient requiring cleaning with balloon). One patient eventually required surgical biliary diversion, and three patients are continuing to require endoscopic plastic stents through the Wallstent to maintain biliary patency *(137)*.

The Amsterdam group reported their results of placing 10-Fr biliary stents in 52 CP patients with cholestasis *(15)*. Jaundice and cholestasis disappeared within 2 weeks after stent insertion in all patients. During a median follow-up of 32 months (range: 3 months to 10 years), 17 patients (33%) had their stent removed without return of cholestasis. Complete resolution of the stricture was seen in 10 of the 17 patients, which suggested that complete resolution of the stricture was unnecessary for long-term relief of symptoms and cholestasis.

A recent exciting development in stent technology utilizing bioabsorbable poly-L lactide (PLLA) polymer strands woven into the tubular mesh design similar to the metallic stent was recently reported by Haber et al. *(111)*. The PLLA stent is unique in that it undergoes slow hydrolytic degradation and disintegration after 6–18 months. In the feasibility study in patients with malignant obstructive jaundice, the endoscopic technique for placement of the bioabsorbable biliary stent was similar to present expandable stents, being technically successful in 48 of 50 patients. The unique feature of this stent is that it may obviate the need for follow-up endoscopy to remove or replace the stent and may potentially be an effective long-term option in benign CP-induced biliary strictures.

The aforementioned studies indicate that plastic biliary stents are a useful alternative to surgery for short-term treatment of CP-induced common bile duct strictures complicated by cholestasis, jaundice, and cholangitis. This therapy should also be considered for high-risk surgical patients. However, because the long-term efficacy of this treatment is much less satisfactory, operative intervention appears to be a better long-term solution for this problem in average-risk patients *(141)*. More data on the long-term outcome, preferably in controlled trials, are necessary before the expandable stents can be advocated for this indication. Trials of membrane-coated metal stents, bioabsorbable stents, and removable coil spring stents are soon to follow.

SPHINCTER OF ODDI DYSFUNCTION

Although sphincter of Oddi dysfunction (SOD) is a known cause of acute recurrent pancreatitis, its role in the pathogenesis of CP is much less certain *(113)*. A direct effect of alcohol on the sphincter of Oddi has been postulated *(114)*. In studies performed in humans with T-tubes, it was demonstrated that intragastric or intravenous *(115)* administration of alcohol increased the sphincter tone. Moreover, Guelrud and colleagues *(106)* showed that local instillation of alcohol on the papilla of Vater produced a significant increase in the basal pancreatic sphincter pressure at sphincter of Oddi manometry in both cholecystectomy patients and patients with CP. The authors postulated that the increased motor activity of the sphincter of Oddi may raise the intraductular pancreatic pressure and result in the disruption of small pancreatic ductules leading to backflow of pancreatic juice into the parenchyma with subsequent injury. Other investigators have refuted these findings by showing that intravenous or intragastric administration of alcohol in humans results in a decrease in sphincter of Oddi basal pressures at manometry *(117)*. In a preliminary study, Morita et al. showed that chronic alcohol administration in the Japanese monkey resulted in an increase in sphincter of Oddi mean basal pressure from 9 to 20 mmHg ($p < 0.01$), whereas phasic amplitude decreased by 75%, and the pancreatic ductal secretory rate nearly doubled *(118)*. More recent studies using modern manometric techniques have shown a high frequency of basal sphincter pressure abnormalities, particularly the pancreatic sphincter, in patients with established CP *(119)*. Results of other studies using sphincter of Oddi manometry negate these findings and have shown no difference in the dynamics of the pancreatic sphincter in patients with CP and controls *(120)*. Such data suggest the sphincter can become dysfunctional as part of the overall general scarring process or has a role in the pathogenesis of CP.

Although limited, the surgical literature suggests that sphincter ablation therapy (both biliary and pancreatic sphincters) alone for patients with CP and manometrically documented or suspected SOD benefits 30–60% of patients *(121,122)*. Bagley and associates reported a surgical series *(123)* of 67 patients with mild-to-moderate CP undergoing empiric biliary and pancreatic sphincterotomy ($n = 33$) or sphincteroplasty ($n = 34$). During a 5-year follow-up, 44% of patients had pain relief. The outcome for patients with ICP was similar to that for patients with alcohol-induced CP. However, 92% (11 of 12) of patients who stopped alcohol consumption were clinically improved when compared with 12.5% (2 of 16) who continued to drink.

Because endoscopic pancreatic sphincterotomy has been performed infrequently in most institutions, its role in the management of pancreatic sphincter stenosis has not been defined. Kozarek et al. reported the resolution of pain and clinical episodes of pancreatitis after pancreatic sphincterotomy in 6 of 10 patients (1-year follow-up) with CP and suspected or manometrically documented pancreatic SOD *(63)*. Okolo et al. retrospectively evaluated 55 patients who had undergone endoscopic pancreatic sphincterotomy over a 4-year period. After a median follow-up of 16 months, 62% of patients reported improvement of pain scores. Patients with pancreatic sphincter dysfunction ($n = 15$) had significant improvement in pain (73%) in comparison to patients with pancreatographic evidence of CP (58%; *138*). The utility of endoscopic sphincter ablation as the only therapy in patients with CP awaits further study, preferably in controlled randomized trials.

PANCREAS DIVISUM

Pancreas divisum is the most common congenital variant of pancreatic ductal anatomy, occurring in 7% of autopsy series *(124)*. Most commonly in the CP setting, minor papilla sphincterotomy is performed to provide access to the duct to affect stone retrieval or facilitate endoprosthesis placement *(9)*. It has been postulated that in a subpopulation of pancreas divisum patients, the minor papilla orifice appears to be critically small, such that excessively high intrapancreatic dorsal duct pressures occur during active secretion *(124)*. This may result in pancreatic pain or pancreatitis *(125)*. Although most authorities agree that pancreas divisum is a definitive cause of acute recurrent pancreatitis, its effect in the pathogenesis of CP is much more controversial. Several lines of evidence favor the association of pancreas divisum and pancreatitis, including (1) the presence of pancreatographic and histologic changes of CP isolated to the dorsal pancreas, (2) an increased incidence

Table 9
Selected Series Reporting the Results of Minor Papilla Therapy
for Pancreas Divisum

Author/ref.	Mean follow-up (months)	Acute recurrent pancreatitis		Pain alone		Chronic pancreatitis	
		N	% Improved	N	% Improved	N	% Improved
Soehendra et al. *(126)*	3	2	100	0	–	4	75
Ligoury et al. *(127)*	24	8	63	0	–	0	–
McCarthy et al. *(21)*	21	19	89	0	–	0	–
Lans et al. *(128)*	30	10	90	0	–	0	–
Lehman et al. *(56)*	22	17	76	23	26	11	27
Coleman et al. *(129)*	23	9	78	5	0	20	60
Sherman et al. *(130)*	28	0	–	16	44	0	–
Kozarek et al. *(131)*	20	15	73	5	20	19	32
Ertan *(138)*	24	25	76	0	–	0	–
Heyries et al. *(139)*	39	24	92	0	–	0	–
Total		129	81	49	29	54	44

of pancreas divisum in patients with idiopathic pancreatitis, and (3) symptomatic benefit following dorsal duct drainage, endoscopically or surgically *(124)*.

Although minor papilla sphincter therapy by endoscopic or surgical techniques has been shown to be effective for patients with pancreas divisum and acute recurrent pancreatitis, the outcome for patients with CP usually has been much less satisfactory *(21,56,126–132,138,139*; Table 9). In summarizing 54 patients undergoing dorsal duct decompressive therapy by minor papilla sphincterotomy and/or dorsal duct stenting, only 44% improved during a mean follow-up of 22 months. A recent 4-year follow-up summary from our institution showed similar 62–70% symptom improvement rate for pancreas divisum patients with and without dorsal duct CP changes. These data suggest that methods to select patients with pancreas divisum and CP who are likely to benefit from endoscopic therapy need further investigation. The role of botulinum toxin use to predict pain relief warrant further study *(133)*. Until such methods are identified, minor papilla sphincterotomy (as the only therapy) for patients with CP should preferably be done in a research setting and restricted to patients who are disabled by pain.

CONCLUSION

Endoscopic therapy of CP is an expanding area for the interventional endoscopist. The techniques employed are very similar to the endoscopic interventions utilized in the biliary tree but tend to be more tedious. The appropriate selection of candidates for the various pancreatic interventions is considered important to obtain optimal results of therapy. The continued improvement in resolution of magnetic resonance cholangiopancreatography may allow for suitable patient selection for endoscopic therapy without performing an initial diagnostic ERCP *(134,135)*. Over the past decade, multiple series that total a few thousand patients have demonstrated the medium-term effectiveness of endoscopic interventions in CP, rivaling the medium-term outcomes from surgery in this disease. ESWL has proven to be indispensable in the management of patients with pancreatic stones. However, well-designed, long-term, and controlled studies comparing endoscopy to surgery in the management of patients with CP are lacking. Further outcome and cost efficacy studies should be done. The inexperienced endoscopist should exercise caution in the application of newer pancreatic techniques, as they are technically demanding and associated with a small, yet significant, complication rate.

REFERENCES

1. Sarles H, Bernard JP, Johnson C. Pathogenesis and epidemiology of chronic pancreatitis. Annu Rev Med 1989; 40: 453–468.
2. Banks PA. Management of pancreatic pain. Pancreas 1991; 6(Suppl 1): S52–S59.
3. Steer ML, Waxman I, Freedman S. Chronic pancreatitis. N Engl J Med 1995; 332: 1482–1490.
4. Widdison AL, Alvarez C, Karanjia ND, Reber HA. Experimental evidence of beneficial effects of ductal decompression in chronic pancreatitis. Endoscopy 1991; 23: 151–154.
5. Karanjia ND, Reber HA. The cause and management of the pain of chronic pancreatitis. Gastrointest Clin North Am 1990; 19: 895–904.
6. Lo SK, Lewis MPN, Reber PU, et al. In-vivo endoscopic trans-sphincteric measurement of pancreatic blood flow (PBF) in humans. Gastrointest Endosc 1996; 43: 409A.

7. Malfertheiner P, Buchler M. Indications for endoscopic or surgical therapy in chronic pancreatitis. Endoscopy 1991; 23: 185–190.

8. Bedford RA, Howerton DH, Geenen JE. The current role of ERCP in the treatment of benign pancreatic disease. Endoscopy 1994; 26: 113–119.

9. Kozarek RA, Traverso LW. Endotherapy of chronic pancreatitis. Int J Pancreatol 1996; 19: 93–102.

10. Kaikaus RM, Geenen JE. Current role of ERCP in the management of benign pancreatic disease. Endoscopy 1996; 28: 131–137.

11. Cavallini G, Tittobello A, Frulloni L, et al. Gabexate for the prevention of pancreatic damage related to ERCP. N Engl J Med 1996; 335: 919–923.

12. Deviere J, Le Moine O, Van Laethem JL, et al. Interleukin-10 reduces the incidence of pancreatitis after therapeutic endoscopic retrograde cholangiopancreatography. Gastroenterology 2001; 120: 498–505.

13. Sherman S, Lehman GA. Endoscopic therapy of pancreatic disease. Gastroenterologist 1993; 1: 5–17.

14. Kozarek RA. Chronic pancreatitis in 1994: Is there a role for endoscopic treatment? Endoscopy 1994; 26: 625–628.

15. Huibregtse K, Smits ME. Endoscopic management of diseases of the pancreas. Am J Gastroenterol 1994; 89(suppl): S66–S77.

16. Jacob L, Geenen JE, Catalano MF, Geenen DJ. Prevention of pancreatitis in patients with idiopathic recurrent pancreatitis: a prospective nonblinded randomized study using endoscopic stents. Endoscopy 2001; 33: 559–562.

17. Cremer M, Deviere J, Delhaye M, et al. Stenting in severe chronic pancreatitis: Results of medium-term follow-up in 76 patients. Endoscopy 1991; 23: 171–176.

18. Grimm H, Meyer WH, Nam VC, Soehendra N. New modalities for treating chronic pancreatitis. Endoscopy 1989; 21: 70–74.

19. Cremer M, Deviere J, Delhaye M, et al. Nonsurgical management of severe chronic pancreatitis. Scand J Gastroenterol 1990; 25(Suppl 175): 77–84.

20. Kozarek RA, Patterson DJ, Ball TJ, Traverso LW. Endoscopic placement of pancreatic stents and drains in the management of pancreatitis. Ann Surg 1989; 209: 261–266.

21. McCarthy J, Geenen JE, Hogan WJ. Preliminary experience with stent placement in benign pancreatic diseases. Gastrointest Endosc 1988; 34: 16–18.

22. Geenen JE, Rolny P. Endoscopic therapy of acute and chronic pancreatitis. Gastrointest Endosc 1991; 37: 377–382.

23. Binmoeller KF, Jue P, Seifert H, et al. Endoscopic pancreatic stent drainage in chronic pancreatitis and a dominant stricture: Long term results. Endoscopy 1995; 27: 638–644.

24. Smits ME, Badiga SM, Rauws EAJ, et al. Longterm results of pancreatic stents in chronic pancreatitis. Gastrointest Endosc 1995; 42: 461–467.

25. Ponchon T, Bory R, Hedelius F, et al. Endoscopic stenting for pain relief in chronic pancreatitis: Results of a standardized protocol. Gastrointest Endosc 1995; 42: 452–456.

26. Rosch T, Daniel S, Scholz M et al. Endoscopic treatment of chronic pancreatitis: A multicenter study of 1000 patients with long-term follow-up. Endoscopy 2002; 34: 765–771.

27. Reber PU, Patel AG, Kusske AM, et al. Stenting does not decompress the pancreatic duct as effectively as surgery in experimental chronic pancreatitis. Gastroenterology 1995; 128: 386A.

28. Nakaizumi A, Uehara H, Takensaka A, et al. Diagnosis of pancreatic cancer by cytology and measurement of oncogene and tumor markers in pure pan-

creatic juice aspirated by endoscopy. Hepatogastroenterology 1999; 46: 31–37.

29. Brandwein SL, Farrell JJ, Centeno BA, Brugge WR. Detection and tumor staging of malignancy in cystic intraductal, and solid tumors of the pancreas by EUS. Gastrointest Endosc 2001; 53: 722–727.

30. Lohr M, Muller P, Mora J, et al. p53 and K-ras mutations in pancreatic juice samples from patients with chronic pancreatitis. Gastrointest Endosc 2001; 53: 734–743.

31. Freeman M, Cass OW, Dailey J. Dilation of high-grade pancreatic and biliary ductal strictures with small-caliber angioplasty balloons. Gastrointest Endosc 2001; 54: 89–92.

32. Van Someran R, Benson M, Glynn M, et al. A novel technique for dilation difficult malignant biliary strictures during therapeutic ERCP. Gastrointest Endosc 1996; 43: 495–498.

33. Baron T, Morgan D. Dilation of a difficult benign pancreatic duct stricture using the Soehendra stent extractor. Gastrointest Endosc 1997; 46: 178–180.

34. Pasricha PJ, Kalloo AN. Successful endoscopic management of complete obstruction of the main pancreatic duct (MPD) in patients with chronic pancreatitis. Gastrointest Endosc 1993; 39: 320A.

35. Ikenberry SO, Sherman S, Hawes RH, et al. The occlusion rate of pancreatic stents. Gastrointest Endosc 1994; 40: 611–613.

36. Cremer M, Suge B, Delhaye M, et al. Expandable pancreatic metal stents (Wallstent) for chronic pancreatitis: First world series. Gastroenterology 1990; 98: 215A.

37. Cremer M, Deviere J, Delhaye M, et al. Endoscopic management of chronic pancreatitis. Acta Gastroenterol Belg 1993; 56: 192–200.

38. Choudari C, Nickl N, Fogel, E et al. Hereditary pancreatitis: clinical presentation, ERCP findings and outcome of endoscopic therapy. Gastrointest Endosc 2002; 56: 66–71.

39. Gabbrielli A, Mutignani M, Pandolfi M, et al. Endotherapy of early onset idiopathic chronic pancreatitis: results with long-term follow-up. Gastrointest Endosc, 2002; 55: 488–93.

40. Ashby K, Lo SK. The role of pancreatic stenting in obstructive ductal disorders other than pancreas divisum. Gastrointest Endosc 1996; 42: 306–311.

41. Burdick JS, Geenen JE, Hogan W, et al. Pancreatic stent therapy in chronic pancreatitis: Which patients benefit? Gastrointest Endosc 1993; 39: 309A.

42. Borel I, Saurin J-C, Napoleon B et. al. Treatment of chronic pancreatitis using definitive stenting of the main pancreatic duct. Gastrointest Endosc 2001; 53: 139A.

43. McHenry L, Gore DC, DeMaria EJ, Zfass AM. Endoscopic treatment of dilated duct chronic pancreatitis with pancreatic stents: Preliminary results of a sham controlled, blinded, crossover trial to predict surgical outcome. Am J Gastroenterol 1993; 88: 1536A.

44. DuVall GA, Scheider DM, Kortan P, Haber GB. Is the outcome of endoscopic therapy of chronic pancreatitis predictive of surgical success? Gastrointest Endosc 1996; 43: 405A.

45. Ammann RW, Akovbiantz A, Larglader F, Schueler G. Course and outcome of chronic pancreatitis: Longitudinal study of a mixed medical-surgical series of 245 patients. Gastroenterology 1984; 86: 820–828.

46. Cotton PB, Lehman G, Vennes J, et al. Endoscopic sphincterotomy complications and their management: An attempt at consensus. Gastrointest Endosc 1991; 37: 383–393.

47. Siegel J, Veerappan A. Endoscopic management of pancreatic disorders: Potential risks of pancreatic prostheses. Endoscopy 1991; 23: 177–180.

48. Leung J. Liu Y, Herrera J et al. Bacteriological and scanning electron microscopy (SEM) analyses of pancreatic stents. Gastrointest Endosc 2001; 53: 138A.
49. Sherman S, Alvarez C, Robert M, et al. Polyethylene pancreatic stent-induced changes in the normal dog pancreas. Gastrointest Endosc 1993; 39: 658–664.
50. Johanson JF, Schmalz MJ, Geenen JE. Incidence and risk factors for biliary and pancreatic stent migration. Gastrointest Endosc 1992; 38: 341–346.
51. Dean RS, Geenen JE, Hogan WJ, et al. Pancreatic stent modification to prevent stent migration in patients with benign pancreatic disease. Gastrointest Endosc 1994; 40: 19A.
52. Kozarek RA. Pancreatic stents can induce ductal changes consistent with chronic pancreatitis. Gastrointest Endosc 1990; 36: 93–95.
53. Derfus GA, Geenen JE, Hogan WJ. Effect of endoscopic pancreatic duct stent placement on pancreatic ductal morphology. Gastrointest Endosc 1990; 36: 206A.
54. Rossos PG, Kortan P, Haber GB. Complications associated with pancreatic duct stenting. Gastrointest Endosc 1992; 38: 252A.
55. Burdick JS, Geenen JE, Venu RP, et al. Ductal morphological changes due to pancreatic stent therapy—A randomized controlled study. Am J Gastroenterol 1992; 87: 155A.
56. Lehman GA, Sherman S, Nisi R, Hawes RH. Pancreas divisum: Results of minor papilla sphincterotomy. Gastrointest Endosc 1993; 39: 1–8.
57. Smith MT, Sherman S, Ikenberry SO, et al. Alterations in pancreatic ductal morphology following polyethylene pancreatic duct stenting. Gastrointest Endosc 1996; 44: 268–275.
58. Eisen G, Coleman S, Troughton A, Cotton PB. Morphological changes in the pancreatic duct after stent placement for benign pancreatic disease. Gastrointest Endosc 1994; 40: 107A.
59. Sherman S, Hawes RH, Savides TJ, et al. Stent-induced pancreatic ductal and parenchymal changes: Correlation of endoscopic ultrasound with ERCP. Gastrointest Endosc 1996; 4: 276–282.
60. Deviere J, Delhaye M, Cremer M. Pancreatic duct stones management. Gastrointest Endosc Clin N Am 1998; 8: 163–179.
61. Sarles A, Bernard JP. Lithostathine and pancreatic lithogenesis. Viewpoints Dig Dis 1991; 23: 7–12.
62. Suda K, Mogaki M, Oyama T, Matsumoto Y. Histopathologic and immunohistochemical studies on alcoholic pancreatitis and chronic obstructive pancreatitis: Special emphasis on ductal obstruction and genesis of pancreatitis. Am J Gastroenterol 1990; 85: 271–276.
63. Kozarek R, Ball TJ, Patterson DJ, et al. Endoscopic pancreatic duct sphincterotomy: Indications, technique, and analysis of results. Gastrointest Endosc 1994; 40: 592–598.
64. Esber E, Sherman S, Earle D, et al. Complications of major papilla pancreatic sphincterotomy: A review of 106 patients. Gastrointest Endosc 1995; 41: 422A.
65. Kim MH, Myung SJ, Kim YS, et al. Routine biliary sphincterotomy may not be indispensable for endoscopic pancreatic sphincterotomy. Endoscopy 1998; 30: 697–701.
66. Delhaye M, Vandermeeren A, Baize M, Cremer M. Extracorporeal shockwave lithotripsy of pancreatic calculi. Gastroenterology 1992; 102: 610–620.
67. Sherman S, Lehman GA, Hawes RH, et al. Pancreatic ductal stones: Frequency of successful endoscopic removal and improvement in symptoms. Gastrointest Endosc 1991; 37: 511–517.
68. Smits ME, Rauws EA, Tytgat GNJ, Huibregtse K. Endoscopic treatment of pancreatic stones in patients with chronic pancreatitis. Gastrointest Endosc 1996; 43: 556–560.

69. Schneider MU, Lux G. Floating pancreatic duct concrements in chronic pancreatitis. Endoscopy 1985; 17: 8–10.
70. Fuji T, Amano H, Ohmura R, et al. Endoscopic pancreatic sphincterotomy— Technique and evaluation. Endoscopy 1989; 21: 27–30.
71. Kozarek RA, Ball TJ, Patterson DJ. Endoscopic approach to pancreatic duct calculi and obstructive pancreatitis. Am J Gastroenterol 1992; 87: 600–603.
72. Sauerbruch T, Holl J, Sackman M, et al. Disintegration of a pancreatic duct stone with extracorporeal shockwaves in a patient with chronic pancreatitis. Endoscopy 1987; 19: 207–208.
73. Soehendra N, Grimm H, Meyer HW, et al. Extrakorporale stobwellen lithotripsie bei chronischer pankreatitis. Dtsch Med Wochenschr 1989; 114: 1402–1406.
74. Neuhaus H. Fragmentation of pancreatic stones by extracorporeal shock wave lithotripsy. Endoscopy 1989; 23: 161–165.
75. den Toom R, Nijs HG, van Blankenstein M, et al. Extracorporeal shock wave lithotripsy of pancreatic duct stones. Am J Gastroenterol 1991; 86: 1033–1036.
76. Sauerbruch T, Holl J, Sackmann M, Paumgartner G. Extracorporeal lithotripsy of pancreatic stones in patients with chronic pancreatitis and pain: A prospective followup study. Gut 1992; 33: 969–972.
77. Schneider HT, May A, Benninger J, et al. Piezoelectric shock wave lithotripsy of pancreatic duct stones. Am J Gastroenterol 1994; 89: 2042–2048.
78. Van der Hul R, Plaiser P, Jeekel J, et al. Extracorporeal shockwave lithotripsy of pancreatic duct stones: Immediate and longterm results. Endoscopy 1994; 26: 573–578.
79. Dumonceau JE, Deviere J, LeMoine O, et al. Endoscopic pancreatic drainage in chronic pancreatitis associated with ductal stones: Longterm results. Gastrointest Endosc 1996; 43: 547–555.
80. Kozarek R, Brandabur J, Ball T, et al. Clinical outcomes in patients who undergo extracorporeal shock wave lithotripsy for chronic pancreatitis. Gastrointest Endosc 2002; 56: 496–500.
81. Farnbacher M, Schoen C, Rabenstein T, et al. Pancreatic ductal stones in chronic pancreatitis: criteria for treatment intensity success. Gastrointest Endosc 2002; 56: 501–506.
82. Alvarez C, Widdison AL, Reber HA. New perspectives in the surgical management of chronic pancreatitis. Pancreas 1991; 6(Suppl 1): 576–581.
83. Fogel EL, Eversman D, Jamidar P, et al. Sphincter of Oddi dysfunction: pancreaticobiliary sphincterotomy with pancreatic stent placement has a lower rate of pancreatitis than biliary sphincterotomy alone. Endoscopy 2002: 325–329.
84. Neuhaus H, Hoffman W, Classen M. Laser lithotripsy of pancreatic and biliary stones via 3.4 mm and 3.7 mm miniscopes: First clinical results. Endoscopy 1992; 24: 208–214.
85. Sahel J, Sarles H. Citrate therapy in chronic calcifying pancreatitis: Preliminary results. In: Mitchell CJ, Keelleheer J, eds. Pancreatic Disease in Clinical Practice. Pitman, London 1981: 346–353.
86. Berger Z, Topa L, Takacs T, Pap A. Nasopancreatic drainage for chronic calcifying pancreatitis (CCP). Digestion 1992; 52: 70A.
87. Noda A, Shibata T, Ogawa Y, et al. Dissolution of pancreatic stones by oral trimethadione in a dog experimental model. Gastroenterology 1987; 93: 1002–1008.
88. Lehman GA, Sherman S. Pancreatic stones: To treat or not to treat? Gastrointest Endosc 1996; 43: 625–626.
89. Grace PA, Williamson RCN. Modern management of pancreatic pseudocysts. Br J Surg 1993; 80: 573–581.

90. Gumaste VV, Pitchumoni CS. Pancreatic pseudocysts. Gastroenterologist 1996; 4: 33–43.
91. Smits ME, Rauws EAJ, Tytgat GNJ, Huibregtse K. The efficacy of endoscopic treatment of pancreatic pseudocysts. Gastrointest Endosc 1995; 42: 202–207.
92. Barthet M, Sahel J, Bodiou-Bertel C, Bernard JP. Endoscopic transpapillary drainage of pancreatic pseudocysts. Gastrointest Endosc 1995; 42: 208–213.
93. Catalano MF, Geenen JE, Schmalz MJ, et al. Treatment of pancreatic pseudocysts with ductal communication by transpapillary pancreatic duct endoprosthesis. Gastrointest Endosc 1995; 42: 214–218.
94. Binmoeller KF, Seifert H, Walter A, Soehendra N. Transpapillary and transmural drainage of pancreatic pseudocysts. Gastrointest Endosc 1995; 42: 219–224.
95. Lehman GA. Endoscopic management of pancreatic pseudocysts continues to evolve. Gastrointest Endosc 1995; 42: 273–275.
96. Howell DA, Lehman GA, Baron TH, et al. Endoscopic treatment of pancreatic pseudocysts: A retrospective multicenter analysis. Gastrointest Endosc 1995; 41: 424A.
97. Howell DA, Lehman GA, Baron TH, et al. Recurrent pseudocyst formation in patients managed with endoscopic drainage: Predrainage features and management. Gastrointest Endosc 1996; 43: 407A.
98. Sahel J. Endoscopic drainage of pancreatic cysts. Endoscopy 1991; 23: 181–184.
99. Cremer M, Deviere J, Engelholm L. Endoscopic management of cysts and pseudocysts in chronic pancreatitis: Long term followup after 7 years' experience. Gastrointest Endosc 1989; 35: 1–9.
100. Kozarek RA, Ball TJ, Patterson DJ, et al. Endoscopic transpapillary therapy for disrupted pancreatic duct and parapancreatic fluid collection. Gastroenterology 1991; 100: 1362–1370.
101. Deviere J, Buseo H, Baize M, et al. Complete disruption of the main pancreatic duct: Endoscopic management. Gastrointest Endosc 1995; 42: 445–451.
102. Espinel J, Jorquera F, Fernandez-Gundin MJ, et al. Endoscopic transpapillary drainage of an infected pancreatic fluid collection in pancreas divisum. Dig Dis Sci 2000; 45: 237–241.
103. Kozarek RA, Jiranek G, Traverso LW. Endoscopic treatment of pancreatic ascites. Am J Surg 1994; 168: 223–228.
104. Kim HS, Lee DK, Kim IW, et al. The role of endoscopic retrograde pancreatography in the treatment of traumatic pancreatic duct injury. Gastrointest Endosc 2001; 54: 49–55.
105. Costamagna G, Mutignani M, Igrosso M, et al. Endoscopic treatment of postsurgical external pancreatic fistulas. Endoscopy 2001; 33: 317–322.
106. Lau ST, Simchuk EJ, Kozarek RA, Traverso LW. A pancreatic ductal leak should be sought to direct treatment in patients with acute pancreatitis. Am J Surg 2001; 181: 411–415.
107. Frey CF, Suzuki M, Isaji S. Treatment of chronic pancreatitis complicated by obstruction of the common bile duct or duodenum. World J Surg 1990; 14: 59–69.
108. Deviere J, Devaere S, Baize M, Cremer M. Endoscopic biliary drainage in chronic pancreatitis. Gastrointest Endosc 1990; 36: 96–100.
109. Davids PHP, Rauws EAJ, Coene PPLO, et al. Endoscopic stenting for postoperative biliary strictures. Gastrointest Endosc 1992; 38: 12–18.
110. Barthet M, Bernard JP, Duval JL, et al. Biliary stenting in benign biliary stenosis complicating chronic calcifying pancreatitis. Endoscopy 1994; 26: 569–572.
111. Haber G, Freeman M, Bedford R, et al. A prospective multi-center study of a bioabsorbable biliary Wallstent in 50 patients with malignant obstructive jaundice. Am J Gastroenterol 1997; 9: A200.

112. Deviere J, Cremer M, Love J, et al. Management of common bile duct strictures caused by chronic pancreatitis with metal mesh self-expandable stents. Gut 1994; 35: 122–126.
113. Kuo W-H, Pasricha P, Kalloo AN. The role of sphincter of Oddi manometry in the diagnosis and therapy of pancreatic disease. Gastrointest Endosc Clin N Am 1998; 8: 79–85.
114. Guelrud M. How good is sphincter of Oddi manometry for chronic pancreatitis? Endoscopy 1994; 26: 265–267.
115. Pirola RC, Davis E. Effects of ethyl alcohol on sphincter resistance at the chole-dochoduodenal junction in man. Gut 1968; 9: 447–560.
116. Guelrud M, Mendoza S, Rossiter G, et al. Effect of local instillation of alcohol on sphincter of Oddi motor activity: Combined ERCP and manometry study. Gastrointest Endosc 1991; 37: 428–432.
117. Viceconte G. Effects of ethanol on the sphincter of Oddi: An endoscopic manometry study. Gut 1983; 24: 20–27.
118. Morita M, Okazaki K, Yamasaki K, et al. Effects of long term administration of ethanol on the papillary sphincter and exocrine pancreas in the monkey. Gastroenterology 1994; 106: 309A.
119. Vestergaard H, Krause A, Rokkjaer M, et al. Endoscopic manometry of the sphincter of Oddi and the pancreatic and biliary ducts in patients with chronic pancreatitis. Scand J Gastroenterol 1994; 29: 188–192.
120. Ugljesic M, Bulajic M, Milosavljevic T, Stimec B. Endoscopic manometry of the sphincter of Oddi and pancreatic duct in patients with chronic pancreatitis. Int J Pancreatol 1996; 19: 191–195.
121. Sherman S, Hawes RH, Madura JA, Lehman GA. Comparison of intraoperative and endoscopic manometry of the sphincter of Oddi. Surg Gynecol Obstet 1992; 175: 410–418.
122. Williamson RCN. Pancreatic sphincteroplasty: Indications and outcome. Ann R Coll Surg 1988; 70: 205–211.
123. Bagley FH, Braasch JW, Taylor RH, Warren KW. Sphincterotomy or sphinctero-plasty in the treatment of pathologically mild chronic pancreatitis. Am J Surg 1981; 141: 418–422.
124. Lehman GA, Sherman S. Pancreas divisum: Diagnosis, clinical significance, and management alternatives. Gastrointest Endosc Clin North Am 1995; 5: 145–170.
125. Cotton PB. Congenital anomaly of pancreas divisum as cause of obstructive pain and pancreatitis. Gut 1980; 21: 105–114.
126. Soehendra N, Kempeneers I, Nam VC, Grimm H. Endoscopic dilation and papillotomy of the accessory papilla and internal drainage in pancreas divisum. Endoscopy 1986; 18: 129–132.
127. Liguory C, Lefebvre JF, Canard JM, et al. Le pancreas divisum: Etude clinique et therapeutique chez l'homme: A propos de 87 cas. Gastroenterol Clin Biol 1986; 10: 820–825.
128. Lans JI, Geenen JE, Johanson JF, Hogan WJ. Endoscopic therapy in patients with pancreas divisum and acute pancreatitis: A prospective, randomized, controlled clinical trial. Gastrointest Endosc 1992; 38: 430–434.
129. Coleman SD, Eisen GM, Troughton AB, Cotton PB. Endoscopic treatment in pancreas divisum. Am J Gastroenterol 1994; 89: 1152–1155.
130. Sherman S, Hawes R, Nisi R, et al. Randomized controlled trial of minor papilla sphincterotomy (MiES) in pancreas divisum (PDiv) patients with pain only. Gastrointest Endosc 1994; 40: 125A.
131. Kozarek RA, Ball TJ, Patterson DJ, et al. Endoscopic approach to pancreas divisum. Dig Dis Sci 1995; 40: 1974–1981.

132. Ertan A. Long term results after endoscopic pancreatic stent placement without pancreatic papillotomy in acute recurrent pancreatitis due to pancreas divisum. Gastrointest Endosc 2000; 52: 9–14.

133. Wehrmann T, Schmitt T, Seifert H. Endoscopic botulinum toxin injection into the minor papilla for treatment of idiopathic recurrent pancreatitis in patients with pancreas divisum. Gastrointest Endosc 1999; 50: 545–548.

134. Farrell RJ, Noonan N, Mahmud N, at al. Potential impact of magnetic resonance cholangiopancreatography on endoscopic retrograde cholangiopancreatography workload and complication rate in patients referred because of abdominal pain. Endoscopy 2001; 33: 668–675.

135. Sahel J, Devonshire D, Yeoh KG, et al. The decision making value of magnetic resonance cholangiopancreatography in patients seen in a referral center for suspected biliary and pancreatic disease. Am J Gastroenterol 2001; 96: 2074–2080.

136. Van Berkel A, Van Westerloo D, Cahen D, et al. Efficacy of wallstents benign biliary strictures due to chronic pancreatitis. Gastrointest Endosc 2003; 57: AB 198.

137. Okolo PI, Pasricha PJ, Kalloo AN. What are the long-term results of endoscopic pancreatic sphincterotomy? Gastrointest Endosc 2000; 52: 15–19.

138. Ertan A. Long-term results after endoscopic pancreatic stent placement without pancreatic papillotomy in acute recurrent pancreatitis due to pancreas divisum. Gastrointest Endosc 2000; 52: 9–14.

139. Heyries L, Barthet M, Delvesto C, et al. Long-term results of endoscopic management of pancreas divisum with recurrent acute pancreatitis. Gastrointest Endosc 2002; 55: 376–381.

140. Baron TH, Harewood GC, Morgan DE, Yates MR. Outcome differences after endoscopic drainage of pancreatic necrosis, acute pancreatic pseudocysts, and chronic pancreatic pseudocysts. Gastrointest Endosc 2002; 56: 7–17.

141. Farnbacher MJ, Rabenstein T, Ell C, Hahn EG. Is endoscopic drainage of common bile duct stenosis in chronic pancreatitis up-to-date? Am J Gastroenterol 2000; 95: 1466–1471.

15 Surgery for Chronic Pancreatitis

Martin D. Smith, MD, Elias Degiannis, MD, and Selwyn M. Vickers, MD

CONTENTS

BACKGROUND

A lack of consensus exists regarding the best treatment for chronic pancreatitis (CP). This condition usually presents with pain and, as little can be done to change the natural history of the disease process, our efforts are directed at improving the quality of life for patients *(1)*. The most common associated etiological factor is alcohol addiction or abuse. The personality type of many of these patients leads commonly to substance abuse, and this significantly impacts on the success of treatment. A nihilistic approach to CP based on evidence suggesting the process burns out in approximately 10 years is difficult to accept when the suffering of these patients is witnessed *(2)*. Surgeons need to guard against the assumption of success without significant involvement and

From: *Pancreatitis and Its Complications*
Edited by: C. E. Forsmark © Humana Press Inc., Totowa, NJ

commitment by the patient. There is proof that pollutants or xenobiotics play a role in the pathophysiology of alcoholic CP *(3)*, and these xenobiotics are often associated with occupations commonly filled by the economically disadvantaged, making rehabilitation more difficult.

Aside from pain, there are other organ-based complications of CP: strictures of the common bile duct, pseudocysts, vascular occlusions, and hollow organ obstruction, which require a more aggressive approach because of their potentially life-threatening nature.

The role of surgery in CP must be viewed against the aforementioned background. Methods to evaluate pain are largely qualitative and, although being developed as research tools, they are not commonly used in clinical practice. There is little standardization in the report of pain and quality-of-life assessment; therefore, comparisons in efficacy of the numerous surgical procedures described in the literature are difficult.

CP is a benign condition; yet, the outcomes of therapy for a palliative procedure must be focused on. Thus, durability of pain relief and improved quality of life are essential. Many reports have relatively short periods of follow-up, encouraging those who do not favor surgery to be skeptical of its benefits. The relationship between the development of various surgical procedures and the understanding of the pathophysiology of pain has not always been linear. Understanding is still largely theoretical, but exciting developments are emerging. Ductal hypertension does not explain the mechanism of pain in all patients *(4)*, which is reflected in the failure of simple duct decompression to relieve the pain in certain cases *(5–7)*. Parenchymal hypertension leads to a compartment syndrome *(8–10)* that is aggravated by pancreatic stimulation, resulting in further ischemia of the neurons or protienaceous infiltrates. Disordered neoproliferation of neurons sensitive to ischemia produces pain *(11)*. Now, there is a growing understanding of noxious agents, such as substance P, serotonin, cytokines, and other substances that stimulate pain receptors on the visceral nerves *(12,13)*. The anatomy of the pain pathways is better understood. The pancreatic head is regarded as the pacemaker for pain based largely on the fact that most of the pancreatic mass is situated in the head *(14)*. There is immunological evidence that the disease in the head of the pancreas may drive the inflammatory process *(15)*.

It is generally thought that the surgical treatment of pain in CP should only be considered when other causes of pain have been excluded and after adequate attempts at medical therapy have failed. Medical therapies have not been adequately proven to make a significant impact on the pain. Enzyme replacement has had moderate success and should be used during the period of patient evaluation *(16)*. Various percutaneous *(17)* and endoscopic *(18)* nerve ablation techniques have also resulted in moderate improvement in pain relief, and there is some evidence that if pain recurs, the severity is increased and the ability to control it is less. Recent reports on minimally invasive thoracoscopic splanchnic nerve ablation procedures have shown promising results *(19)*. Whether they should be used as a primary or as salvage procedure after failed surgery is debated *(20)*. Some recent evidence suggests that pain relief from this procedure is not durable with a 50% failure rate at 5 years *(21)*.

DIAGNOSTIC TESTS FOR SURGICAL EVALUATIONS

The diagnostic tests utilized for CP are discussed in Chapter 12. From the surgeon's perspective, the goal of these diagnostic tests is not only to reliably confirm the diagnosis, but also to look for surgically correctable complications (e.g, common bile duct obstruction) and to assess for the suitability of surgery. The commonly used diagnostic tests are discussed from this viewpoint.

Ultrasonography

Ultrasonography is used frequently and more commonly in Europe than in the United States with an overall sensitivity of 60–70% in detecting pancreatic duct dilation, pancreatic inflammatory masses, cysts, and calculi *(22)*. However, the accuracy of this study remains very dependent on the examiner. False-negative findings are reported in the range of 25% *(22)*. It may provide some benefit in the cachectic and pregnant patient in determining potential complications of CP.

Computed Tomography Scan

Multidetector ("spiral") CT with bolus contrast enhancement and a pancreas protocol (so-called thin cuts through the pancreas) provide a highly detailed image of the pancreas and have a false-negative rate less than 5% in many series *(23)*. This study frequently provides valuable information regarding the morphological changes within the gland for the diagnosis of CP and particularly the morphological requirements for successful surgical intervention. In most institutions, CT scans are seen as a complement to endoscopic retrograde cholangiopancreatography (ERCP). In the decision-making process of evaluating patients for surgical intervention, these two methods provide greater than 95% accuracy in determining the morphological criteria necessary for surgical treatment of CP.

Endoscopic Retrograde Cholangiopancreatography

ERCP frequently reveals the subtle and overt findings of pancreatic and biliary ductal dilatation, defines filling defects caused by calculi, detects cystic collections, and determines their communication with the pancreatic ductal system. From a surgical standpoint, ERCP may be crucial in determining whether resection or drainage is appropriate and deciding whether additional procedures, such as biliary drainage or pseudocyst drainage, may be required at the time of surgical intervention. In a series from the University of Alabama at Birmingham and Baraguanath Hospital in South Africa, the majority of patients who had surgical intervention had ERCP prior to their surgical treatment to evaluate the anatomy of their pancreatic duct. However, ERCP does fail to outline the ductal system in approximately 5–10%, but it is more than adequate and accurate in greater than 90% of patients who are evaluated *(23a)*.

Newer Imaging Techniques

MAGNETIC RESONANCE CHOLANGIOPANCRENTOGRAPHY

Magnetic resonance cholangiopancrentography appears to provide sufficient gross imaging of the main pancreatic duct of Wirsung, but it is limited in detecting side branches in mild CP. Thus far, it seems to be a complement to CT and ERCP and does provide evidence of severe CP in those patients who may have contraindications to contrast-enhanced CT scans *(24,25)*.

ENDOSCOPIC ULTRASOUND

Endoscopic ultrasound (EUS) is a promising new tool for the diagnosis of CP. The principle advantage of this method is to visualize both parenchemal and ductal changes with a high-frequency linear transducer. Wiersema et al. have described and investigated positive predictive values for parenchymal and ductal signs of CP detected by EUS *(26,27)*. Although EUS may provide high sensitivity for detecting disease, it does not provide a great deal of additional information beyond CT or ERCP in determining what patients have met the surgical criteria for resection or drainage for CP. However, EUS is quite helpful in distinguishing patients with CP from those patients who have intraductal mucinous papillary tumors of the pancreas. Thus, EUS does play a critical role in many patients with ductal dilatation and pancreatitis. These patients with intraductal mucinous papillary tumors are sometimes mistakenly confused with patients who have a history of pancreatitis and are diagnosed by CT scans *(26,27)*.

INDICATIONS FOR OPERATION

Surgical therapy for patients with CP is indicated when medical treatment fails, which generally consists of analgesics, dietary restriction, and enzyme therapy (*see* Chapter 13). Patients referred to surgical

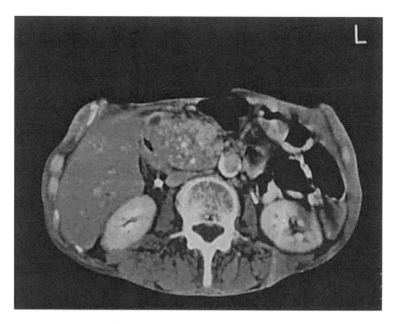

Fig. 1. Enlarged head of pancreas.

clinics that view a significant number of patients with CP consistently demonstrate that only 40–50% of those patients referred will be candidates for surgery. Patients may be disqualified owing to either comorbid illnesses or lack of morphological criteria for operative treatment. In patients who do proceed to surgery, there are usually four major goals for the surgical treatment:

1. Eliminate or reduce intractable pain.
2. Address end-organ or associated complications of CP (biliary obstruction, and pseudocyst formation).
3. Rule out the presence of pancreatic adenocarcinoma.
4. Conserve as much functional pancreatic tissue as possible.

Along with these objectives, there are three morphological criteria that clearly predict the likelihood of surgical success and relief of intractable pain:

1. Segmental (distal or proximal) fibrosis (*see* Figs. 1 and 2).
2. Diffuse ductal dilatation (length of dilatation >10 cm, diameter of ductal dilatation >5–7 mm; *see* Figs. 3 and 4).
3. Associated or adjacent organ obstruction or occlusion (biliary obstruction, duodenal obstruction, or pseudocyst compression).

These anatomic criteria are usually defined by CT and/or ERCP and allow the surgeon and patient to expect a positive result in addressing

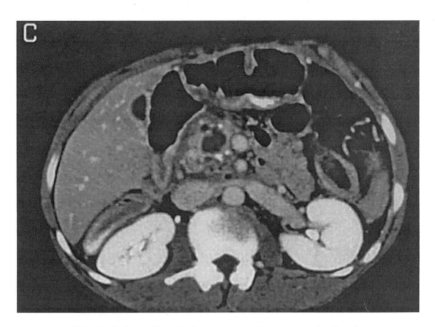

Fig. 2. Enlarged head of pancreas with a cyst in the head.

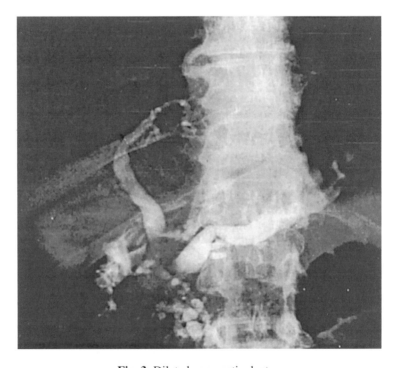

Fig. 3. Dilated pancreatic duct.

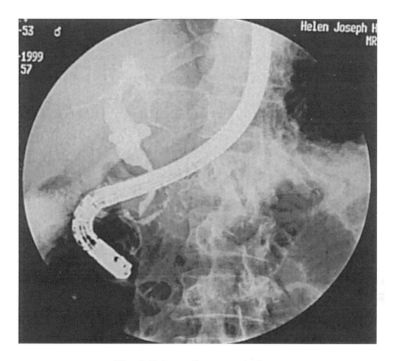

Fig. 4. Sclerosed pancreatic duct.

intractable pain in the CP setting. Patients failing to meet these criteria who receive operative intervention short of total pancreatectomy usually have a less than desirable result in the treatment of their pain. Thus, surgery is generally performed in those with "big-duct" CP rather than "small-duct" CP (*see* Chapter 12).

SURGERY

There is a long menu of surgical procedures to choose from for the surgical treatment of CP and include three major categories of operations: drainage procedures, resection procedures, and a combination of the two.

Drainage Procedures

LATERAL PANCREATICOJEJUNOSTOMY (FIG. 5)

Ductal drainage procedures were first described by Du Val *(28)* and included a distal pancreatic resection. Peustow *(29)*, with whose name this operation is usually associated, described a distal pancreatectomy and a side-to-side pancreaticojejunostomy. It is the Partington–Rochelle procedure *(30)* that is commonly performed currently. For this procedure, a dilated duct is essential, but authors differ as to the definition of

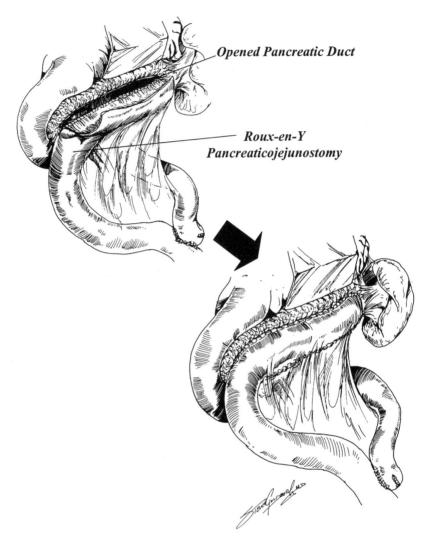

Opened Pancreatic Duct

Roux-en-Y
Pancreaticojejunostomy

Fig. 5. Operative drawing of lateral pancreaticojejunostomy for chronic pancreatitis with a dilated duct.

duct dilation *(31)*. Most regard 8 mm as acceptable *(32)*. This operation requires opening the gastrocolic omentum and identifying the anterior surface of the neck, body, and tail of the pancreas. Defining the duct can be problematic in some patients, but once found, it is opened along the anterior surface of the pancreas. The duct is opened for a variable length—usually for 10–15cm—extending as far into the head (right side) as possible. A Roux-en-Y limb is fashioned and sutured side-to-side to the pancreas using monofilament suture material.

This is a relatively simple operation; early pain relief is good but decreases with time, and eventually, only 50–80% of patients remain pain-free *(5,7)*. It has the advantage of a low morbidity and mortality (<5%; *7,33–35)*. Because there is no resection of pancreatic parenchyma, there is a low rate of new endocrine and exocrine insufficiency. However, a deterioration of function has been shown over a period of time, likely unrelated to surgery but instead to disease progression *(15,16,35)*. One study has shown this may be retarded if early duct drainage is performed even in the asymptomatic patient, but this analysis remains controversial *(35)*. The disadvantage of this operation is the lack of durability in regard to pain relief. This is explained partly because of an undrained obstructed segment of duct in the head of the pancreas and uncinate process. The extent of the dissection to define the pancreatic head may be incomplete with resulting inadequate decompression of the ducts in this region. In addition, the parenchymal hypertension and disordered neoproliferation of nerves are not addressed *(36)*. The authors believe that as our understanding of the pathophysiology of pancreatic pain increases, the role of this procedure will decrease and will be replaced by combination procedures.

CYSTENTEROSTOMY

Cystgastrostomy, cystduodenostomy, and cystjejunostomy for symptomatic pseudocysts are simple procedures with excellent perioperative results. CP recurrence of the inflammatory cyst and ongoing pain occurs in 20–50% of cases *(37)*. These pseudocyst operations address the pseudocyst, not the underlying pancreatic disease; therefore, if the symptoms or cause of the cyst is not addressed, failure is likely. At present, the trend is endoscopic drainage, which is based on a similar principle and has a low complication rate (17%), as well as a relatively low recurrence rate of 5–19% *(38–41)*. However, the durability of symptom relief remains uncertain. In some series, cystenterostomy is the predominant procedure for undifferentiated pseudocysts associated with acute pancreatitis, but the author believes that this is inadequate for inflammatory cysts in CP, and the underlying pancreatic disease should be addressed.

RESECTION PROCEDURES

Proximal Resections

The classical Whipple's operation or pancreaticoduodenectomy (PD) was originally performed for malignant disease (Fig. 6). However, as the mortality for this procedure was reduced in major

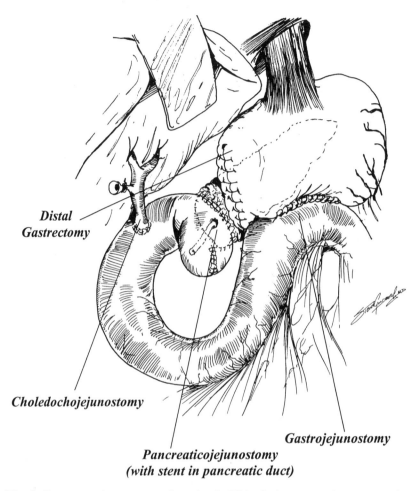

Distal Gastrectomy

Choledochojejunostomy

Gastrojejunostomy

*Pancreaticojejunostomy
(with stent in pancreatic duct)*

Fig. 6. Reconstruction sequence in a classic Whipple (antrectomy) or pancreatic-oduodenectomy for chronic pancreatitis.

centers (<5%), it also became acceptable as a procedure for benign disease *(42–44)*. In big-duct disease, the lateral pancreaticojejunostomy (LPJ) is still the procedure of choice. However, in 20–40% of patients, a sclerosing form of the disease is found with a nondilated duct. This is known as small-duct disease. In these patients, duct drainage procedures are not appropriate, and medical therapy is usually preferred. In many series for CP, the need to exclude malignancy is the main indication for surgery in up to 43% *(14)*. Even with intra-operative ultrasound and fine-needle aspiration cytology, it is found that malignancy cannot always be unequivocally excluded, and resection is required.

A low-operative mortality for PD is reported from high-volume centers, but morbidity in some studies is up to 50%. The extent of the parenchymal loss also results in a new diabetic rate of up to 30% and a similar new exocrine insufficiency rate *(45–48)*. The problem is that in performing this operation, uninvolved organs like the stomach and distal common bile duct are resected. The loss of normal gastrointestinal continuity can result in significant weight loss. Only 80% of patients will regain up to 90% of their preoperative weight *(49)*. This loss of continuity may also explain the new diabetic rate in predominantly head resections. In an attempt to improve the nutritional status of patients, the pylorus-preserving pancreaticoduodenectomy (PPPD) was described. This operation has become the preferred procedure in many centers. Its most significant disadvantage is a significantly higher postoperative delayed gastric-emptying rate (30%) *(49)*. This is an important problem that delays discharge. In some studies, the nutritional benefit is minimal *(49)*. For these reasons, the performance of PPPD has been stopped in favor of the PD.

Either operation has the advantage of excluding malignancy. Both address all aspects related to the pathophysiology of pain (i.e., it resects the mass in the head, removes the pacemaker and disordered nerves, and relieves the compartment syndrome in the head). Technically, this procedure for CP follows the same principles as for malignancy. The fibrosis is often concentrated around the confluence of the veins at the inferior border of the pancreas at the point where the superior mesenteric vein (SMV) passes posterior to the neck of the pancreas. This makes the mobilization of the neck in preparation for division very difficult. In the absence of jaundice, the biliary tree is not dilated. In this situation, a 2-cm side-to-side choledochojejunostomy is performed. Alternatively, a hepaticojejunostomy can be performed by extending the incision in the common hepatic duct onto the left hepatic duct as described by Hepp and Couinaud *(49a)*. Reconstruction of pancreatic continuity in our practices is achieved with a pancreaticogastrostomy to the posterior wall of the stomach. Although pancreaticojejunostomy is still commonly performed *(50)*, there is evidence to support a lower incidence of leaks with the gastric anastomosis and a lower morbidity associated with leaks of inactivated pancreatic enzymes from the pancreaticogastrostomy *(51)*.

The results for pain relief are good with 80% of patients pain-free at 5 years *(45–48)*. Because of the presence of fibrosis, this operation is extremely difficult and should only be performed in centers experienced in this procedure. In North America, the PD and PPPD remain the procedures of choice when surgery is contemplated for small duct CP and to exclude malignancy.

Distal Resections

Localized fibrosis is unusual in CP, especially in the body and tail (52,53). Distal pancreatectomy has been shown to be a poor operation with high recurrence rates for pain (54). There is also a high incidence of new diabetes related to the predominance of β islet cells in the tail. However, there are two circumstances in which distal resections have been shown to be of benefit. First, patients with pseudocysts localized to the tail, distal resection has good results (54). Second, in the disconnected duct syndrome resulting from a complete major duct disruption following severe acute pancreatitis or trauma, resection of the gland distal to the obstruction results in effective pain relief (55,56).

In CP, it is possible to do a splenic-preserving distal resection (57,58). This can be a very challenging procedure, requiring longer operating times and significant blood loss, but certainly in regions with high prevalence of diseases, such as malaria, it is thought that splenic preservation is important (59). Attempts at splenic preservation are recommended but not always possible (57). The spleen should be mobilized before the pancreatic resection. This is performed as for a splenectomy by dividing the ligaments around the spleen, but the short gastric vessels are preserved. The pancreatic neck is mobilized and divided using a stapling device. Owing to fibrosis, the splenic artery is often incorporated into this staple line. The pancreas is then mobilized from the splenic vein by division of the pancreatic branches.

Total Pancreatectomy

Total pancreatic resections are still described, and most series contain only a few patients undergoing this procedure (1). The results for pain relief are poor, possibly because by the time this operation is performed, pain is neuronal or central in origin (similar to phantom limb pain) and not only the result of local factors in the pancreatic bed, such as fibrosis and inflammation (60,61). Additionally, patients develop brittle diabetes with rapid onset of diabetic ketoacidosis and coma. This can be prevented by the various options in pancreatic transplantation presently available and increasingly being shown to have good functional results (36,62). Total resections should not be preformed as a primary operation for CP and should be limited to salvage operations (15). Other salvage procedures like the thoracoscopic splanchnicectomy offer a far less invasive approach to pain in this group of patients.

COMBINATION PROCEDURES

Duodenal Preserving Resections of the Head of the Pancreas

As has been discussed, the previous options do not always adequately address the pain or involve resection of healthy organs. Although the failure rate for duct drainage is of concern and its use limited to dilated ducts, the results of proximal head resections are good, but it involves removing significant organs unnecessarily. In the late 1980s, Beger described the duodenal-preserving resection of the head (DPRH) *(63)*. The results of this operation showed it to be similar to that of PD regarding pain control but with a lower morbidity rate. As it involves a lesser resection and preserves gastrointestinal continuity, the functional results are better, and nutritional status is preserved *(64)*. This procedure has been reported with long follow-up periods (>5 years) and has also been compared in randomized trials to the PD, as well as other duodenal-preserving resections *(65)*. In all these studies, it has been consistently shown to have beneficial results with durable pain relief in more than 80% *(45,66,67)*. The procedure addresses the mass in the head, the compartment syndrome in the gland, and is suitable for small and large duct disease.

This operation also manages the complications in neighboring organs. It addresses the narrowing in the distal common bile duct from fibrosis and can relieve duodenal obstruction. Mobilization of the SMV and portal vein (PV) can help restore blood flow in this venous complex and may theoretically reduce the segmental portal hypertension in the left upper quadrant.

Mobilization of the pancreatic neck of the pancreas over the superior mesenteric-splenic and PV complex is required. In the presence of significant fibrosis, this is a taxing maneuver, even more difficult than for malignant disease. After dividing the neck of the pancreas, the head is resected, leaving a very narrow rim of pancreatic tissue containing the arterial blood supply on the duodenum. A Roux-en-Y limb is then anastomosed to the distal pancreatic remnant, and the same limb is sutured to the pancreatic capsule that is left on the duodenum. Conceptually, this operation addresses most aspects of the pathophysiology of pain. Many authors believe that this procedure requires further evaluation. However, the evidence is compelling, and in many European centers, this operation has replaced the PD.

Local Resection of the Head of the Pancreas and Lateral Pancreaticojejunostomy (Fig. 7)

Charles Frey reported a variation of the DPRH *(68)*, which also involves a lesser resection of the head of the pancreas and also includes a LPJ to decompress the ductal hypertension in the remaining

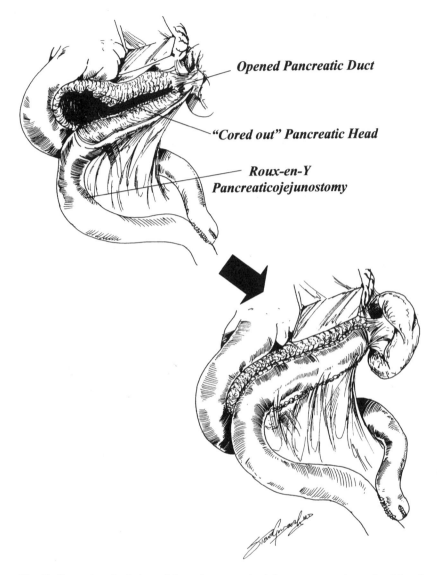

Opened Pancreatic Duct

"Cored out" Pancreatic Head

**Roux-en-Y
Pancreaticojejunostomy**

Fig. 7. Operative depiction of lateral pancreaticojejunostomy and proximal head resection or "Frey Procedure."

gland *(69)*. This operation involves coring out of the pancreatic head, leaving a narrow rim of pancreatic capsule on the duodenum and the posterior aspect of the head. No dissection of the SMV/PV complex is required. However, to adequately core out the head and uncinate process, the head needs to be completely exposed, which is the challenge in this operation. The head must be adequately kocherized and anterior surface well-defined. Failure to sufficiently expose the head leads to incomplete coring out and thereby undrained segments of the main pancreatic duct, santorini duct, or the duct to the uncinate process.

Initially, this operation was described for patients with an enlarged head of the pancreas. However, we now routinely include patients without large fibrous masses in the head of the pancreas. There is also no need for a dilated duct, as the pancreaticojejunal anastomosis is performed to the pancreatic capsule. Following on from this, identification of the duct is not required initially. After adequate exposure of the pancreatic head, the coring out process begins by radially removing thin slices of pancreatic tissue. In the presence of a dilated duct, this is identified in the head, then followed into the neck and body. It serves to identify the posterior aspect of the dissection in the neck and thereby protects the SMV/PV. The dilated duct is opened as far to the left as possible, allowing the body and tail to be decompressed. Palpation helps define the posterior aspect of the dissection in the head, as well as identifying undrained segments of the head. This is particularly helpful in the uncinate process, where the tendency is to under-resect the diseased gland. The pancreaticojejunostomy is performed using monofilament suture and is done as a single-layer anastomosis. The left corner of the anastomosis is the area where leaks occur, and meticulous suture placement is of paramount importance.

Debate continues in how to address the distal common bile duct (CBD) obstruction with this procedure. Coring out in the right upper quadrant of the head threatens the integrity of the CBD. A choledochotomy with a sound placed in the CBD identifies the anatomy; however, it is a concern that the incision in the nondilated CBD may result in delayed stricture formation. In the nonobstructed patient, the choice is to avoid the right upper quadrant and preserve biliary integrity. However, in the event that CBD is breached in the head of the pancreas, two approaches have been proposed. The duct can be left to drain into the pancreaticojejunostomy *(36)*, or an attempt to suture the CBD to the pancreatic capsule to maintain drainage has been suggested *(70)*. Our preference is the former option, but avoidance of the area makes this problem unusual in our experience.

In patients with obstruction of the biliary tree because of pancreatic fibrosis, Frey suggests that adequate coring out of the head and skeletonizing the distal CBD relieves the obstruction. We are concerned that there may be an element of ischemia owing to the skeletonizing of the duct that could lead to secondary stricture formation. We prefer to use the same Roux-en-Y to perform a side-to-side choledochojejunostomy.

The benefit of this procedure, particularly when compared to the DPRH, is the evasion of the vascular dissection. In a randomized study comparing these two procedures, the outcomes were very similar, but there was a significant difference in morbidity rates in favor of the local resection of the head of the pancreas and lateral pancreatiojejunostomy (LR LPJ) *(71)*. The long-term follow-up of this procedure is less well-defined, and most of the reported experience is from the original author's center. Yet, a broader experience from other centers is being reported, and the longer term results are very good. We no longer perform the LPJ but rely on the LR LPJ for all patients—when malignancy is not of concern—regardless of the status of the duct. We are unaware of any evidence that the sclerosing form of the disease is pathologically different from the dilated duct form, requiring a different management approach.

The concept of a lesser resection should theoretically reduce the functional losses experienced with the classic head resections. There is a lesser incidence of new diabetic and exocrine insufficiency with both the DPHR and LR LPJ procedures *(32)*, but new diabetic rates of less than 15% are reported, and similar deterioration in exocrine insufficiency is seen *(36)*.

It may be too early to suggest that the combined lesser resection and drainage procedures should replace the LPJ and PD, but the emerging perspective suggests that these could be the procedures of choice in the future. It is our belief that the LR LPJ is a lesser procedure with effective results for pain relief. Also, combining it with a choledochojejunostomy is considered appropriate for the management of biliary obstruction. However, further reports are required before a definite consensus can be reached.

"V" Plasty

Recently, Izbicki et al. described the "V" plasty *(72)*, which is a variation in the concept of limited resection and drainage procedures. In this operation, a V-shaped excision of the anterior aspect of the body and head is performed, including the region of the main pancreatic duct. This addresses the parenchymal hypertension and removes the nondilated sclerosed duct. A Roux-en-Y pancreaticojejunostomy is then performed in a side-to-side manner. This lesser procedure certainly requires a far smaller pancreatic resection, preventing functional deterioration and conceptually dealing with the parenchymal compartment syndrome. However, the limited coring of the head region may not decompress all the ducts in the head of the pancreas. Conceptually, it is a beneficial procedure, and the results reported are good, but the follow-up is not adequate to yet incorporate this procedure into routine use.

Open Celiac Axis Block

This well-described procedure is usually reserved for patients with unresectable pancreatic cancer. Its role in benign conditions is less well-defined. It can be performed in association with other surgical procedures for pain relief, including the LPJ, but the additional benefit this affords is not well-established. There is concern that the disordered nerve regeneration that can possibly occur will result in worse pain, which may be more difficult to control *(73)*. It is unclear whether it improves the initial pain control or if it adds to the durability of pain control from other procedures on the pancreas.

SPECIAL CIRCUMSTANCES

Suspected Malignancy

CP can present with a mass in the head of the pancreas in 18–50% *(74)*. In addition, there is an increased association between CP and malignancy, particularly in familial pancreatitis. Therefore, in this scenario, the possibility of malignancy in the presence of CP should always be considered. As previously mentioned, up to 43% of proximal resections are performed to exclude malignancy (a large biopsy), and malignancy is found in 6–16% *(53,66)*. If the approach to CP in these cases is routine proximal resection, then the goal of excluding malignancy will be achieved. However, with the development of lesser resection procedures, the ability to exclude malignancy becomes mandatory. Most preoperative methods are of limited benefit. EUS can be particularly helpful if available to differentiate malignancy from CP. Positron emission tomography scan also has been shown to make a significant contribution to exclude malignancy in these patients. Unfortunately, the costs have prevented it from becoming widely available *(75)*.

Our own approach relies on intraoperative cytology. A combination of intraoperative ultrasound to identify suspicious lesion, then trans-duodenal fine-needle aspiration cytology of these lesions, has excluded malignancy in the vast majority of our cases. There are a few instances where a false-positive result has led to a proximal resection, but certainly this policy reduces the number of nontherapeutic proximal resections. Unfortunately, the dense calcification that is often present makes the ultrasound less reliable in establishing suspicious areas. In these cases, after mobilizing the head of the pancreas, palpation is relied on to guide the site of aspiration. With the pathologist in the operating room, repeated aspiration is performed if necessary. In all equivocal situations, if judged to be resectable, a proximal resection is performed.

Pseudocysts

The management of pseudocysts is not well-defined. Most authors follow the Atlanta classification, but there is no universal consensus on their classification *(76)*. Three types are recognized based on the likelihood of pathogenesis: the postnecrotic fluid collection in acute pancreatitis, retention cyst in CP, and necrotic fluid collection following acute pancreatitis in a patient with underlying CP. Theoretically, the three should be managed differently; however, the challenge lies in classifying the individual collection. In the well-defined retention cyst, which is symptomatic, the authors approach is to initially perform endoscopic drainage. If this is successful, no further treatment is required. If this approach fails either initially or at follow-up, and the patient remains symptomatic, surgery is indicated. Cystoenterostomy is an easy procedure with low morbidity and mortality and good early results. However, the recurrence rate is fairly high *(37,77)*, and particularly in CP, it does not address the disease in the pancreas itself. It is not possible to determine if the pain is originates from the cyst or is a result of the pathology in the pancreas *(78)*. A failed endoscopic approach could also be interpreted as a failed trial of therapy for cyst drainage alone. Therefore, our opinion is that for all other patients with CP, the morphology of the pancreas and the pancreatic duct should be defined, and the appropriate procedure chosen to address the disease in the gland itself.

The approach to patients with acute pancreatitis is not as clear. In these cases, the classification is difficult. It is our tendency to be conservative and initially employ percutaneous aspiration or endoscopic procedures. However, when this fails, the decision making must be individualized and should be driven by the underlying pancreatic pathology.

SUMMARY

There is no single operation for all patients with CP. As yet, there is no uniform method of reporting results for the available modalities of treatment *(79)*. The natural history of this disease suggests that there is an ongoing inflammatory process; therefore, the benefit of a procedure must be evaluated in the long term. Pain relief and quality of life must both be assessed. Function is affected by the ongoing inflammation, but there can be little doubt that surgery usually accelerates the progression to functional insufficiency. Malignancy must be excluded. The choice between PD and LR LPJ/DPRH is presently based on individual preference, but it is our belief that with time, the lesser resections will probably replace the PD because of their lower morbidity rates. As the understanding of the pathophysiology of pain in CP increases, the ability to choose the most appropriate operation will improve. Total pancreatectomy should be avoided and distal pancreatic resections limited to a few well-defined patients.

ACKNOWLEDGMENT

We would like to thank Dr. Steve Goldberg for his original drawings.

REFERENCES

1. Stone WM, Sarr MG, Nagorney DM, et al. Chronic pancreatitis: Results of Whipple resection and total pancreatectomy. Arch Surg 1998; 123: 815–819.
2. Ammann RW, Akovbiantz A, Largiarder F, et al. Course and outcome of chronic pancreatitis. Gastroenterol 1984; 86: 820–828.
3. Uden S, Bilton D, Nathan L, et al. Antioxidant therapy for recurrent pancreatitis: placebo-controlled trial. Aliment Pharmacol Ther 1990; 4: 357–371.
4. Ebbehoj N, Svendsen LB, Madsen P. Pancreatic tissue pressure in chronic obstructive pancreatitis. Scand J Gastroenterol 1984; 19: 1066–1068.
5. Adams DB, Ford MC, Anderson MC. Outcome after lateral pancreaticojejunostomy for chronic pancreatitis. Ann Surg 1994; 219: 481–489.
6. Markowitz JS, Rattner DW, Warshaw AL. Failure of symptomatic relief after pancreaticojejunal decompression for chronic pancreatitis. Arch Surg 1994; 129: 374–380.
7. Prinz RA, Greenlee HB. Pancreatic duct drainage in 100 patients with chronic pancreatitis. Ann Surg 1981; 194: 313–320.
8. Ebbehoj N, Borly J, Madsen P, et al. Pancreatic tissue pressure and pain in chronic pancreatitis. Pancreas 1990; 4: 556–558.
9. Karanjia ND, Widdison AL, Leung F, et al. Compartment syndrome in experimental chronic obstructive pancreatitis: Effect of decompressing the main pancreatic duct. Br J Surg 1994; 81: 259–264.
10. Manes G, Buchler M, Pieramico O, et al. Is increased pancreatic pressure related to pain in chronic pancreatitis? Int J Pancreatol 1994; 15: 113–117.
11. Bockmann DE, Buechler M, Malfertheimer P, et al. Analysis of nerves in chronic pancreatitis. Gastroenterol 1988; 94: 1459–1469.
12. Keith RG, Keshavie SH, Kerenvi NR. Neuropathology of chronic pancreatitis in humans. Can J Surg 1985; 28: 207–211.
13. Friess H, Zhu ZW, di Mola, FF, et al. Nerve growth factors and its high affinity receptor in chronic pancreatitis. Ann Surg 1999; 230: 615–624.
14. Traverso LW, Kozarek RA. Pancreatoduodenectomy for chronic pancreatitis: Anatomic selection criteria and subsequent long-term outcome analysis. Ann Surg 1997; 226: 429–439.
15. Anonymous. AGA technical review. Treatment of pain in chronic pancreatitis. Gastroenterology 1998; 115: 765–776.
16. Ammann RW, Heitz PU, Kloppel G. Course of alcoholic chronic pancreatitis: a prospective clinicomorphological long-term study. Gastroenterology 1996; 111: 224–231.
17. Leung JW, Bowen-Wright M, Aveling W, et al. Coeliac plexus block for pain in pancreatic cancer and chronic pancreatitis. Br J Surg 1983; 70: 730–732.
18. Gress F, Ikenberry S, Gottlieb K. A randomized prospective trial of endoscopic ultrasound (EUS) guided celiac plexus block (CB) for the control of pain due to chronic pancreatitis (CP). Gastrintest Endosc 1996; 43 (Abstract): 423.

19. Maher JW, Johlin FC, Pearson D. Thoracoscopic splanchnicectomy for chronic pancreatitis pain. Surg 1996; 131: 233–234.
20. Stone HH, Chauvin EJ. Pancreatic denervation for pain relief in chronic alcohol associated pancreatitis. Br J Surg 1990; 77: 303–305.
21. Buscher HC, Jansen JB, van Dongen R, et al. Long-term results of bilateral thoracoscopic splanchnicectomy in patients with chronic pancreatitis. Br J Surg 2002; 89: 158–162.
22. Bolondi L, Bassi SL, Gaiani S, et al. Sonography of chronic pancreatitis. Radiological Clin North Am 1989; 27: 815.
23. Luetmer PH, Stephens DH, Ward EM. Chronic pancreatitis: reassessment with current CT. Radiology 1989; 171: 353.
23a. Swobodnik W, Meyer W, Brecht-Kraus D, et al. Ultrasound, computed tomography and endoscopic retrograde cholangiopancreatography in the morphologic diagnosis of pancreatic disease. Klinische Wochenschrift 1983; 61: 291.
24. Merkle EM, Nussle K, Glasbrenner B, et al. MRCP—current status. Z Gastroenterol 1998; 36: 215–224.
25. Soto JA, Yucel EK, Barish MA, et al. Cholangiopancreatography after unsuccessful or incomplete ERCP. Radiology 1996; 199: 91–98.
26. Wiersema MJ, Hawes RH, Lehman GA, et al. Prospective evaluation of endoscopic ultrasonography and endoscopic retrograd cholangiopancreatography in patients with chronic abdominal pain of suspected pancreatic origin. Endoscopy 1993; 25: 555–564.
27. Wiersema MJ, Wiersema LM. Endosonography of the pancreas: normal variation verses changes of early chronic pancreatitis. Gastrointest Endosc Clin North Am 1995; 5: 487–496.
28. Du Val MK. Caudal pancreatico-jejunostomy for chronic relapsing pancreatitis. Ann Surg 1954; 140: 775–785.
29. Puestow CB, Gillesby WJ. Retrograde surgical drainage of pancreas for chronic pancreatitis. Arch Surg 1958; 76: 898–906.
30. Partington PE, Rochelle RE. Modified Puestow procedure for retrograde drainage of the pancreatic duct. Ann Surg 1960; 152: 1037–1042.
31. Delcore R, Rodriguez FJ, Thomas JH, et al. The role of pancreatojejunostomy in patients without dilated pancreatic ducts. Am J Surg 1994; 168: 598–602.
32. Izbicki JR, Bloechle C, Knoefel WT, et al. Surgical treatment of chronic pancreatitis and quality of life after operation. Surg Clin North Am 1999; 79: 913–944.
33. Holmberg JT, Isaksson G, Ihse I. Long-term results of pancreaticojejunostomy in chronic pancreatitis. Surg Gynecol Obstet 1985; 160: 339–346.
34. Adolff M, Schloegel M, Arnaud JP, Ollier JCI. Role of pancreatojejunostomy in the treatment of chronic pancreatitis: study of 105 operated patients. Chirurgie 1991; 117: 251–257.
35. Nealon WH, Thompson JC. Progressive loss of pancreatic function in chronic pancreatitis is delayed by main pancreatic duct compression. Ann Surg 1993; 217: 458–468.
36. Frey CF, Amikura K. Local resection of the head of the pancreas combined with longitudinal pancreaticojejunostomy in the management of patients with chronic pancreatitis. Ann Surg 1994; 220: 492–507.
37. Lohr-Happe A, Peiper M, Lankisch PG. Natural course of operated pseudocysts in chronic pancreatitis. Gut 1994; 35: 1479–1482.
38. Cremer M, Deviere J, Engelholm L. Endoscopic management of cysts and pseudocysts in chronic pancreatitis: long-term follow-up after 7 years of experience. Gastrointest Endosc 1989; 35: 1–9.

39. Kozarek RA, Ball TJ, Patterson DJ, et al. Endoscopic trans-papillary therapy for disrupted pancreatic duct and peripancreatic fluid collections. Gastroenterology 1991; 100: 1362–1370.
40. Smits ME, Rauws EAJ, Tytgat GN, et al. The efficacy of endoscopic treatment of pancreatic pseudocysts. Gastrointest Endosc 1991; 42: 202–207.
41. Barthet M, Sahel J, Bodiou-Bertel, et al. Endoscopic transpapillary drainage of pancreatic pseudocysts. Gastointest Endosc 1995; 42: 208–213.
42. Grace PA, Pitt HA, Tompkins RK, et al. Decreased morbidity and mortality after pancreatoduodenectomy. Am J Surg 1986; 151: 141–148.
43. Pellegrini CA, Heck CF, Raper S, Way LWE. An analysis of the reduced morbidity and mortality rates after pancreaticoduodenectomy. Arch Surg 1989; 124: 778–781.
44. Fernandez-del Castillo C, Rattner DW, Warshaw AL. Standards for pancreatic resection in the 1990s. Arch Surg 1995; 130: 295–300.
45. Buechler M, Friess H, Mueller MW, et al. Randomized trial of duodenum preserving pancreatic head resection versus pylorus preserving Whipple in chronic pancreatitis. Am J Surg 1995; 169: 65–70.
46. Martin RF, Rossi RL, Leslie KA. Long-term results of pylorus- preserving pancreatoduodenectomy for chronic pancreatitis. Arch Surg 1996; 131: 247–252.
47. Stapleton GN, Williamson RCN. Proximal pancreatoduodenectomy for chronic pancreatitis. Br J Surg 1996; 83: 1433–1440.
48. Saeger HD, Schwall G, Trede M. Standard whipple in chronic pancreatitis. In: Beger HG, Buechler M, Malfertheimer P, eds. Standards in Pancreatic Surgery. Springer-Verlag, Berlin, 1993, 385–391.
49. Jimenez RE, Fernandez-del Castillo C, Rattner DW. Outcome of pancreaticoduodenectomy with pylorus preservation or with antrectomy in the treatment of chronic pancreatitis. Ann Surg 2000; 231: 293–300.
49a. Hepp J, Couinaud C. L'abord et l' utilisation du canal hépatique gauche dans les réparations de la voie biliaire principale. Press Md. 1956; 64: 947.
50. Yeo CJ, Cameron JL, Maher MM, et al. A prospective randomized trial of pancreaticogastrostomy versus pancreaticoduodenectomy. Ann Surg 1995; 222: 580–592.
51. Sauvanet A, Belghiti J, Panis Y, et al. Pancreaticogastrostomy after pancreatoduodenectomy. HPB Surg 1992; 6: 91–98.
52. Prinz RA. Surgical options in chronic pancreatitis. Ital J Pancreatol 1993; 14: 97–105.
53. Hakain AG, Brougham TA, Vogt DP, Herman RE. Long term results of the surgical management of chronic pancreatitis. Am Surg 1994; 60: 306–308.
54. Rattner DW, Fernandez-del Castillo C, Warshaw AL. Pitfalls of distal pancreatectomy for relief of pain in chronic pancreatitis. Am J Surg 1996; 171: 142–146.
55. Degiannis E, Levy RD, Potokar T, et al. Distal pancreatectomy for gunshot injuries of the distal pancreas. Br J Surg 1995; 82: 1240–1242.
56. Sakorafas GH, Sarr MY, Rowland CM, Farnell MB. Post obstructive chronic pancreatitis. Arch Surg 2001; 136: 643–648.
57. Degiannis E, Bowley DM, Smith, MD. Non-operative management of splenic injury in adults: Current management status and controversies. S Afr J Surg 2003; 41: 33–34.
58. Aldridge MC, Williamson RCN. Distal pancreatectomy with and without splenectomy. Br J Surg 1991; 78: 976–979.
59. Boone KE, Watters DA. The incidence of malaria after splenectomy in Papua New Guinea. Br Med J 1995; 311: 1273.
60. Braasch JW, Vito L, Nugent FW. Total pancreatectomy for end stage chronic pancreatitis. Ann Surg 1978; 188: 317–322.
61. Cooper MJ, Williamson RCN, Benjamin IS, et al. Total pancreatectomy for chronic pancreatitis. Br J Surg 1987; 74: 912–915.

62. Rossi RL, Soeldner JS, Braasch JW, et al. Long-term results of pancreatic resection and segmental pancreatic autotransplantation for chronic pancreatitis. Am J Surg 1990; 159: 51–58.
63. Beger HG, Buechler M, Bittner R, et al. Duodenum-preserving resection of the head of the pancreas in severe chronic pancreatitis. Ann Surg 1989; 209: 273–278.
64. Beger HG, Krautzberger W, Bittner R, et al. Duodenum-preserving resection of the head of the pancreas in patients with severe chronic pancreatitis. Surgery 1985; 97: 467–473.
65. Izbicki JR, Bloechle C, Broering DC, et al. Extended drainage versus resection in surgery for chronic pancreatitis: Prospective randomized trial comparing the longitudinal pancreaticojejunostomy combined with local pancreatic head excision with the pylorus preserving pancreatoduodenectomy. Ann Surg 1998; 228: 771–779.
66. Buechler MW, Friess H, Bittner R, et al. Duodenum-preserving pancreatic head resection: Long-term results. J Gastrointest Surg 1997; 1: 13–19.
67. Beger HG, Schlosser W, Helmut M, et al. Duodenum-preserving head resection in chronic pancreatitis changes the natural course of the disease. Ann Surg 1999; 230: 512–523.
68. Frey CF, Smith GJ. Description and rationale of a new operation for chronic pancreatitis. Pancreas 1987; 2: 701–707.
69. Ho HS, Frey CF. The Frey procedure. Arch Surg 2001; 136: 1353–1358.
70. Izbicki JR, Bloechle C, Broering DC, Broelsch CE. Reinsertion of the distal common bile duct into the resection cavity during duodenum-preserving resection of the head of the pancreas for chronic pancreatitis. Br J Surg 1997; 84: 791–792.
71. Izbicki JR, Bloechle C, Knoefel WT, et al. Duodenum-preserving resection of the head of the pancreas in chronic pancreatitis: a prospective, randomized trial. Ann Surg 1995; 221: 350–358.
72. Izbicki JR, Bloechle C, Broering DC, et al. Longitudinal V-shaped excision of the ventral pancreas for small duct disease in severe chronic pancreatitis. Ann Surg 1998; 227: 213–219.
73. Leung JW, Bowen-Wright M, Aveling W, et al. Coeliac plexus block for pain in pancreatic cancer and chronic pancreatitis. Br J Surg 1983; 70: 730–732.
74. Traverso LW, Kozarek RA. Pancreticoduodenectomy for chronic pancreatitis. Ann Surg 1999; 236: 429–436.
75. Delbeke D, Rose D, Chapman WC, et al. Optimal interpretation of FDG PET in the diagnosis, staging and management of pancreatic carcinoma. J Nucl Med 1999; 40: 1784–1791.
76. Bradley EL 3rd. A clinically based classification system for acute pancreatitis. Summary of the International Symposium on Acute Pancreatitis, Atlanta, GA, September 11 through 13, 1992. Arch Surg 1993; 128: 586–590.
77. Jordan PH, Pikoulis M. Operative treatment for chronic pancreatitis pain. J Am Coll Surg 2001; 192: 498–509.
78. Di Magno ED. Towards understanding (and management) of painful chronic pancreatitis. Gastroenterology 1999; 116: 1252–1256.
79. Frey CF, Pitt HA, Yoe CJ, Prinz RA. A plea for uniform reporting in patient outcome in chronic pancreatitis. Arch Surg 1996; 131: 233–234.

16 Treatment of Exocrine Pancreatic Insufficiency

Supot Pongprasobchai, MD and Eugene P. DiMagno, MD

CONTENTS

INTRODUCTION

Exocrine pancreatic insufficiency is the reduced secretion of exocrine pancreatic enzymes into the duodenum. Its severity can range from mild to moderate insufficiency, causing no symptoms to severe

From: *Pancreatitis and Its Complications*
Edited by: C. E. Forsmark © Humana Press Inc., Totowa, NJ

($\geq$90% reduction of maximal enzyme secretion), which causes malabsorption *(1)* and malnutrition and may significantly impact on morbidity and mortality *(2)*. Causes of exocrine insufficiency include cystic fibrosis, pancreatic cancer, surgical removal of the pancreas, trauma to the pancreas and chronic pancreatitis (CP). In principle, treatment of exocrine insufficiency is simple: replace enzyme secretion by ingesting adequate amounts of pancreatic enzymes with meals. Unfortunately, in practice, although carbohydrate and protein malabsorption can be easily abolished, fat malabsorption or steatorrhea is rarely abolished *(3)*. Reasons for inadequate treatment of fat malabsorption include giving an insufficient amount of pancreatic enzymes, improper timing and dosing of enzymes, and destruction of the ingested enzymes by acid denaturation and proteolytic digestion. All these problems will be summarized and the treatment recommendations will be discussed in this chapter.

PATIENTS WHO NEED TREATMENT OF EXOCRINE PANCREATIC INSUFFICIENCY

The exocrine pancreas has a large reserve for exocrine secretion. Malabsorption of fat (steatorrhea), protein (azotorrhea), and carbohydrate do not occur until lipase, trypsin, and amylase secretion are reduced by 90% of normal value *(1,4*; Fig. 1). However, in clinical practice, fat malabsorption is the most pronounced problem, because lipase secretion decreases more rapidly than the secretion of other enzymes, and steatorrhea often occurs before and is more severe than azotorrhea *(5*; Fig. 2). For example, in alcoholic CP, severe exocrine insufficiency occurs in a mean of 13 years after onset of CP symptoms *(5,6)*. In contrast, in early-onset and late-onset idiopathic CP, severe exocrine insufficiency occurs in a mean of 26 and 17 years, respectively, after the onset of symptoms *(6)*.

Although there is no data available to precisely define when treatment of pancreatic insufficiency should be initiated, oral pancreatic enzyme replacement should begin when there is more than a 90% reduction of enzyme secretion and/or when there is malabsorption or weight loss.

PANCREATIC ENZYME REPLACEMENT

Dose

To abolish malabsorption, the minimum total amount of enzymes that should be postprandially delivered into the duodenum is 5–10% of normal enzyme outputs *(1,7)*. This quantity is approximately 30,000 IU

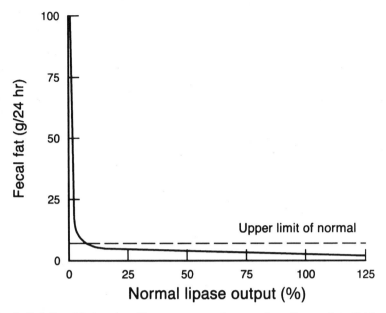

Fig. 1. Relationship between lipase output and steatorrhea. Steatorrhea (24-hour fecal fat more than 7 g per day when 100 g of fat is ingested daily) does not occur until lipase output is reduced below 5–10% of normal. (Modified from ref. *3* with permission.)

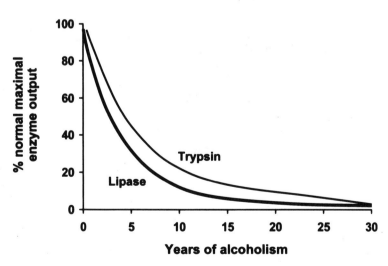

Fig. 2. Relationship between reduction of enzyme outputs and years of alcoholism in patients with alcoholic pancreatitis. Note the earlier and more reduction of lipase output than trypsin output. (Modified from ref. *5* with permission.)

of lipase per meal (by triolein assay; *2,8*) or 90,000 United States Pharmacopoeia (USP) units. This is the ideal amount required when there is no inactivation of orally ingested enzymes by gastric acid. Currently, all pancreatic enzyme preparations in the United States are labeled in USP units, which are approximately three times the lipolytic activity obtained with the triolein assay *(9)*. Thus, at least 90,000 USP units of lipase are required per meal. Suboptimal doses will decrease, but they will not abolish steatorrhea. This minimum amount of lipase should be given to assess the efficacy of treatment before deciding to change treatment to either enteric-coated preparations or adjunctive acid suppression treatments (*see* those sections below). Similarly, this dose should be used to compare the efficacy of different treatment options.

The quantity of lipase varies among tablets and capsules of preparations. Thus, the number to achieve a dose of 90,000 USP units differs among commercial preparations (Table 1). However, usually this dose reduces steatorrhea by approximately 50% and seldom abolishes steatorrhea. Most patients, therefore, still excrete 10–20 g per day of fat *(3,7,10*; normal <7 g/24 hours), because up to 90% of the ingested lipase is destroyed by acid in the stomach *(10,11)* and by luminal chymotrypsin and trypsin *(12–14)*.

Another problem is that the amount of enzymes in each preparation differs among lots. Lower amounts than labeled have been reported as a cause of treatment failure *(15)*. However, when we actually measured lipolytic activity *(9)*, we found that activity exceeds what is listed in the Physicians Desk Reference (PDR). For example, the measured amount of lipolytic activity in USP units for Viokase was 14,000 instead of the 8000 listed in the PDR. Therefore, to achieve ingestion of 90,000 USP units, the Viokase dose is 6 tablets instead of the 11–12 tablets calculated on the basis of the units listed in the PDR. From these data *(9)*, the minimal dose to achieve ingestion of 90,000 USP units of lipolytic activity calculated on the basis of amounts given in the PDR (Table 1) are likely about twice the number of capsules, tablets, or teaspoons needed.

Protein malabsorption or azotorrhea is more easily corrected than steatorrhea because: (1) azotorrhea usually occurs later and is less severe than steatorrhea *(5)*; (2) pancreatic protease deficiency can be compensated for by gastric proteases and intestinal brush-border peptidases to maintain protein absorption *(16)*; and (3) trypsin and other proteases are much more resistant to acid denaturation than lipase. In contrast, fat digestion mainly depends on pancreatic lipase *(17)*, and ingested pancreatic lipolytic activity is lost more often than tryptic activity. Gastric lipases incompletely compensate for lack of pancreatic lipase, and about 90% of lipolytic activity is lost during transit through

Table 1
Commercial Pancreatic Enzymes Preparations and Minimal Dose
for Treating Steatorrhea

Preparation	Type[b]	Content (USP units) Lipase	Protease	Amylase	Minimal dosage per meal for treating steatorrhea
Cotazyme	C	8,000	30,000	30,000	11–12 capsules
Cotazyme-S	ECMS	5,000	20,000	20,000	18 capsules
Creon 10	ECMS	10,000	37,500	33,200	9 capsules
Creon 20	ECMS	20,000	75,000	66,400	4–5 capsules
Creon 25	ECMS	25,000	62,500	74,700	3–4 capsules
Ilozyme	UCT	11,000	30,000	30,000	8–9 tablets
Ku-zyme HP	ECMS	8,000	30,000	30,000	11–12 capsules
Pancrease	ECMS	4,000	25,000	20,000	22–23 capsules
Pancrease MT-4	ECMT	4,000	12,000	12,000	22–23 capsules
Pancrease MT-10	ECMT	10,000	30,000	30,000	9 capsules
Pancrease MT-16	ECMT	16,000	48,000	48,000	5–6 capsules
Pancrease MT-20	ECMT	20,000	44,000	56,000	4–5 capsules
Protilase	ECMT	4,000	25,000	20,000	22–23 capsules
Ultrase MT-12	ECMT	12,800	39,000	39,000	7 capsules
Ultrase MT-18	ECMT	18,000	50,500	50,500	5 capsules
Ultrase MT-20	ECMT	20,000	65,000	65,000	4–5 capsules
Viokase	UCT	8,000	30,000	30,000	11–12 tablets
Viokase	Powder	[a]16,800	[a]70,000	[a]70,000	1.5 teaspoonfuls
Zymase	ECMS	12,000	24,000	24,000	7–8 capsules

[a]Contents per one-fourth teaspoonful (0.7 g).
[b]C, capsule; UCT, uncoated tablets; ECMS, enteric-coated microspheres, ECMT, enteric-coated microtablets.
The content in United States Pharmacopeia (USP) units is the amount listed in the Physicians Desk Reference (PDR). The minimal dose represents the number of capsules, tablets, or teaspoons needed to ingest 90,000 USP units of lipase calculated on the basis of the amount of lipolytic activity given in the PDR. This number is likely approximately twice the number of tablets capsules or teaspoons actually needed (see text for explanation).

the stomach and duodenum, whereas only approximately 75% of tryptic activity is lost (10). In a patient with CP, if azotorrhea persists after adequate enzyme replacement, especially if there is hypoproteinemia (an unusual finding in CP), protein-losing enteropathy or concomitant liver disease may be present (18).

Dose Schedule

Controversy exists about the best schedule for pancreatic enzyme administration. Taking enzymes with meals is as effective as an hourly schedule (enzymes every hour throughout the day) in correcting steatorrhea, but the prandial schedule is more practical *(10)*. The hourly schedule is more effective only when postprandial gastric pH is above 4.0 for more than 1 hour, which occurs in some CP patients *(3,10)*. Therefore, we recommend administrating pancreatic enzymes with meals (e.g., two tablets of Viokase® after the first few bites, four tablets during meals, and two tablets at the end of the meal). A common error is to instruct patients to take enzymes before the meal, which does not promote the mixing of enzymes with food and may cause excessive acid denaturation of lipolytic activity because of the unbuffered gastric acid.

Choice of Pancreatic Enzymes: Nonenteric-Coated or Enteric-Coated?

The first decision in treating a patient with exocrine pancreatic insufficiency is to select the pancreatic enzyme replacement preparation. At present, there are three types: nonenteric-coated, enteric-coated tablets, and microencapsulated enteric-coated preparations (Table 1). The enteric-coated preparations have been developed to circumvent the problem of acid inactivation of enzymatic activity during gastro-duodenal transit.

Enteric-coated enzyme preparations do not disintegrate or release enzymes until the pH is more than 5.5–6.0, which is assumed to be the pH within the duodenum in patients with exocrine insufficiency. Theoretically, the preparations should traverse the stomach without being inactivated by acid and liberate their enzymatic activity within the duodenum and improve the treatment of malabsorption. However, in most studies, when adequate dosages of lipolytic activity were used, enteric-coated enzymes were generally no better than conventional enzymes in alleviating steatorrhea *(7,19–21)*.

There are several reasons for enteric-coated preparations failing to significantly improve treatment of exocrine insufficiency. First, in CP, gastric and duodenal pH rise above 5.0 in the early postprandial period because of the buffering effects of food, then drop to less than 4.0 after 40 minutes. During 24-hour gastric and duodenal pH studies in CP, the 2-hour postprandial duodenal pH also was below 5.0 for 15–25% of time when compared with 0–6% in healthy person and gastric pH was below 3.0 for 75% when compared with 50% in healthy persons *(22)*. Thus, some enzymatic activity is initially liberated from the enteric-coated preparations, then inactivated when gastric and duodenal pH fall below 4.0. Second, because upper gastrointestinal pH is low for so long, enteric-coated enzymes are released in the ileum *(13,20,23)*. In vitro data also support these in vivo findings. At pH 5.0–5.5, only 13–40% of enzymatic activity of the enteric-coated enzymes are released in 2 hours; in contrast, at pH

6.0, 90% of the enzymatic activity is released within 15 minutes *(24)*. Third, enteric-coated preparations may be delayed in emptying from the stomach until several hours after meals *(25)*. This problem has been partly solved by the development of 1–2 mm enteric-coated microspheres (ECMS), which empty from the stomach with meals but varying the size of the microspheres does not affect the treatment of malabsorption *(26)*.

ECMS may benefit patients with hyperchlorhydria or when post-prandial gastric pH and duodenal pH are below 4.0 for a long period of time, e.g., cystic fibrosis patients *(3,7,27)*. In cystic fibrosis, conventional enzymes, even taken with cimetidine, are sometimes ineffective from the inactivation of lipase by the overwhelming acid *(28–30)*. Other advantages of ECMS are: (1) some ECMS contain a relatively high amount of lipase and may permit taking a smaller number of capsules, which may improve patient compliance, particularly in children; (2) ECMS may be taken without the gelatin capsule (but they must not be crushed or chewed) and may be used by young children who cannot swallow the capsules or patients with conditions that may impair gastric mixing (e.g., postgastric resection or gastro-duodenal bypass surgery; *31)*. However, enteric-coated preparations are more expensive than nonenteric preparations, and are associated with colonic strictures in cystic fibrosis children who received high-dose ECMS *(32–34)*, perhaps because the enteric-coated prepara-tions deliver enzymes and the enteric coating to the distal small intestine *(13,17,20,23)*.

Currently, it is our recommendation that treatment should start with conventional enzymes because of the lower cost and a comparable effi-cacy to the more expensive ECMS. ECMS are appropriate if the patients: (1) do not respond to the adequate dose of conventional enzymes with or without acid suppression therapy; (2) are unable to tolerate or poorly compliant to taking tablets or capsules of conventional preparations; and (3) have persistent gastric and duodenal pH below 4.0 documented by a gastric and duodenal pH study, despite acid suppression therapy (*see* below). ECMS should not be used if patients are hypochlorhydric (e.g., total gastrectomy or on long-term acid suppression therapy for other gastrointestinal diseases).

Adjunctive Acid Suppression Therapy

In patients who do not have a satisfactory response to enzyme therapy, adjunctive acid neutralization or acid suppression therapy should be considered. For these adjunctive therapies to be successful, postprandial gastric and duodenal pH must be maintained above 4.0 for at least 60 and 90 minutes, respectively *(3)*.

Magnesium-containing antacids and calcium carbonate are of no benefit (7) and even increase steatorrhea (35) as a result of the formation of magnesium and calcium soaps and the precipitation of glycine-conjugated bile salts (36). Aluminum hydroxide antacid only slightly reduces steatorrhea. Although it increases pH, it also increases gastric volume secretion and duodenal volume flow, consequently reducing the concentration of duodenal lipolytic activity (7,8). Sodium bicarbonate is ineffective at a low dose of 2.5 g postprandially (7) and only minimally effective when 16.6 g per day is given in divided doses with meals (35).

Adjuvant therapy with H_2-receptor antagonists will abolish steatorrhea in 40–50% of persons with pancreatic exocrine insufficiency if increased gastric and duodenal pH are maintained more than 4.0 (7). Even if this pH is not obtained, especially if patients have hyperchlorhydria (e.g., cystic fibrosis), H_2-receptor antagonists with conventional enzymes reduce steatorrhea 25–30% more than conventional enzymes alone (28–30). Before each meal, 300 mg cimetidine orally for 30 minutes was the initial H_2-receptor antagonist and dose (7). In this study, gastric and duodenal pH were successfully maintained above 4.0, and cimetidine increased the duodenal concentration of lipase, because cimetidine inhibited gastric acid secretion and reduced duodenal volume flow (7). Similar results with cimetidine have been reported by others (28–30,37,38) and with other H_2-receptor antagonists, such as ranitidine (39) and famotidine (40). Although cimetidine was ineffective in some studies (35,41), the dose of lipase in these studies was not enough to abolish steatorrhea, which is the likely reason for its ineffectiveness (8). Additionally, it is possible that there was inadequate inhibition of gastric acid secretion (gastric and duodenal pH was not measured in either study) (8). Proton pump inhibitors (PPIs), 20 mg/day omeprazole or 15 mg/day lansoprazole, also significantly reduce steatorrhea (38,42–44). In cystic fibrosis, adjuvant therapy with PPIs reduce steatorrhea by 25–50% when compared to pancreatic enzymes alone (43,44). However, adjuvant therapy with PPIs may not be better than H_2-receptor antagonists (38). Yet, PPIs once daily may be more convenient for patients.

Adjunctive acid suppression therapy may also reduce steatorrhea because it corrects bile acid malabsorption. In CP, the amount of bile acids in the micellar phase is significantly reduced because bile acids precipitate owing to the low duodenal pH (45), and this is corrected only by increasing duodenal pH by using acid suppression therapy.

Although adjunctive acid suppression therapy is beneficial, routine use may not be justified because of cost, drug interactions, and long-term safety. Therefore, it should be used only when abolition of steatorrhea is not achieved following treatment with sufficient dosage of conventional enzymes.

Summary of the conditions preferred for each pancreatic enzyme preparation is shown in Table 2.

DIET MODIFICATION

Current recommendations indicate that patients who do not decrease steatorrhea with enzyme therapy and remain symptomatic should ingest a diet containing a moderate quantity of fat (50–75 g/day), high amount of protein, and low intake of carbohydrate. These suggestions are supported by in vitro studies that show lipolytic activity is maximally preserved by the presence of nutrients high in protein and low in starch (46–48). However, in careful studies done with a controlled diet of four meals per day containing 25 g fat per meal (100 g fat/day), steatorrhea was abolished by pancreatic enzymes with cimetidine (7). Additionally, dogs with exocrine insufficiency increase fat absorption when pancreatic enzymes are given with high-fat diets (49,50). Whether a high-fat diet improves fat absorption in humans with exocrine insufficiency is unknown. However, if there is difficulty in correcting steatorrhea, it might be useful to test a diet of four meals per day with 25 g of fat per meal.

NOVEL TREATMENTS AND FUTURE RESEARCH

Acid Stable Lipases

The ideal lipase to treat exocrine insufficiency should be resistant to denaturation by acid and luminal proteases and maintain lipolytic activity in the upper small intestine. Gastric lipase and fungal lipase (from fungi *Aspergillus niger* and *Rhizopus arrhizus*) are acid-resistant, but they are inactivated by physiological concentrations of bile acids in the intestinal lumen (51). Bacterial lipase isolated from *Burkholderia plantarii*, previously called *Pseudomonas glumae* (52), is resistant to acid denaturation, protease digestion, and does not require colipase for lipolytic activity. In vitro lipolytic activity of bacterial lipase survives better than porcine lipase in human gastric and duodenal juice at conditions most likely present postprandially, as well as in the presence of physiological concentrations of bile acids (53). In canine exocrine insufficiency, bacterial lipase at 300,000 IU (120 mg) is as effective as porcine lipase at 300,000 IU (18 g pancreatin) in correcting steatorrhea, but requires administering 75 times less (120 mg versus 18 g). A higher dosage of bacterial lipase (600,000 IU [240 g]) abolishes steatorrhea without any use of adjunctive acid suppression (49,50). Thus, bacterial lipase

Table 2
Summary of the Indications Contraindications for each Pancreatic Enzyme Preparation

Preparation	Indication(s)	Contraindication(s)	Comment
Powdered pancreatic extracts	Conditions that impair gastric mixing e.g., postgastrectomy or gastroduodenal bypass surgery	Patient intolerant to the taste	Unpleasant taste
Conventional nonenteric-coated enzyme		Conditions associated with hyperchlorhydria. Poorly compliant patient	Widely available and less expensive
Enteric-coated enzyme	Conditions likely associated with hyperchlorhydria. Poorly compliant patient	Conditions likely associated with hypochlordydria e.g., total gastrectomy, achlorhydria, on long-term acid suppression therapy	More expensive
Enteric-coated enzyme taken without gelatin capsule	Conditions that impair gastric mixing e.g., post gastrectomy or gastroduodenal bypass surgery	Same as enteric-coated enzyme	More acceptable taste than powdered pancreatic extract More expensive
Conventional nonenteric-coated enzyme with adjunctive acid suppression		Conditions likely associated with hypochlordydria e.g., total gastrectomy, achlorhydria	Additional expense Long-term safety Drug interactions Effects on patient compliance

is a promising treatment for human exocrine insufficiency and should be further explored.

Decreasing Protease Content in Preparations

Degradation within intestinal chyme of lipase by protease in the same preparation might limit the efficacy of pancreatic enzyme treatment *(17)*. Decreasing the proteolytic activity of preparations increases lipolytic activity following enzyme ingestion and is associated with improving decreased fat absorption *(54)*. Thus, reduction of protease contents in pancreatic enzyme preparations might improve treatment of steatorrhea.

MONITORING THE EFFICACY OF TREATMENT

Response to treatment with pancreatic enzymes varies among patients and is not predictable. The etiology of pancreatic insufficiency (alcoholic or cystic fibrosis), the inconsistent amount of enzymes between lots or preparations with equally labeled doses, and differences in the gastroduodenal acidity among patients cause different responses to treatment. Clinical indicators, such as weight gain, reduction in the number of stools, lessening of abdominal pain, and bloating, are all indications of effective treatment. Reduction or normalization of fecal fat measured by 72-hour fecal fat determination during treatment is the best method to evaluate efficacy. The qualitative microscopic examination of fat globules in stool is simpler, more practical, and nearly as sensitive as the gold-standard 72-hour fecal fat *(55)*.

WHAT WE SHOULD DO WITH NONRESPONSIVE PATIENTS

Most patients improve with treatment. If patients' symptoms and steatorrhea do not improve despite appropriate treatment, several possibilities should be considered, such as reviewing compliance and the diagnosis. If a patient possibly has CP, but exocrine insufficiency is not severe enough to cause steatorrhea, which may be the result of a complication of CP (bacterial overgrowth) or nonpancreatic disease (nontropical sprue). A direct pancreatic function test is the best way to confirm pancreatic malabsorption. Many conditions have been reported to occur with an increased prevalence in CP. Giadiasis *(56,57)* or bacterial overgrowth syndrome can occur in 25–40% of patients with CP *(58–61)*. Menetrier's disease should be excluded if there is no improvement of azotorrhea. Specific treatment of these conditions will improve or abolish the steatorrhea.

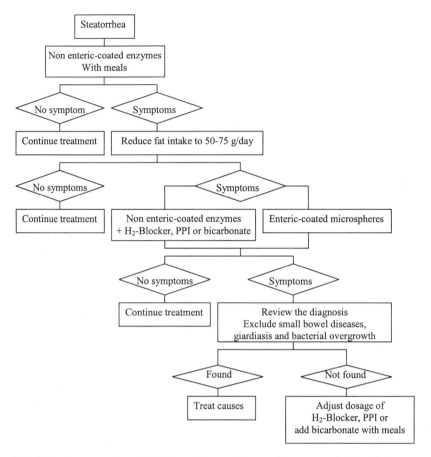

Fig. 3. Treatment approach for the patients with exocrine pancreatic insufficiency.

If none of the previous causes has been identified, a gastric acid study might be necessary to guide treatment. If postprandial gastric pH is below 4.0, acid suppression should be adjusted to achieve gastric pH above 4.0 by changing the H_2-receptor antagonist to a PPI, increasing dosage of PPI, adding bicarbonate with meals, or changing to an enteric-coated preparation. In contrast, if gastric pH is above 4.0, an hourly schedule of pancreatic enzymes is an option, but this schedule is impractical.

RECOMMENDATION FOR TREATMENT OF EXOCRINE PANCREATIC INSUFFICIENCY

A step-by-step approach (Fig. 3) for the treatment of exocrine pancreatic insufficiency should begin by giving nonenteric-coated conventional enzymes containing 90,000 USP units of lipolytic activity with meals. If the response to treatment is unsatisfactory, reduce dietary fat to 50–75 g per day. If steatorrhea is still not improved, combine adjuvant therapy with H_2-receptor antagonists or PPIs. Alternatively, change to the enteric-coated preparations. We prefer using adjuvant acid suppression therapy to enteric-coated enzymes because of the benefit on bile acids malabsorption, as mentioned earlier. Most patients are much improved and do well with these treatments.

If these treatments fail, compliance must be checked, and diagnosis of exocrine pancreatic insufficiency should be verified as a cause of malabsorption. A pancreatic function test may be necessary. Causes of small bowel malabsorption and bacterial overgrowth syndrome should be excluded and, if present, treated appropriately. If a cause for treatment failure is not found and, if tests of gastric and duodenal pH are unavailable, increasing the dose of the H_2-receptor antagonists, changing to PPIs, or elevating the dose of PPI should be attempted. If patients are still unimproved, they may need referral to centers with expertise in pancreatic diseases.

GOALS OF THE TREATMENT OF EXOCRINE INSUFFICIENCY

The goal for pancreatic enzyme replacement is controversial. Our belief is that it should be the abolition of steatorrhea. Pancreatic enzymes usually reduce steatorrhea by 50% (but not abolish it), improve stool symptoms, nutritional status, the sense of well-being, and weight gain, despite persistence of steatorrhea. Adults with exocrine insufficiency have a significantly shortened life span (6), partly from an increase in atherosclerotic cardiovascular disease (62). The reason for the association with cardiovascular disease is unknown, but malabsorption, malnutrition, and metabolic derangement might be involved. Whether long-term outcomes differ between patients with continued mild steatorrhea when compared to patients with complete abolition of steatorrhea is unknown. The answer to this question may help clarify the optimal goal in the treatment of exocrine insufficiency.

SIDE EFFECTS OF PANCREATIC ENZYMES REPLACEMENT

Most side effects of pancreatic enzymes (Table 3; 63) are minor and require no treatment. Pancreatic extracts form insoluble complexes with folic acid (64) and long-term treatment might cause folic acid deficiency. Hyperuricosuria has been described in children with cystic fibrosis treated with high doses of conventional enzymes (65,66), but is more likely associated with the severity of cystic fibrosis rather than

Table 3
Side Effects of Pancreatic Enzymes Replacement

Soreness of mouth
Perianal irritation
Abdominal pain
Abdominal distention
Diarrhea
Constipation (in infants)
Hyperuricemia
Folic acid deficiency
Allergy to porcine protein
Hypersensitivity reactions following inhalation (powdered forms)
Colonic strictures

Taken from ref. *63*.

pancreatic enzyme treatment *(67)*. The most important and severe complication is fibrosing colonopathy or colonic strictures. Originally described in 1994, this complication is mostly associated with high-dose pancreatic enzymes in children with cystic fibrosis *(32–34)*. However, two cases of fibrosing colonopathy have also been reported in adults, one with and the other without cystic fibrosis *(68,69)*. Relative risks of fibrosing colonopathy were 10.9 with a dose of lipase 24,000–50,000 U/kg/day and 199.5 with a dose of lipase more than 50,000 U/kg/day *(70)*. Thus, a 1995 consensus conference on the use of pancreatic-enzyme supplements sponsored by the US Cystic Fibrosis Foundation recommended the daily dose of lipase should not exceed 10,000 U/kg/day *(70)*.

SUMMARY

Treatment of exocrine pancreatic insufficiency is necessary if patients have symptoms of malabsorption secondary to severe exocrine pancreatic insufficiency, steatorrhea, or weight loss. Nonenteric-coated pancreatic enzymes at a dose of at least 90,000 USP lipolytic activity units should be given with meals. Reduction of dietary fat to 50–75 g per day may be an option. Addition of H_2-receptor antagonists or PPIs will improve steatorrhea in most cases and abolish steatorrhea in about half of patients. If patients do not respond to these measures, compliance and diagnosis should be checked; a small intestinal disease or bacterial overgrowth may be present and require treatment. Eventually, increasing the dose of acid suppression treatment may be needed. In difficult cases, referral to a pancreatic center may be necessary for tests, such as gastric and duodenal pH, along with direct pancreatic function tests.

REFERENCES

1. DiMagno EP, Go VL, Summerskill WH. Relations between pancreatic enzyme outputs and malabsorption in severe pancreatic insufficiency. N Engl J Med 1973; 288: 813–815.
2. Gaskin K, Gurwitz D, Durie P. Improved respiratory prognosis in cystic fibrosis patients with normal fat absorption. J Pediatr 1982; 100: 857–862.
3. DiMagno EP. Medical treatment of pancreatic insufficiency. Mayo Clin Proc 1979; 54, 435–442.
4. Hiele MI, Ghoos YF, Rutgeerts PJ, Vantrappen GR. Starch digestion in normal subjects and patients with pancreatic disease, using a $^{13}CO_2$ breath test. Gastroenterology 1989; 96: 503.
5. DiMagno EP, Malagelada JR, Go VL. Relationship between alcoholism and pancreatic insufficiency. Ann NY Acad Sci 1975; 252: 200–207.
6. Layer P, Yamamoto H, Kalthoff L, et al. The different courses of early- and late-onset idiopathic and alcoholic chronic pancreatitis. Gastroenterology 1994; 107: 1481–1487.
7. Regan PT, Malagelada JR, DiMagno EP, et al. Comparative effects of antacids, cimetidine and enteric coating on the therapeutic response to oral enzymes in severe pancreatic insufficiency. N Engl J Med 1977; 297: 854–858.
8. DiMagno EP. Controversies in the treatment of exocrine pancreatic insufficiency. Dig Dis Sci 1982; 27: 481–448.
9. Egberts JH, DiMagno EP. What is the dose of lipolytic activity that corrects human pancreatic steatorrhea? Gastroenterology 2000; 118(Suppl I), A420.
10. DiMagno EP, Malagelada JR, Go VL, Moertel CG. Fate of orally ingested enzymes in pancreatic insufficiency. Comparison of two dosage schedules. N Engl J Med 1977; 296: 1318–1322.
11. Heizer WD, Cleaveland CR, Ibert FL. Gastric inactivation of pancreatic supplements. Bull Johns Hopkins Hosp 1965; 116: 261–270.
12. Layer P, vd Ohe M, Groger G, et al. Luminal availability and digestive efficacy of substituted enzymes in pancreatic insufficiency. Pancreas 1992; 7: 745.
13. Layer P, Go VL, DiMagno EP. Fate of pancreatic enzymes during small intestinal aboral transit in humans. Am J Physiol 1986; 251(4 Pt 1): G475–G480.
14. Thiruvengadam R, DiMagno EP. Inactivation of human lipase by proteases. Am J Physiol 1988; 255: G476–G481.
15. Hendeles L, Dorf A, Steckenko A, Weinberger M. Treatment failure after substitution of generic pancrealipase capsules: correlation with in vitro lipase activity. JAMA 1990; 263: 2459–2461.
16. Layer P, Baumann J, Hellmann C, et al. Effect of luminal protease inhibition on prandial nutrient digestion during small intestinal chyme transit. Pancreas 1990; 5: 718.
17. Layer P, Holtmann G. Pancreatic enzymes in chronic pancreatitis. Int J Pancreatol 1994; 15: 1–11.
18. Regan PT, Phillips SF, DiMagno EP. Pancreatic insufficiency and Menetrier's disease. Report of a case with clinical response to pancreatic enzyme replacement. Am J Dig Dis 1978; 23: 759–762.
19. Graham DY. An enteric-coated pancreatic enzyme preparation that works. Dig Dis Sci 1979; 24: 906–909.
20. Dutta SK, Rubin J, Harvey J. Comparative evaluation of the therapeutic efficacy of a pH-sensitive enteric coated pancreatic enzyme preparation with conventional pancreatic enzyme therapy in the treatment of exocrine pancreatic insufficiency. Gastroenterology 1983; 84: 476–482.

21. Gouerou H, Dain MP, Parrondo I, et al. A lipase versus nonenteric-coated enzymes in pancreatic insufficiency. A French multicenter crossover comparative study. Int J Pancreatol 1989; 5(Suppl): 45–50.
22. Geus WP, Eddes EH, Gielkens HA, et al. Post-prandial intragastric and duodenal acidity are increased in patients with chronic pancreatitis. Aliment Pharmacol Ther 1999; 13: 937–943.
23. Guarner L, Rodrigues R, Guarner F, Malagelada J. Fate of oral enzymes in pancreatic insufficiency. Gut 1993; 34: 708–712.
24. Lenaerts C, Beraud N, Castaigne JP. Pancrease gastroresistance: in vitro evaluation of pH-determined dissolution. J Pediatr Gastroenterol Nutr 1988; 7(Suppl 1): S18–S21.
25. Layer P, Groger G, Dicke D, et al. Enzyme pellet size and luminal nutrient digestion in pancreatic insufficiency. Digestion 1992; 52: 100.
26. Halm U, Loser C, Lohr M, et al. A double-blind, randomized, multicentre, crossover study to prove equivalence of pancreatin minimicrospheres versus microspheres in exocrine pancreatic insufficiency. Aliment Pharmacol Ther 1999; 13: 951–957.
27. Youngberg CA, Berardi RR, Howatt WF, et al. Comparison of gastrointestinal pH in cystic fibrosis and healthy subjects. Dig Dis Sci 1987; 32: 472–480.
28. Cox KL, Isenberg JN, Osher AB, Dooley RR. The effect of cimetidine on maldigestion in cystic fibrosis. J Pediatr 1979; 94: 488–492.
29. Durie P, Bell L, Linton W, et al. Effect of cimetidine and sodium bicarbonate on pancreatic replacement therapy in cystic fibrosis. Gut 1980; 21: 778–786.
30. Boyle BJ, Long WB, Balistreri WF, et al. Effect of cimetidine and pancreatic enzymes on serum and fecal bile acids and fat absorption in cystic fibrosis. Gastroenterology 1980; 78(5 Pt 1): 950–953.
31. Dobrilla G. Management of chronic pancreatitis. Focus on enzyme replacement therapy. Int J Pancreatol 1989; 5(Suppl); 17–29.
32. Lebenthal E. High strength pancreatic exocrine enzyme capsules associated with colonic strictures in patients with cystic fibrosis: "more is not necessarily better". J Pediatr Gastroenterol Nutr 1994; 18: 423–425.
33. Smyth RL, van Velzen D, Smyth AR, et al. Structures of ascending colon in cystic fibrosis and high-strength pancreatic enzymes. Lancet 1994; 343: 85–86.
34. Taylor CJ. Colonic strictures in cystic fibrosis. Lancet 1994; 343: 615–616.
35. Graham DY. Pancreatic enzyme replacement: the effect of antacids or cimetidine. Dig Dis Sci 1982; 27: 485–490.
36. Graham DY, Sackman JW. Mechanism of increase in steatorrhea with calcium and magnesium in exocrine pancreatic insufficiency: an animal model. Gastroenterology 1982; 83: 638–644.
37. Lankisch PG, Lembcke B, Goke B, Creutzfeldt W. Therapy of pancreatogenic steatorrhoea: does acid protection of pancreatic enzymes offer any advantage? Z Gastroenterol 1986; 24: 753–757.
38. Bruno MJ, Rauws EA, Hoek F, Tytgat GN. Comparative effects of adjuvant cimetidine and omeprazole during pancreatic enzyme replacement therapy. Dig Dis Sci 1994; 39: 988–992.
39. Heijerman HG, Lamers CB, Dijkman JH, Bakker W. Ranitidine compared with the dimethyprostaglandin E2 analogue enprostil as adjunct to pancreatic enzyme replacement in adult cystic fibrosis. Scand J Gastroenterol 1990; 178: 26–31.
40. Carroccio A, Pardo F, Montalto G, et al. Use of famotidine in severe exocrine pancreatic insufficiency with persistent maldigestion on enzymatic replacement therapy. A long-term study in cystic fibrosis. Dig Dis Sci 1992; 37: 1441–1446.

41. Staub JL, Sarles H, Soule JC, et al. No effect of cimetidine on the therapeutic response to oral enzymes in severe pancreatic insufficiency. N Engl J Med 1981; 304: 1364–1365.

42. Nakamura T, Arai Y, Tando Y, et al. Effect of omeprazole on changes in gastric and upper small intestine pH levels in patients with chronic pancreatitis. Clin Ther 1995; 17: 448–459.

43. Heijerman HG, Lamers CB, Bakker W. Omeprazole enhances the efficacy of pancreatin (pancrease) in cystic fibrosis. Ann Intern Med 1991; 114: 200–201.

44. Tran TMD, Van den Neucker A, Hendriks JE. Effects of a proton-pump inhibitor in cystic fibrosis. Acta Paediatr 1998; 87: 553–558.

45. Regan PT, Malagelada JR, Dimagno EP, Go VL. Reduced intraluminal bile acid concentrations and fat maldigestion in pancreatic insufficiency: correction by treatment. Gastroenterology 1979; 77: 285–289.

46. Kelly DG, Sandberg RJ, Bentley KJ, et al. Protection of lipolytic activity (L) by nutrients in simulated pancreatic insufficiency. Pancreas 1988; 3(Abstract): 601.

47. Kelly DG, Sternby B, DiMagno EP. How to protect human pancreatic enzyme activities in frozen duodenal juice. Gastroenterology 1991; 100: 189–195.

48. Holtmann G, Kelly DG, Sternby B, DiMagno EP. Survival of human pancreatic enzymes during small bowel transit: effects of nutrients, bile acids, and enzymes. Am J Physiol 1997; 273: G553–G558.

49. Suzuki A, Mizumoto A, Sarr MG, DiMagno EP. Bacterial lipase and high-fat diets in canine exocrine pancreatic insufficiency: a new therapy of steatorrhea? Gastroenterology 1997; 112: 2048–2055.

50. Suzuki A, Mizumoto A, Rerknimitr R, et al. Effect of bacterial or porcine lipase with low- or high-fat diets on nutrient absorption in pancreatic-insufficient dogs. Gastroenterology 1999; 116: 431–437.

51. Zentler-Munro PL, Assoufi BA, Balasubramanian K, et al. Therapeutic potential and clinical efficacy of acid-resistant fungal lipase in the treatment of pancreatic steatorrhea due to cystic fibrosis. Pancreas 1992; 7: 311–319.

52. Cleasby A, Garman E, Egmond MR, Batenberg M. Crystallization and preliminary X-ray study of a lipase from Pseudomonas glumae. J Mol Biol 1992; 224: 281–282.

53. Raimondo M, DiMagno EP. Lipolytic activity of bacterial lipase survives better than that of porcine lipase in human and duodenal content. Gastroenterology 1994; 107: 231–235.

54. Layer P, vd Ohe M, Groger G, et al. Intraluminal proteolytic degradation of lipase and fat malabsorption in pancreatin-treated pancreatic insufficiency. Pancreas 1992; 7: 745.

55. Newcomer AD, Hofmann AF, DiMagno EP, et al. Triolein breath test: A sensitive and specific test for fat malabsorption. Gastroenterology 1979; 76: 6–13.

56. Sheehy TW, Holley HP, Jr. Giardia-induced malabsorption in pancreatitis. JAMA 1975; 233: 1373–1375.

57. Wright JA, Lopez J, Daum RS, Ertan A. Chronic pancreatitis is associated with a high prevalence of giardiasis. Gastroenterology 1988; 94: A503.

58. Lembcke B, Kraus B, Lankisch PG. Small intestinal function in chronic relapsing pancreatitis. Hepatogastroenterology 1985; 32: 149–151.

59. Balgha V, Pap A. Bacterial overgrowth of small intestine demonstrated by H2 test in patients with chronic pancreatitis. Digestion 1991; 49: A6.

60. Casellas F, Guarner L, Vaquero E, et al. Hydrogen breath test with glucose in exocrine pancreatic insufficiency. Pancreas 1998; 16: 481–486.

61. Trespi E, Ferrieri A. Intestinal bacterial overgrowth during chronic pancreatitis. Curr Med Res Opin 1999; 15: 47–52.

62. Gullo L, Stella A, Labriola E, et al. Cardiovascular lesions in chronic pancreatitis: a prospective study. Dig Dis Sci 1982; 27: 716–722.
63. Lebenthal E, Rolston DD, Holsclaw DS, Jr. Enzyme therapy for pancreatic insufficiency: present status and future needs. Pancreas 1994; 9: 1–12.
64. Russell RM, Dutta SK, Oaks EV. Impairment of folic acid absorption by oral pancreatic extracts. Dig Dis Sci 1980; 25: 369–373.
65. Stapleton FB, Kennedy J, Nousia-Arvanitakis S, Linshaw MA. Hyperuricosuria due to high-dose pancreatic extract therapy in cystic fibrosis. N Engl J Med 1976; 295: 246–248.
66. Nouisa-Arvanitakis S, Stapleton FB, Linshaw MA, Kennedy J. Therapeutic approach to pancreatic extract-induced hyperuricosuria in cystic fibrosis. J Pediatr 1977; 90: 302–305.
67. Niessen KH, Wolf A. Studies on the cause of hyperuricosuria in cystic fibrosis patients. J Pediatr Gastroenterol Nutr 1982; 1: 349–354.
68. Hausler M, Mellicke R, Biesterfeld S, Heimann G. First adult patient with fibrosing colonopathy. Am J Gastroenterol 1998; 93: 1171–1172.
69. Bansi DS, Price AR, Russell CG, Sarner M. Fibrosing colonopathy in an adult owing to overuse of pancreatic enzyme supplements. Gut 2000; 46: 283–285.
70. FitzSimmons SC, Burkhart GA, Borowitz D, et al. High-dose pancreatic-enzyme supplements and fibrosing colonopathy in children with cystic fibrosis. N Engl J Med 1997; 336: 1283–1289.

17 Complications of Chronic Pancreatitis

John Petersen, DO, FACP, FACG and Chris E. Forsmark, MD

CONTENTS

INTRODUCTION

Chronic pancreatitis (CP) is a disease characterized by the progressive and irreversible loss of pancreatic structure and exocrine and endocrine function. Various complications can develop that require medical evaluation and intervention. The vast majority of patients with

From: *Pancreatitis and Its Complications*
Edited by: C. E. Forsmark © Humana Press Inc., Totowa, NJ

CP have the disease because of alcohol intake, and these patients often develop symptoms related to alcohol abuse, as well as problems directly attributable to pancreatitis. CP is burdened with numerous complications, but only a fraction (~20%) is directly the result of pancreatitis or one of its direct effects. Most patients with CP die of respiratory and other digestive malignancies, coexistent chronic liver disease, cardiovascular causes, or postoperative complications. This chapter examines some of the more unusual complications of CP, including pancreatic diabetes, nutritional issues, pleuropulmonary influences, panniculitis and arthritis, gastroparesis, venous thromboses, biliary and duodenal obstruction, pancreatic fistulae, and pancreatic malignancy. (Exocrine insufficiency is discussed in Chapter 16.)

PANCREATIC DIABETES

Histologic damage to the pancreas eventually destroys ductal and acinar tissue and islet cells. If this damage is significantly extensive, endocrine and exocrine insufficiency can develop. This degree of damage usually takes many years. Generally, pancreatic exocrine or endocrine insufficiency appears to develop more slowly in the early-onset form of idiopathic pancreatitis rather than in the alcoholic and late-onset idiopathic forms of CP (1,2). Endocrine failure with diabetes typically begins 20 years after disease onset in the alcoholic form, 12 years in late-onset, and nearly 27 years in the early-onset CP subset (1–3). Although abstinence from alcohol does not arrest the deterioration of exocrine and endocrine function, it is commonly agreed that the decline rate is slower in those patients that abstain. The islets of Langerhans account for only 1–2% of the total cellular mass of the pancreas. In CP, fibrotic infiltration into the islets splits the islets into small lobules and dysfunctional units (4). These islets may even undergo hyperplasia in the CP setting. Fasting insulin levels in CP may be decreased, normal, or even mildly elevated, whereas insulin release after glucose stimulation is markedly reduced. Most patients with diabetes resulting from CP have decreased insulin activity, yet some may have a pattern of insulin resistance, such as that seen in type II diabetes mellitus. Endocrine insufficiency ultimately occurs in 30–50% of patients with CP. The factors responsible for the development of pancreatic diabetes include the loss of islet cell mass and function, a reduced incretin affect (decreased secretion of hormones, e.g., gastric inhibitory polypeptide), and the consequences of pancreatic surgery (5).

Insulin-secreting β-cells seem to exhibit more susceptibility to destruction by the sclerotic changes than do glucagon-secreting α-cells

(6), but both may be eventually destroyed. There is a substantial reserve of insulin secretory capacity, and diabetes does not develop until damage to the islets is substantial. The usual time of diabetes onset is from 5 to more than 25 years after the initial diagnosis of CP. Although there is significant variability, diabetes is often a feature of far-advanced and long-standing CP.

Unlike patients with type II diabetes, patients with diabetes because of CP may develop quite profound and prolonged hypoglycemia, which is secondary to inadequate glycogen release, coexistent liver disease, or malnutrition *(6)*. Glucagon release is usually impaired in CP and may contribute to profound hypoglycemic episodes. Hypoglycemia frequently complicates pancreatic diabetes as a result of inadequate glycogen stores from irregular caloric intake related to ongoing alcohol abuse and/or malabsorption. Finally, severe and prolonged hypoglycemia may develop as a consequence of excessively vigorous insulin therapy. These patients often lack a glucagon surge in response to treatment-induced hypoglycemia, and the prolonged hypoglycemia that ensues can be fatal. Ketosis in CP patients is rare, and if coma ensues, it is usually the hyperosmolar nonketotic variant. Patients with CP have a "brittle" diabetes characterized by decreased insulin requirements, resistance to ketosis, increased levels of circulating gluconeogenic amino acids, and susceptibility to insulin-induced hypoglycemia *(7–10)*.

Diabetes mellitus can disturb the metabolism of zinc, copper, and selenium in the setting of CP *(11)*. Diabetes from CP has been shown to be associated with decreased plasma zinc and selenium concentrations, as well as with increased urinary copper excretion. Currently, there is no concrete evidence that suggests differences in these trace elements contribute to the clinical expression of the disease. Zinc is a cofactor in many enzymatic processes, e.g., collagen synthesis, and a deficiency may possibly be involved in the pathophysiology of CP. Urinary zinc excretion is invariably high in diabetes mellitus. The excretion of copper in the bile and pancreatic juice is also altered in CP, which could explain its high-plasma concentration in these patients. However, malabsorption and concomitant diabetes mellitus may also affect the metabolism of copper. Decreased exocrine pancreatic flow may lead to an increase in copper absorption, which could be the reason for the very high urinary excretion of copper in patients with CP that is not typically observed in idiopathic type I diabetic patients *(11)*.

Treatment of diabetes in the CP setting with the use of insulin can bring about sudden and prolonged hypoglycemia owing to the inability of the damaged α cells to release glucagon as a counter-regulatory mechanism against hypoglycemia. Normally, glucagon stimulates gluconeogenesis and glycogenolysis in the liver, restoring blood glucose to close to normal level. Absent from this effect, some of these patients may experience severe or even fatal hypoglycemia as a consequence of extremely strict attempts at glucose control. However, some patients with CP may have characteristics of type II diabetes mellitus with profound insulin resistance. These patients tend to be those with CP caused by hypertriglyceridemia, and diabetes is a primary, not secondary condition. In this subgroup of patients, tighter control of blood sugar is appropriate, as this is required to adequately maintain lipid levels.

End-organ complications of diabetes occur in CP as much as it does in type I and type II diabetes mellitus. These include the development of neuropathy, microvascular damage, retinopathy, and nephropathy as that seen in primary diabetes mellitus *(12)*. In general, management of pancreatic diabetes should be individualized, and treatment may be with insulin and/or oral hypoglycemics. It is important to educate the patient on how to suspect and self-treat hypoglycemic episodes. Optimal glucose control can delay or prevent microvascular problems, but firmer control of blood sugar leads to the higher risk of treatment-induced hypoglycemia. These patients should always have identification as being diabetics and taking therapy. Periodic measurement of glycoslated hemoglobin tests should be performed regularly to determine long-term glucose control. Additionally, attention to details, such as astute skin and podiatric care, as well as yearly ophthalmologic visits for the diagnosis and treatment of diabetic retinopathy, is vital. Urine should be checked for albumin at regular intervals. As in all diabetics, treatment of hyperlipidemia and hypertension is also necessary, as is encouraging patients to stop smoking.

An additional and fascinating aspect of diabetes and CP is worth discussing. Patients with diabetes mellitus appear to develop impaired pancreatic exocrine function and may even develop structural damage to the pancreas. Several studies have noted decreases in fecal elastase-1 in patients with primary diabetes *(13,14)*, and one study even noted abnormalities reminiscent of CP in the pancreatic duct in patients with primary diabetes mellitus *(15)*. The clinical importance and frequency of these findings remains to be determined.

PANCREATIC MALDIGESTION AND MALNUTRITION

Exocrine insufficiency is discussed in Chapter 16. This section focuses on other nutritional problems and deficiencies that may be encountered. Patients with CP may suffer from maldigestion and malnutrition. Abdominal pain, sitophobia, nausea, vomiting, postprandial satiety, and ongoing alcohol abuse may all contribute to poor oral intake. Chronic inflammation of the pancreas interferes with both its exocrine

and endocrine function. The metabolic demands of CP create a challenge for the clinician pertaining to the nutritional support requirements
in this disease. Poor oral intake, coupled with a hypercatabolic state,
often results in negative energy balance and malnutrition *(16)*. These
patients may experience profound maldigestion with marked steatorrhea
and weight loss. Gastric dysmotility and mechanical outlet obstruction
from disease in the pancreatic head may contribute to their malnutrition
and decline. Small-bowel bacterial overgrowth, which commonly
occurs in patients with CP *(17)*, is characterized by 10^4 or more organisms
per milliliter of small bowel contents. This overabundance of bacteria
leads to the deconjugation of bile salts that impair micelle formation
and cause more problems with maldigestion. As many as 40% of patients
with CP have coexistent small-bowel bacterial overgrowth owing to
either previous surgery, hypomotility from the use of narcotics, or other
currently undefined causes.

Deficiencies of vitamins and trace elements may complicate CP, particularly when there is inadequate intake from pain or alcohol abuse.
Abnormalities in zinc, copper, and selenium are discussed previously, as
they most commonly occur in the setting of CP and coexistent diabetes.
Fat-soluble vitamin deficiency can also occur. Specifically malabsorption of vitamin D and calcium can be associated with osteopenia and
osteoporosis, a frequent finding in patients with CP *(18)*. The absorption of fat-soluble vitamins A, E, and K is often preserved in pancreatic
disease as opposed to primary mucosal diseases. Water-soluble vitamin
absorption is also usually maintained. Especially in chronic alcoholics
with advanced CP, such features of malnutrition as peripheral edema, skin
breakdown, decubitus formation, glossitis, profound hypoproteinemia,
hypovitaminosis, and essential fatty acid deficiencies can be observed.

PLEUROPULMONARY COMPLICATIONS
OF CHRONIC PANCREATITS

There are three main categories of pleuropulmonary complications
of CP, which include the following:

1. Pleural effusion.
2. Diffuse pulmonary injury (adult respiratory distress syndrome
   [ARDS]).
3. Nonspecific complications: atelectasis, bibasilar infiltrates, elevated
   diaphragm, pleural reaction, bronchopleural fistula, aspiration
   pneumonia.

Pleural effusions may occur in the setting of an acute flare of CP,
similarly to that possibly seen in any episode of acute pancreatitis (AP).
In this setting, they are often hemorrhagic and occur from 4 to 17% of

cases *(19)*. Most of these effusions are painless and occur three times more often on the left when compared to the right pleural space. Several theories have been proposed regarding the mechanism of pleural effusions in acute flares of pancreatitis. These include: (1) amylase-rich fluid that leaks from the vascular space into the pleural space; (2) holes in the diaphragm or hiatus that allow inflammatory fluid to traverse from the abdomen to the pleural space; and (3) via lymphatics carrying products of inflammation that traverse the abdomen, travel to the mediastinum, and eventually reach the pleural space. Pleural effusions may also occur without an associated acute attack of pancreatitis caused by the leakage of pancreatic juice from the pancreatic duct or a ruptured pseudocyst. This fluid can reach the peritoneal or pleural compartment and can cause pancreatic ascites or a pancreatic pleural effusion (*see* the following section).

ARDS characterized by a capillary leak syndrome in the lungs may also complicate a severe acute flare of CP. ARDS and other nonspecific pulmonary consequences, which may occur in a severe episode of AP, are discussed in Chapter 6.

PANCREATIC FISTULAE

Patients with CP may develop fistulae that reach either the pleural space (producing a pancreatic pleural effusion) or the abdominal cavity (creating pancreatic ascites). This most often occurs when an established pseudocyst ruptures, and the fluid tracks to one of these compartments. Both of these complications are relatively rare, but up to 15% of patients with pseudocyts will have ascites. The ductal leak is often contained by the back wall of the stomach, transverse colon, and other adjacent structures, which results in a pseudocyst. In those patients where this process is unsuccessful, pancreatic juice may directly reach the peritoneal cavity. Fluid within the abdominal cavity can also track through the esophageal hiatus or aortic hiatus into the mediastinum or erode through the diaphragm into the pleural space. As a consequence, unilateral or bilateral pleural effusions can be found. The majority of patients with these internal fistulae are chronic alcoholics with long-standing CP. In children, trauma is the most common cause of ductal disruption with internal fistulae.

Patients with pancreatic ascites may have no history or signs to suggest an internal fistula. Most often, they note abdominal distension and typically do not have a history of a recent episode of pancreatitis, although they are often known to suffer from CP *(20)*. In some patients, there may be abdominal pain, weight loss, or dyspnea. Also, in a number of patients, the presentation may mimic intra-abdominal carcinomatosis with weakness, weight loss, and even false-positive ascitic fluid cytology. It has been hypothesized that pancreatic enzymes can induce metaplasia of serosal cells, and this might be mistaken by less-experienced cytopathologists as malignant cells. When the ascites is sampled, the amylase in the fluid is usually greater than 1000 IU/L and averages 4000 IU/L (19). The fluid is usually "exudative" with albumin levels typically over 3 g. Serum amylase is often elevated, but a normal serum amylase does not eliminate pancreatic ascites or pancreatic pleural effusion.

Those patients with pancreatic pleural effusion also commonly lack a history of a recent flare of pancreatitis and may mainly complain of dyspnea or chest pain rather than pancreatic-type abdominal pain. Like pancreatic ascites, there is mainly anecdotal data. Most reviews note that the majority of patients are chronic alcoholics, and at least half involve ruptured pseudocysts (21,22). The fluid is also generally exudative, and the amylase level is often more than 4000 IU/L.

In those with pancreatic ascites or a pancreatic pleural effusion, a high-quality computed tomography (CT) with pancreatic protocol may define the presence or absence of a residual pseudocyst and may occasionally define the fistula track. There are also reports of accurate localization of the fistula track using magnetic resonance pancreatography. In most cases, however, an endoscopic retrograde cholangiopancreatography (ERCP) is required to localize the site of the leak and assess for downstream pancreatic duct strictures, both of which must be known for appropriate therapeutic planning.

Medical therapy for internal pancreatic fistulae includes making the patient null *per os*, paracentesis or thoracentesis, and hyperalimentation. The use of the somatostatin analog, octreotide, has been used with anecdotal success. Medical therapy by itself has only moderate efficacy but may be worth the attempt in some patients. In one recent review, octreotide or somatostatin was effective in 12 of 17 patients (20). Efforts at external drainage are usually met with failure and/or recurrence.

If medical therapy is undertaken, and ascites or pleural effusions do not resolve, ERCP should be performed if not already done. Endoscopic therapy can be an option at the same setting. The placement of pancreatic duct stents has become more widely used as therapy of these fistulae. In one recent review, stent placement was as successful as surgery (20). In those with a leak from the pancreatic head or body, a stent that covers the site of the leak is often used, but some have advocated that a shorter pancreatic duct stent across the ampulla is adequate. Pancreatic duct sphincterotomy is also used, usually in conjunction with stent placement. Leaks from the tail of the gland are only able to be treated with these shorter stents. Even if endoscopic therapy is not possible, ERCP should be done in all of these patients with pancreatic ascites or pancreatic pleural effusion to assist the surgeon. The anatomy of the duct and site of the leak allow the surgeon to plan the operative approach, shorten operative time, avoid enterotomy if possible, and aid in the design of optimal operation directed at the duct, pseudocyst, or parenchyma alone. If endoscopic therapy is impossible or unsuccessful, the surgical management of a direct leak in the absence of a persistent or residual pseudocyst is to cap the leak with a defunctionalized jejunal limb and roux anastamosis. If the leak is in the tail, distal pancreatectomy may suffice. In those with a dilated pancreatic duct, therapy may include the addition of a duct decompression surgery, such as the Peustow procedure. In the presence of a pseudocyst, it may be possible to perform a cystjejunostomy or cystgastrostomy.

ARTHRITIS AND PANNICULITIS IN PANCREATITIS

Patients with AP and/or CP can suffer from significant arthropathy. This disease may be mono- or polyarticular with the involvement of small and large joints. Joint aspiration of these patients reveals fat globules, and the fluid is typically milky, sterile, with a very high free-fatty acid content and elevated levels of glycerol (23). Circulating lipase levels are typically quite high, and fat necrosis develops in the soft tissues of periarticular regions, producing the arthritis. The spectrum of panniculitis is also quite fascinating in this disease. Panniculitis can occur in the setting of both AP and CP, as well as associated with pancreatic neoplasms. These lesions may often mimic erythema nodosum or the Weber-Christian disease. The panniculitis may precede the clinical onset of pancreatic disease by up to 13 weeks. The vast majority of patients with panniculitis from fat necrosis will have associated pancreatitis or pancreatic carcinoma. The legs are the most commonly involved sites, thighs and buttocks also being quite frequent, and arms being involved very rarely. These areas of fat necrosis are typically found in regions of pressure or contact in the body. In the skin, one sees liquefaction necrosis as well as fibrinoid necrosis. Other classic histological findings are necrotic adipose cells and fat lobules surrounded by lipophages, numerous polymorphonuclear cells, and "ghost cells," which are cells with absent nuclei composed of amorphous granular debris. Saponified calcium can be found in the panniculitis inflammatory reaction. These nodules are red, quite painful, and may coalesce into subcutaneous nodules typically more than 5 cm in size much similar to that viewed in erythema nodosum. They may occasionally progress to sterile abscesses. Panniculitis is believed to occur in 3% of pancreatic disorders, including both benign inflammatory and malignant disease. Pancreatic ductal obstruction is considered to be crucial to the release of exocrine factors, particularly lipase, which causes metastatic fat necrosis. The higher the lipase levels, the greater the risk of panniculitis, but it is essential to note that this disorder can be found with normal levels of lipase. Interestingly, drainage of an associated pseudocyst or relief of the pancreatic duct obstruction by pancreatic stenting, Whipple resection, lithotripsy, and even dilation of the pancreatic duct, can all improve this panniculitis process (24,25).

GASTROPARESIS IN CHRONIC PANCREATITIS

Although not widely appreciated, gastroparesis may complicate CP. This may complicate clinical management, because gastroparesis may produce similar symptoms (nausea, vomiting, and abdominal pain), and gastroparesis may interfere with the delivery of pancreatic enzymes used for the treatment of pain or exocrine insufficiency. The overall prevalence of gastroparesis in patients with CP is not completely defined. One study from the authors' institution examined 56 patients with small duct CP (26), and 44% of these patients had gastroparesis. The cause of gastroparesis was probably multifactorial. Many patients with chronic pancreatitis have elevated levels of choleystokinin (CCK). CCK is thought to cause delayed gastric emptying in humans. Gastroparesis could also be produced by many independent factors, such as the effect of unabsorbed nutrients reaching the ileum, coexistent diabetes, pancreatic inflammation affecting the antrum of the stomach, and the influence of narcotics used to treat chronic pain.

Another study (27) evaluated postprandial motility of patients with CP and their response to a liquid meal and placebo versus a liquid meal with a pancreatic enzyme supplement. A multilumen catheter was used to record contractions, and markers were used to measure transit. In CP, a liquid meal induced a much shorter migratory motor pattern that was associated with increased gastric emptying and rapid intestinal transit. Added exogenous enzymes reversed these changes, and delivery of unabsorbed nutrients to the ileum reproduced the changes.

The difference between the two studies may relate to the variety in patient populations (the second study included only patients with advanced CP and exocrine insufficiency) or to modifications in methodology (liquid versus solid meal). A more recent study (28) used antroduodenal manometry and a liquid meal and documented a prolongation of the postprandial motor pattern in patients with CP along with a significant reduction in the antral motility index. The addition of exogenous enzymes improved these changes. Interestingly, these changes were only significantly different from controls in patients with advanced CP and exocrine insufficiency, again suggesting that the nature and severity of motility disorders may differ in patients with advanced disease when compared to those with small duct disease. The clinical implications of these findings are not entirely clear, but in the author's experience, it is valueable to measure gastric emptying in patients with CP who experience significant nausea and vomiting or do not respond to enzyme therapy. In these patients with coexistent gastroparesis, the combination of a prokinetic, such as erythromycin ethyl succinate, can markedly improve symptoms.

VENOUS THROMBOSIS IN CHRONIC PANCREATITIS

The inferior mesenteric vein that drains the left colon and rectum joins the splenic vein to the left of the ligament of Treitz behind the pancreas. The splenic vein is closely associated with the posterior aspect of the pancreas, whereas the superior mesenteric vein and splanchnic vein form the portal vein behind the neck of the gland. In the acute phase, these patients also often develop a hypercoagulable state, contributing to the venous thrombotic tendency. The development of pseudocysts, peripancreatic fluid collections, and necrosis of the gland all contribute to an inflammatory venulitis predisposed to thrombosis and its complications *(29)*. As a result, acute and/or chronic inflammation in the pancreas can lead to venous thrombosis.

Given its close apposition to the pancreatic body and tail, splenic vein thrombosis is not surprisingly the most common. The rate of splenic vein thrombosis in CP is estimated to be 11% *(29,30)*. Splenic vein obstruction produces a left-sided or sinistrial portal hypertension with gastric varices in the absence of esophageal varices or gastric varices out of proportion to esophageal varices *(30)*. Consequently, ascites, splenomegaly, and bleeding from gastric varices may occur in a dramatic manner. The risk of a variceal bleed in these patients is in the range of 6% *(29–31)*. Therefore, not all patients require therapy, because the risk of bleeding is relatively low. The use of duplex ultrasonography to identify the magnitude and direction of the venous flow is useful in diagnosing venous thrombosis. Also, CT and magnetic resonance venography can clarify the presence or absence of venous thrombosis in this critical region.

Splenectomy is curative for splenic vein thrombosis *(29–31)*. Thromboses of other splanchnic veins poses much more challenging therapeutic options, and mortality is very high *(32)*. Surgical shunt, transjugular intrahepatic portocaval shunt, and regional thrombolysis have all been attempted with limited success.

BILIARY OR DUODENAL OBSTRUCTION IN CHRONIC PANCREATITIS

Fibrosis within the pancreatic head or compression by a pseudocyst in the same location can obstruct the distal common bile duct as it passes behind the head of the pancreas *(19)*. This can lead to cholestasis, jaundice, and even secondary biliary cirrhosis, and is most commonly seen in the setting of chronic alcoholic pancreatitis in patients with advanced big-duct disease. These patients present with jaundice after a very indolent and prolonged clinical course typified by postprandial pain, nausea, or low-grade fever. Elevations of transaminases can be quite subtle for years, and only later do the alkaline phosphatase or γ-glutamyl transpeptidase begin to rise. It is at the late stage of this disease that bilirubin levels may rise above three and become clinically detectable as scleral icterus or jaundice *(33,34)*.

These patients may also develop abnormal liver chemistries for other reasons, particularly alcoholic hepatitis or cirrhosis. The pattern of abnormal liver chemistries is not an accurate method in differentiating common bile duct stenosis from intrinsic alcoholic liver disease *(35)*. Liver biopsy is usually helpful in distinguishing these conditions so that appropriate therapy can be planned *(35)*. There is now increasing evidence that relief of the obstruction not only can prevent hepatic fibrosis, but that pre-existing hepatic fibrosis may actually improve after relief of obstruction *(36)*.

Operative biliary bypass is the treatment of choice with choledochoduodenostomy or a Roux-en-Y jejunal bypass *(33,34)*. The Roux procedure is generally favored, because this technique prevents reflux of lumenal contents up into the biliary tree. In those with an associated pseudocyst, decompression of the pseudocyst may relieve biliary obstruction, but often a biliary bypass is also required. In those patients with an associated inflammatory mass in the head of the pancreas or coexistent duodenal obstruction, more extensive surgical procedures may be required, including pancreaticoduodenectomy or duodenum-preserving pancreatic head resection *(37,38)*. Endoscopic stent placement allows the prompt decompression of the obstructed biliary tree, but it is usually not effective as a permanent solution *(39–41)*. It is usually needed as a temporizing measure, especially in the setting of concomitant cholangitis. Long-term stenting is associated with significant complications *(40)*, often owing to noncompliance with scheduled stent changes. Permanent metal biliary stents have also been used *(39,42)*. Presently, the long-term results of removable or permanent endoscopic stenting remains unknown, and these therapies are generally used as temporizing measures. In patients considered poor surgical candidates, endoscopic management is utilized, but this usually frequently obligates the patient to multiple return visits for stent changes.

Some patients with bile duct obstruction also have concomitant duodenal obstruction from fibrosis in the pancreas and surrounding tissues. Not uncommonly, these patients have a large inflammatory mass in the head of the pancreas, which can even mimic carcinoma *(34)*. These patients develop symptoms of gastric outlet obstruction with postprandial satiety, bloating, nausea, and periods of violent vomiting of poorly digested food remnants. As a result, they may develop a fear of the sight and smell of food and can lose a significant amount of weight. It is not unusual to appreciate gastric distension clinically with a succussion "splash." The diagnosis is best made with upper gastrointentestinal barium radiography, as the endoscopic findings may be subtle. Surgery remains the preferred treatment. This is usually a gastric bypass with gastrojejunostomy, but some patients require a more extensive resection (pancreaticoduodenectomy and duodenum preserving head resection). These more extensive resections are generally undertaken for patients with a large inflammatory mass in the head of the gland with duodenal (and often biliary) obstruction *(34,37,38,43)*. For the patient who is not an operative candidate, dilation of the duodenum and pyloric channel may provide temporary relief. On rare occasions, enteral metallic stents to maintain patency of the postbulbar region and descending portion of the duodenum can be considered for patients with extreme fibrosis and encasement who have other severe underlying medical conditions, but this is usually considered for those with malignant obstruction *(44)*.

PSEUDOCYSTS

Pseudocysts and fluid collections are discussed in Chapter 8. A few additional comments are related specifically to CP. Some patients with CP develop pseudocysts from the evolution of peripancreatic fluid collections that complicate a severe episode of pancreatitis. Pseudocysts may also develop without this series of events. In some patients, an obstruction of the pancreatic duct or one of its side branches leads to a "retention"-type cyst upstream of the obstruction. In this situation, there is no preceding history of a severe flare of AP complicating pre-existing CP. Therapy of pseudocysts is often undertaken when the wall of the collection is mature. This may take several weeks for pseudocysts that evolve from acute fluid collections, but these retention-type cysts are usually mature when discovered, and there is no need for therapy to be delayed *(19)*.

A second issue that merits specific discussion is the pseudocyst complication of a bleeding pseudoaneurysm, which is found almost exclusively in patients with CP and a pseudocyst. These pseudoaneurysms form in visceral arteries *(45)* with the splenic artery being most common, followed by gastroduodenal arteries and pancreaticoduodenal arteries. The most frequent presentation is bleeding into the associated pseudocyst. Blood may remain in the pseudocyst, rupture the pseudocyst, and reach the peritoneal cavity, or reach the gut lumen through the pancreatic duct (hemosuccus pancreaticus; *30*). The usual clinical scenarios include sudden onset of pain associated with unexplained anemia or gastrointestinal bleeding. The diagnosis is usually established with a CT that demonstrates the pseudocyst containing a contrast-enhancing vascular structure. Urgent angiography is indicated with embolization of the pseudoaneurysm. Some patients require definitive surgery, but the majority can be initially managed with embolization alone.

PANCREATIC CANCER IN CHRONIC PANCREATITIS

Pancreatic cancer, one of the most lethal of all human malignancies, ranks within the five most common causes of cancer mortality in the United States. Evidence shows that some forms of pancreatitis are associated with a high risk of pancreatic cancer. The duration and etiology of pancreatitis appears to be key factors. Although CP is a risk factor for pancreatic malignancy, most cases of pancreatic adenocarcinoma do not arise in patients with pre-existing pancreatitis.

A multicenter study that examined an excess of 2000 patients from clinical centers located around the United States and Europe revealed that the excess risk of carcinoma was observed in both alcoholic and idiopathic CP in both sexes and in all countries *(46)*. Older patients with CP appeared to be at greater risk than younger patients, likely because of the longer duration of their disease. Twenty years after the diagnosis of pancreatitis, the cumulative risk of pancreatic cancer was 4%. Pancreatic malignancy is obviously only one cause of death in these patients. In one large natural history study, smoking, alcohol intake, or development of cirrhosis increased the risk of death during the observation period *(47)*. At 10 years after the diagnosis of CP, the crude survival rate was 70% when compared with an expected 93%; at 20 years, more than half of the group had expired. In distinction, diabetes and calcification of the pancreas were associated with increased survival. This connection is likely because of the fact that both factors often indicate longer duration of disease, yielding an apparent survival advantage for subjects who live long enough to develop either one of these complications. As this cohort was followed, many of the patients developed cancers outside the pancreas, such as cancer of the mouth, oropharynx, larynx, and lung (47).

The risk of pancreatic cancer developing in the background of CP varies with the duration of disease but also with the etiology of disease. Patients with hereditary pancreatitis are particularly prone to the development of pancreatic adenocarcinoma. One study followed a large international cohort of these patients and noted a marked increase in risk (48). In these patients, the mean age of diagnosis of pancreatic cancer was 54 years, and the cumulative risk of cancer to an age of 70 was close to 40%. In the subgroup with a paternal inheritance pattern, the risk was even greater. Smoking appeared to be a major cofactor; smokers had double the risk in comparison to nonsmokers (48). Tropical pancreatitis, another rare form of CP, also brings particular risk for pancreatic adenocarcinoma. In one report of 185 cases followed for an average of less than 5 years, six pancreatic cancers were observed when compared to an expected number of 0.06 with a risk ratio of 100 (49). Cystic fibrosis, another cause of pancreatic exocrine insufficiency, is also linked with an excessive risk of all forms of digestive cancers, including pancreatic malignancy.

Although chronic inflammation in the pancreas is a risk factor for malignancy (like chronic colonic inflammation is a risk factor for colonic carcinoma), there are undoubtedly numerous cofactors that influence the risk of malignancy. Age is unquestionably the strongest known risk factor for pancreatic carcinoma. Pancreatic cancer is nearly 20 times more common in patients older than age 50 than in younger patients. Additionally, smoking, a well-established risk factor for pancreatic cancer, is the single factor most amenable to preventative measures. A 20-pack-per-year smoking history leads to an approximately twofold increased risk of pancreatic cancer. In the United States, African-American men and women have higher rates of pancreatic cancer than whites. Indeed, there may be racial differences in nicotine metabolism and the susceptibility to tobacco-related carcinogens. Racial differences and the ability to detoxify tobacco-related carcinogens could explain the excess of both lung and pancreatic cancer (50). Several dietary factors are also suspected to be risk factors for pancreatic carcinoma, including high-fat diets, high-carbohydrate diets, and diets deficient in fruits, vegetables, and fiber. The alcoholic with chronic pancreatitis may fit into this category.

The clinical ramifications in the relationship between pancreatic cancer and pancreatitis are substantial. Most patients with pancreatic carcinoma present with abdominal pain, anorexia, and weight loss. However, some may present with an initial episode of AP. In one study from the Veterans Administration database, patients with pancreatic cancer commonly had pre-existing admissions with the diagnosis of pancreatitis. This study revealed a clear excess of prior hospitalization for pancreatitis in patients who subsequently developed pancreatic malignancy when compared to a matched control group *(51)*. The new onset of diabetes mellitus is also an occasional harbinger of pancreatic cancer, particularly if the onset is sudden, the patient is thin, and there is no family history of diabetes *(52)*. The symptoms of CP, such as anorexia, weight loss, and persistent abdominal pain, may also mimic the symptoms of carcinoma; therefore, it is essential for the clinician to consider the possibility of malignancy as a frequent and often lethal complication in these patients. Not only can pancreatic cancer mimic CP, but the two conditions can occur simultaneously. Distinguishing pancreatic cancer from an inflammatory "pseudotumor" in CP can be difficult. Presently, multidetector CT with "thin slices" through the pancreas is most useful. Endoscopic ultrasonography (EUS) with fine-needle aspiration biopsy (FNA) of any visible masses is also frequently used, but the changes of CP within the gland make the identification of a tumor difficult (Fig. 1). In one study of 102 patients with negative cytology via CT-guided FNA or ERCP, 57 of 102 patients had positive EUS-guided FNA cytology aspirates *(53)*. EUS-guided FNA can also assess vascular invasion and sample suspicious peripancreatic nodes—critical components of accurate tumor staging. ERCP can also be beneficial in differentiating CP from pancreatic malignancy with the definition of ductal strictures or mass effect *(54,55)*. Brush cytology obtained at ERCP of pancreatic or biliary strictures is diagnostic in only one half of cases; combining biopsy of ductal stricture substantially improves accuracy. It is worth noting that the small cytologic specimens obtained under CT, ERCP, or EUS guidance require substantial skill in pathological interpretation. Distinguishing well-differentiated carcinoma from CP can be difficult for even the best cytopathologist.

The sensitivity and specificity of several serum tumor markers may be insufficient to differentiate CP from pancreatic carcinoma. CA 19-9 remains the most well-studied marker with the best accuracy. The positive predictive value of CA19-9 in the diagnosis of early pancreatic cancer in the CP setting is still inadequate owing to the fact that CA19-9 can be elevated in approximately 20% of patients with benign CP *(56)*. New technologies, including positron emission tomography utilizing flouro-deoxy glucose (PET-FDG), are also being studied. One recent study of 48 patients with CP and 27 with pancreatic carcinoma compared

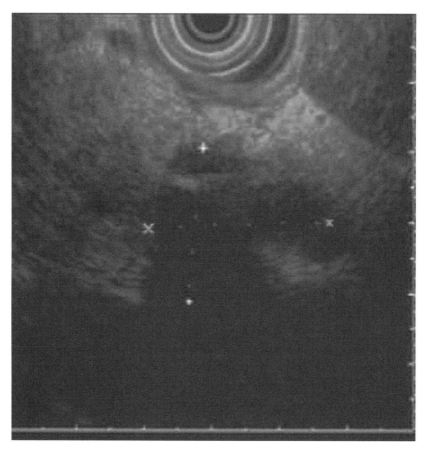

Fig. 1. An endosonographic image of the pancreatic head reveals a hypoechoic mass within the pancreatic parenchyma—a feature of pancreatic carcinoma. The markers identify the margins of the mass. A fine-needle aspiration biopsy can be obtained by endoscopic ultrasound to verify the diagnosis.

the results of PET-FDG with CT, ultrasound, ERCP, operative findings, and histology *(57)*. The sensitivity and specificity of PET was 98% and 100%, respectively, for carcinoma, and 100% and 97% for CP. FDG-PET assesses glycolysis in tumorous tissue and must be interpreted with caution in diabetics.

New methods to examine cytologic specimens and analyze pancreatic secretions are also being evaluated. These analyses are generally based on an understanding of the genetic alterations that commonly occur in pancreatic malignancy *(58)*. Various malignant markers can be studied in this regard, such as k-*ras*-2, telomerase, mucin gene (MUC), and tissue polypeptide-specific antigen. It remains to be known whether these markers add to the accuracy of cytologic examination, but initial studies do show promise. A mucin termed MUC 4 may be extremely sensitive and specific for adenocarcinoma; in one study, none of the CP patients displayed this mucin *(59)*. K-*ras* mutation is an early event in carcinogenesis. Measurement of k-*ras*-2 can be performed in pancreatic secretions and brush cytology collected at the time of ERCP. However, k-*ras* mutations do not improve the diagnostic yield of cytology, nor does it act as a marker of potential malignant transformation, as it can be present in patients with benign CP *(60)*. Finally, telomerase activity in ductal brushings as measured by the telomeric repeat amplification protocol assay may become a useful adjunct in differentiating CP from malignancy. Only 3% of CP patients display telomerase activity. It is postulated that telomerase activity is a marker of cell immortalization and malignant change *(61)*. Whether new markers or a combination of these markers noted previously ultimately become clinically useful remains to be determined. With current technology, the differentiation of pancreatic cancer from CP remains a difficult clinical challenge.

REFERENCES

1. Apte MV, Keogh GW, Wilson JS. Chronic pancreatitis: Complications and management. J Clin Gastroenterol 1999; 29: 225–240.
2. Layer P. The different courses of early- and late-onset idiopathic and alcoholic chronic pancreatitis. Gastroenterology 1994; 107: 1481–1487.
3. Lankisch PG. Natural course in chronic pancreatitis: pain, exocrine and endocrine pancreatic insufficiency and prognosis of the disease. Digestion 1993; 54: 148–155.
4. Kloppel G, Maillet B. Pathology of acute and chronic pancreatitis. Pancreas 1993; 8: 659–670.
5. Malka D, Hammel P, Sauvenet A, et al. Risk factors for diabetes mellitus in chronic pancreatitis. Gastroenterology 2000; 119: 1324–1332.
6. Wakasugi H, Funakoshi A, Iguchi H. Clinical assessment of pancreatic diabetes caused by chronic pancreatitis. J Gastroenterol 1998; 33: 254–259.
7. Marks V. The enteroinsular axis. J Clin Path 1980; 33: 38–42.
8. Ebert R, Creutzfeldt W. Reversal of impaired GIP and insulin secretion in patients with pancreatic steatorrhea following enzyme substitution. Diabetologica 1980; 19: 198–204.
9. Larsen S, Hilsted J, Phillipsen EK, et al. Glucose counter-regulation in diabetes secondary to chronic pancreatitis. Metabolism 1990; 39: 138–143.
10. Sjoberg RJ, Kidd GS. Pancreatic diabetes mellitus. Diabetes Care 1989; 12: 715–724.
11. Quilliot D, Dousset B, Guerci B, et al. Evidence that diabetes mellitus favors impaired metabolism of zinc, copper, and selenium in chronic pancreatitis. Pancreas 2001; 22: 299–306.
12. Couet C, Genton P, Pointel JP, et al. The prevalence of retinopathy is similar in diabetes mellitus secondary to chronic pancreatitis with or without pancreatectomy and in idiopathic diabetes mellitus. Diabetes Care 1985; 8: 323–328.

13. Icks A, Haastert B, Giani G, Rathman W. Low fecal elastase-1 in type I diabetes mellitus. Z Gastroenterol 2001; 39: 823–830.
14. Hardt PD, Krauss A, Bretz L, et al. Pancreatic exocrine function in patients with Type 1 and 2 diabetes mellitus. Acta Diabetol 2000; 37: 105–110.
15. Hardt PD, Killinger A, Nalop J, et al. Chronic pancreatitis and diabetes mellitus. A retrospective analysis of 156 ERCP investigations in patients with insulin-dependent and non-insulin dependent diabetes mellitus. Pancreatology 2002; 2: 30–33.
16. Hebuterne X, Hastier P, Peroux J-L, et al. Resting energy expenditure in patients with chronic pancreatitis. Dig Dis Sci 1996; 41: 533–539.
17. Trespi E, Ferrieri A. Intestinal bacterial overgrowth during chronic pancreatitis. Curr Med Res Opin 1999; 15: 47–52.
18. Haaber AB, Rosenfalck AM, Hansen B, et al. Bone mineral metabolism, bone mineral density, and body composition in patients with chronic pancreatitis and pancreatic exocrine insufficiency. Int J Pancreatol 2000; 27: 21–27.
19. Forsmark CE, Grendell JH. Complications of pancreatitis. Semin Gastrointest Dis 1991; 2: 165–176.
20. Gomez-Cerezo J, Barbado Cano A, Suarez I, et al. Pancreatic ascites: study of therapeutic options by analysis of case reports and case series between the years 1975 and 2000. Am J Gastroenterol 2003; 98: 568–577.
21. Bedingfield JA, Anderson MC. Pancreatopleural fistula. Pancreas 1986; 1: 283–290.
22. Rockey DC, Cello JP. Pancreaticopleural fistula. Report of 7 patients and a review of the literature. Medicine 1990; 69: 332–344.
23. Tannenbaum H, Anderson LG, Schur PH. Polyarthritis, subcutaneous nodules, and pancreatic disease. J Rheum 1975; 2: 14–20.
24. Dahl PR, Su WPD, Cullimore KC, Dicken CH. Pancreatic panniculitis. J Am Acad Derm 1995; 33: 415–417.
25. Mehringer S, Vogt T, Tabusch H-C, et al. Treatments of panniculitis in chronic pancreatitis by interventional endoscopy following extracorporeal lithotripsy. Gastrointest Endosc 2001; 53: 234–238.
26. Chowdhury RC, Forsmark CE, Davis RH, et al. Prevalence of gastroparesis in patients with chronic pancreatitis. Pancreas 2003; 26: 235–238.
27. Layer P, Vonderohe MR, Holst JJ, et al. Altered postprandial motility in chronic pancreatitis: Role of malabsorption. Gastroenterology 1997; 112: 1624–1634.
28. Vu MK, Vecht J, Eddes EH, et al. Antroduodenal motility in chronic pancreatitis: are abnormalities related to exocrine insufficiency? Am J Physiol 2000; 278: G 458–466.
29. Bernades P, Baetz A, Levy P, et al. Splenic and portal vein obstruction in chronic pancreatitis. A prospective longitudinal study of a medical-surgical service of 266 patients. Dig Dis Sci 1992; 37: 340–346.
30. Forsmark CE, Wilcox CM, Grendell JG. Endoscopy-negative upper gastrointestinal hemorrhage in a patient with chronic pancreatitis. Gastroenterology 1992; 102: 320–329.
31. Saforkas GH, Sarr MG, Farley DR, et al. The significance of sinistrial portal hypertension complicating chronic pancreatitis. Am J Surg 2000; 179: 129–133.
32. Fogartie JA, Adams DB, Vujic I, et al. Splanchnic venous obstruction. A complication of chronic pancreatitis. Am Surg 1989; 55: 191–197.
33. Warshaw AL, Rattner DW. Facts and fallacies of common bile duct obstruction by pancreatic pseudocysts. Ann Surg 1979; 192: 33–37.
34. Rattner DW, Warshaw AL. Venous, biliary, and duodenal obstruction in chronic pancreatitis. Hepatogastroenterol 1990; 37: 301–306.
35. Lesur G, Levy P, Flejou JF, et al. Factors predictive of liver histological appearance in chronic alcoholic pancreatitis with common bile duct stenosis and increased serum alkaline phosphatase. Hepatology 1993; 18: 1078–1081.

36. Hammel P, Couvelard A, O'Toole D, et al. Regression of liver fibrosis after biliary drainage in patients with chronic pancreatitis and stenosis of the common bile duct. N Engl J Med 2001; 344: 418–423.
37. Schlosser W, Siech M, Gorich J, et al. Common bile duct stenosis in complicated chronic pancreatitis. Scand J Gastroenterol 2001; 36: 214–219.
38. Schlosser W, Poch B, Beger HG. Duodenum-preserving pancreatic head resection leads to relief of common bile duct stenosis. Am J Surg 2002; 183: 37–41.
39. Ng C, Huibregtse K. The role of endoscopic therapy in chronic pancreatitis-induced common bile duct stricture. Gastrointest Endosc Clin N Am 1998; 8: 181–193.
40. Kiehne K, Folsch UR, Nitsche R. High complication rate of bile duct stents in patients with chronic alcoholic pancreatitis due to noncompliance. Endoscopy 2000; 32: 377–380.
41. Eickhoff A, Jakobs R, Leonhardt A, et al. Endoscopic stenting for common bile duct stenoses in chronic pancreatitis: results and impact on long term outcome. Eur J Gastroenterol Hepatol 2001; 13: 1161–1167.
42. Kahl S, Zimmerman S, Glasbrenner B, et al. Treatment of benign biliary strictures in chronic pancreatitis by self-expandable metal stents. Dig Dis 2002; 20: 199–203.
43. Izbicki JR, Bloechle C, Knoefel WT, et al. Complications of adjacent organs in chronic pancreatitis managed by duodenum preserving resection of the head of the pancreas. Br J Surg 1994; 81: 1351–1355.
44. Nassif T, Pratt F, Meduri B, et al. Endoscopic palliation of malignant gastric outlet obstruction using self-expandable metallic stents: results of a multicenter study Endoscopy 2003; 35: 483–489.
45. Stabile BE, Wilson SE, DeBas HT. Reduced mortality from pseudocysts and pseudoaneurysms caused by pancreatitis. Arch Surg 1983; 118: 45–51.
46. Lowenfels AB, Maisonneuve P, Cavallini G, et al. Pancreatitis and the risk of pancreatic cancer. N Engl J Med 1993; 328:1433–1437.
47. Lowenfels AB, Maissonnueve P, Cavalini G, et al. Prognosis of chronic pancreatitis: An international multicenter study. Am J Gastroenterol 1994; 89: 1467–1471.
48. Lowenfels AB, Maissonnueve P, DiMagno EP, et al., for the International Hereditary Pancreatitis Study Group. Hereditary pancreatitis and the risk of pancreatic carcinoma. J Natl Cancer Inst 1997; 89: 442–446.
49. Chari ST, Mohan V, Pitchumoni CS, et al. Risk of pancreatic carcinoma in tropical calcifying pancreatitis. Pancreas 1994; 9: 62–66.
50. Perez-Stable EJ, Herrera B, Jacobs P III, et al. Nicotine metabolism and intake in black and white smokers. JAMA 1998; 280: 152–156.
51. Bansal P, Sonnenberg A. Pancreatitis as a risk factor for pancreatic carcinoma. Gastroenterology 1995; 109: 247–241.
52. Everhar J, Wrigh D. Diabetes mellitus as a risk factor for pancreatic carcinoma. JAMA 1995; 273: 1605–1609.
53. Gress F, Gottlied K, Sherman S, Lehman G. Endoscopic ultrasonography guided fine needle aspiration biopsy of suspected pancreatic carcinoma. Ann Intern Med 2001; 134: 459–464.
54. Jowell PS. Assessment of pancreatic duct strictures. Gastrointest Endosc Clin N Am 1995; 5: 125–143.
55. Yusuf TE, Bhutani MS. Differentiating pancreatic cancer from pseudotumorous chronic pancreatitis. Curr Gastroenterol Rep 2002; 4: 135–139.
56. Steinberg W. Clinical utility of the CA 19-9 tumor associated antigen. Am J Gastroenterol 1990; 85: 350–355.

57. Imdahl A , Nitzsche E, Krautmann F, et al. Evaluation of PET with FDG for the differentiation of chronic pancreatitis and pancreatic carcinoma. Br J Surg 1999; 86: 194–199.
58. Schneider G, Schmid RM. Genetic alterations in pancreatic carcinoma. Mol Cancer 2003; 2: 15, 1–7.
59. Andrianifahanana M, Moniaux N, Schmied BM, et al. Mucin (MUC) gene expression in human pancreatic carcinoma and chronic pancreatitis. A potential role of MUC 4 as a tumor marker of diagnostic significance. Clin Cancer Res 2001; 7: 4033–4040.
60. Pugliese V, Puji N, Saccomanno S, et al. Pancreatic intraductal sampling during ERCP in patients with chronic pancreatitis and pancreatic carcinoma: Cytologic studies of k-ras-2 codon 12 molecular analysis in 47 patients. Gastrointest Endosc 2001; 54: 595–599.
61. Bueltler P, Conejo-Garcia JR, Lehman G, et al. Real-time quantitative PCR of telomerase mRNA is useful in differentiation of benign and malignant pancreatic disorders. Pancreas 2001; 22: 337–340.

INDEX

A

Abscess, pancreatic, 83
Acinar cell
  and acute pancreatitis, 10
  and cytosolic calcium, 10
Acute pancreatitis
  alcoholic, 5, 8, 52
  autoimmune, 58–59
  chemokines and, 12
  and CT grading system, 27
  cystic fibrosis transmembrane
     conductance regulator, 57
  cytokines and, 12
  C-reactive protein and, 28
  drug-induced, 5
  diagnosis, 17–23
  epidemiology, 7–8
  ERCP-induced, 69–76
  etiology of, 4–7
  fluid collections and, 113–134
  gallstone-induced, 5, 8, 31–50
    complications of, 38–40
    prognosis of, 40–41, 45
    treatment, 41–45, 91–93
  hemoconcentration and, 28
  hereditary, 56–7
  hyperlipidemic, 5, 52–53
  hypercalcemia-induced, 53
  idiopathic, 51, 57
  incidence of, 7, 59
  infections causing, 59
  interstitial pancreatitis, 27
  medication-induced, 53
  microlithiasis, 5
  mild acute pancreatitis
    treatment, 64–69
      acid suppression, 66
      analgesics, 65–66
      calcitonin, 68
      fluid resuscitation, 64

      gabexate, 67
      nasogastric suction, 66
      nutrition, 65–66
      octreotide, 66–67
      peritoneal lavage, 67
      pirenzipine, 68
      somatostatin, 66–67
  miscellaneous causes, 59
  mortality from, 7, 9
  natural history, 9
  necrosis, 5, 9, 27, 83, 85–88,
    99–112
    definition, 100
    diagnosis, 100, 102–103
    infected necrosis, 87, 93–94,
      100, 103
      antibiotics and, 104
      treatment, 104–109
    quality of life, 110
    sequelae, 109–10
  and obesity, 28, 101
  organ failure and, 13–14
  pancreas divisum and, 6, 55–56
  pancreatic adenocarcinoma and,
    6
  pathophysiology, 9, 12–14
  and Purtscher's retinopathy,
    39
  recurrent acute, 8, 163–164
  risk stratification, 23–29
  scorpion venom and, 53
  severe acute pancreatitis, 9, 27,
    81–98
    definition, 82
    and local complications, 83,
      85–88
      fluid collections, 113–134
        definition, 113
        necrosis, 87–88, 99–112,
          120